Penile Implant Surgery

Eduardo P. Miranda • John P. Mulhall
Editors

Penile Implant Surgery

Contemporary Challenges and Controversies

Springer

Editors
Eduardo P. Miranda
Urology Division
Universidade Federal do Ceará
Fortaleza, Ceará, Brazil

John P. Mulhall
Urology Service
Memorial Sloan Kettering Cancer Center
New York, NY, USA

ISBN 978-3-030-82362-7 ISBN 978-3-030-82363-4 (eBook)
https://doi.org/10.1007/978-3-030-82363-4

This Springer imprint is published by the registered company Springer Nature Switzerland AG
The registered company address is: Gewerbestrasse 11, 6330 Cham, Switzerland

Preface

For decades penile implants have been considered the most effective treatment for severe and medication-refractory erectile dysfunction. There remains great interest in this treatment modality as the number of procedures is expected to increase over time with our aging population globally. However, implant surgery is associated with the potential for complications, and a high level of expertise is required to identify and manage these problems during and after surgery.

This book provides a comprehensive and illustrated resource to the most salient aspects of penile implant surgery, ranging from indications to long-term complications. Having an international authorship of world authorities, chapters are aimed to address common concerns, such as patient and device selection, key steps in operative technique, pain control, management of residual penile deformity, and prevention and management of infection. It also provides a step-by-step guide for specific scenarios such as penile fibrosis and neophalloplasty. Rarely discussed issues such as lengthening procedures, operating on anticoagulated patients, and medicolegal aspects are also discussed.

Penile Implant Surgery: Contemporary Challenges and Controversies is intended for both beginners and the most advanced audience, which includes, but is not limited to, residents and fully trained urologists, fellows, and practitioners in sexual medicine and reconstructive urology.

Ceará, Brazil — Eduardo P. Miranda
New York, NY, USA — John P. Mulhall

Contents

Contributors

Hussain M. Alnajjar Institute of Andrology, University College London Hospital, London, UK

Division of Surgery and Interventional Science, UCL, London, UK

Petar Bajic Glickman Urological and Kidney Institute, Cleveland Clinic, Cleveland, OH, USA

Gideon A. Blecher The Alfred Hospital, Melbourne, VIC, Australia

Department of Surgery, Monash University, Melbourne, VIC, Australia

Kristina Buscaino Morsani College of Medicine, University of South Florida, Tampa, FL, USA

Rafael Carrion Morsani College of Medicine, University of South Florida, Tampa, FL, USA

Nathan A. Chertack, MD Department of Urology, UT Southwestern Medical Center, Dallas, TX, USA

Nim Christopher University College London Hospitals & St Peter's Andrology, London, UK

Jonathan Clavell-Hernández St Joseph Medical Center, Houston, TX, USA

McGovern Medical School at Houston, University of Texas Health Science Center, Houston, TX, USA

Brian Dick Department of Urology, Tulane University School of Medicine, New Orleans, LA, USA

Benjamin M. Dropkin, MD Department of Urology, UT Southwestern Medical Center, Dallas, TX, USA

Raul E. Fernandez-Crespo Morsani College of Medicine, University of South Florida, Tampa, FL, USA

Esaú Fernández-Pascual Lyx Institute of Urology, Universidad Francisco de Vitoria, Madrid, Spain

Department of Urology, Hospital Universitario La Paz, Madrid, Spain

Giulio Garaffa The Institute of Urology, University College London Hospitals, London, UK

Eiftu Haile Glickman Urological and Kidney Institute, Cleveland Clinic, Cleveland, OH, USA

Kevin J. Hebert Mayo Clinic, Rochester, MN, USA

Wayne J. G. Hellstrom Department of Urology, Tulane University School of Medicine, New Orleans, LA, USA

Gerard D. Henry WK Advanced Urology, Bossier City, Louisiana, USA

Gregory A. Joice, MD Department of Urology, UT Southwestern Medical Center, Dallas, TX, USA

Tobias S. Köhler Mayo Clinic, Rochester, MN, USA

Pramod Krishnappa Andrology Division, Department of Urology, NU Hospitals, Bangalore, India

Gabe Leinwand Department of Urology, Tulane University School of Medicine, New Orleans, LA, USA

Laurence A. Levine Division of Urology, Rush University Medical Center, Chicago, IL, USA

Juan Ignacio Martinez-Salamanca Lyx Institute of Urology, Universidad Francisco de Vitoria, Madrid, Spain

Department of Urology, Hospital Universitario Puerta de Hierro, Majadahonda, Madrid, Spain

Eduardo P. Miranda Sexual & Reproductive Medicine Program, Urology Service, Memorial Sloan Kettering Cancer Center, New York, NY, USA

Division of Urology, Federal University of Ceara, Fortaleza, Brazil

Allen F. Morey, MD Department of Urology, UT Southwestern Medical Center, Dallas, TX, USA

John P. Mulhall Sexual & Reproductive Medicine Program, Urology Service, Memorial Sloan Kettering Cancer Center, New York, NY, USA

Asif Muneer Institute of Andrology, University College London Hospital, London, UK

Division of Surgery and Interventional Science, UCL, London, UK

Bruno C. G. Nascimento Sexual & Reproductive Medicine Program, Urology Service, Memorial Sloan Kettering Cancer Center, New York, NY, USA

Sexual Medicine Group, Division of Urology, Hospital das Clinicas – University of Sao Paulo Medical School, Sao Paulo, Brazil

Caleb Natale Department of Urology, Tulane University School of Medicine, New Orleans, LA, USA

Samantha W. Nealon, MD Department of Urology, University of South Florida, Tampa, FL, USA

Daniar Osmonov University Medical Center Schleswig Holstein, Kiel, Germany

Michael Polchert Department of Urology, Tulane University School of Medicine, New Orleans, LA, USA

Mirko Preto A.O.U. Città della Salute e della Scienza di Torino – Clinica Urologica – Presidio Molinette, Torino, Italy

Ahmed M. Ragheb Department of Urology, Beni-Suef University, Beni Suef, Egypt

Bedaya Fertility & IVF Hospitals, Cairo, Egypt

IHUN, Cairo, Egypt

David J. Ralph University College London Hospitals & St Peter's Andrology, London, UK

Karina Evelyn Sidabutar Regional Urology, Jakarta, Indonesia

Ayman Soubra Department of Urology, Tulane University School of Medicine, New Orleans, LA, USA

Jared J. Wallen YOU & WEE Urologic Surgery and Wellness, Sarasota, FL, USA

Run Wang McGovern Medical School at Houston, University of Texas Health Science Center, Houston, TX, USA

University of Texas MD Anderson Cancer Center, Houston, TX, USA

David Y. Yang Mayo Clinic, Rochester, MN, USA

Chapter 1
Patient and Device Selection

Pramod Krishnappa, Esaú Fernández-Pascual, and Juan Ignacio Martinez-Salamanca

Penile prosthesis (PP) has become the standard of care in the management of refractory erectile dysfunction (ED). The success of a surgery is half completed even before the start of the surgery if one knows how to select the patients and devices diligently.

There are several aspects which need to be considered before doing the PP surgery to maximise the patient-partner satisfaction and to be medicolegally safe. Patients should be given a realistic overview of the entire procedure, outcomes and possible complications so that they know what to expect following the surgery.

A legal database review published in 2014 by Sunaryo et al. [1] about PP malpractice litigation revealed that 42% of cases (17/40) led to indemnity payment to the plaintiff with a mean settlement of US$335,000 and a mean indemnity award of US$831,050. The other important and alarming findings were error in surgical decision-making (48% of cases), informed consent (31%) and postoperative infection (31%) which were the top three reasons for above claim.

A detailed preoperative discussion about the entire surgical procedure and taking signature on a detailed informed consent form is of major importance. This chapter gives a detailed outline of the issues that need to be resolved before attempting a PP surgery to make the outcomes better for the patient and also for the treating doctor.

P. Krishnappa
Andrology Division, Department of Urology, NU Hospitals, Bangalore, India

E. Fernández-Pascual
Lyx Institute of Urology, Universidad Francisco de Vitoria, Madrid, Spain

Department of Urology, Hospital Universitario La Paz, Madrid, Spain

J. I. Martinez-Salamanca (✉)
Lyx Institute of Urology, Universidad Francisco de Vitoria, Madrid, Spain

Department of Urology, Hospital Universitario Puerta de Hierro, Majadahonda, Madrid, Spain

E. P. Miranda, J. P. Mulhall (eds.), *Penile Implant Surgery*,
https://doi.org/10.1007/978-3-030-82363-4_1

Patient Selection

Modifiable Risk Factors

Identifying risk factors of the patient is a top priority as some of these can be optimised before the planned PP surgery.

Smoking

There is level 1 evidence to say that smoking increases surgical site infections (SSI) [2].

As there is no published data on the adverse effects of smoking in PP surgery outcomes, we have derived established conclusions from other surgical specialities. Smokers with 11 or more pack-years had significantly increased deep surgical-site infection ($p < 0.01$) and reoperations in plastic surgery procedures [3].

Adding onto this data, studies from gastrointestinal surgery group have shown that smoking (odds ratio = 1.506, 95% confidence interval 1.131–2.004, $P = 0.005$) was an independent risk factor for postoperative complications [4].

Smoking cessation should ideally be done 4 weeks prior to the planned surgery to reduce the complications [2].

Diabetes Mellitus (DM)

A high-quality population-based data reiterated the fact that DM is an increased risk for inflatable penile prosthesis (IPP) infection [5]. The New York State-wide Planning and Research Cooperative System (SPARCS) database was searched from 1995 to 2014, and 14,969 patients underwent initial IPP insertion. Infectious complications were experienced by 3% (133/4478) of diabetic patients and 2% (210/10,491) of non-diabetic patients ($P < 0.001$) controlling for age, race, comorbidities, insurance status, annual surgeon volume and era of implantation.

The reasons for the higher implant infection rates among diabetics have been numerous. Le et al. have shown in diabetic animal models that adverse tissue healing and subsequent fibrosis around the implants can prevent the optimal functioning of the implants [6].

In a biochemical model of penis/prosthesis complex, Gefen et al. noted poor corporal elasticity of diabetic penis leading to persistent penile pain due to nerve stimulation or ischaemia in regions of compressed vascular tissue [7].

A multicentric study assessed the relation between HbA1C levels and PP infection rates in 902 PP procedures [8]. They found that infection rates were 1.3% with HbA1c level of <6.5%, 1.5% for 6.5–7.5%, 6.5% for 7.6–8.5%, 14.7% for 8.6–9.5% and 22.4% for >9.5% ($P < 0.001$). The study concluded that a threshold HbA1c level of 8.5% is suggested for clinical use to identify patients at increased infection risk.

Most authors agree that HbA1c below 8.5% is reasonably good level for PP surgery [9, 10].

Obesity

Lifestyle changes are associated with improvement in sexual function in about one third of obese men with erectile dysfunction at baseline [11].

Before attempting PP surgery, patient should be advised to lose at least 10% of body weight and to observe any spontaneous improvement in erectile function.

Chronic inflammation and dysmetabolism observed in visceral obese patients negatively influence postoperative outcomes [12].

There may be technical challenges in an obese individual with respect to placing the skin incision, operating table dimensions and appropriate placement of scrotal pump for the patient to handle it comfortably in postoperative period.

Akin-Olugbade et al. noted that those men with body mass index >30 undergoing PP surgery have lower satisfaction rates than the general PP population [13].

Pre-existing Basic Infection Screening

Fungal Infection in the Groin

Penoscrotal and groin examination should involve examining specifically for active fungal infections [14]. Candida infections were seen in 11.1% of cultures isolated from infected PP in a multicentric study, and fungal flora can be eliminated with oral fluconazole before surgery [15].

Nasal Swab Testing for Staphylococcus aureus

The commonest organism isolated from PP infection is *Staphylococcus aureus* [16].

More than 80% of healthcare-associated *S. aureus* infections are endogenous [17, 18].

In a randomised, double-blind, placebo-controlled, multicentre trial published in 2010, patients prior to surgery were randomly assigned in a 1:1 ratio to either active treatment with mupirocin ointment 2% in combination with chlorhexidine gluconate soap, 40 mg/mL or placebo ointment in combination with placebo soap. The infection rates were significantly lesser in mupirocin-chlorhexidine group (3.4% vs 7.7%) [19].

But there is no study that has analysed the role of nasal screening treatment and its benefits in reduction of PP infection. Hence it would be difficult to make a statement on this aspect. Not many prosthetic urologists do nasal screening routinely.

Urine Culture

The common sense in any prosthetic surgery is not to have any focus of infection anywhere in the body. It is practically difficult to rule out all asymptomatic infections.

It would be advisable to do preoperative urine culture in all PP surgeries from medicolegal standpoint although there is some controversy about its true value [20]. Kavoussi et al. found only a 20% (1/5) match between the germ isolated in the urine culture and that obtained from the infected PP. [21] It should be noted that all these patients were intervened with artificial urinary sphincter (AUS) implants, and not with PP. The surgical site in the case of PP surgery is closer to the urinary catheter, while in the case of AUS, the access route is usually perineal.

Katz et al. did a survey which revealed that routine urine culture was not performed by 40% and 50% of Sexual Medicine Society of North America (SMSNA) and International Society of Sexual Medicine (ISSM) members, respectively [22].

Despite this, the current prosthetic implant guidelines recommend preoperative urine culture [23].

Age

Elderly age should not be a restricting factor for penile implant surgery.

Multivariate analysis by Shabsigh et al. on a cross national survey on male health issues noted that older men (60–75 years) consistently reported that they did not seek treatment because they felt ED was a normal part of ageing [24].

Chung E et al. reported that men aged ≥75 years had satisfactory outcome with IPP surgery with no statistically significant difference identified across device survival and satisfaction rates compared to men aged <75 years [25].

Adolescent and teen cancer rates are increasing, particularly thyroid, testicular and non-Hodgkin lymphoma (NHL) cancer. Ultrasound evidence of corporal fibrosis has been observed in adolescent with NHL following cyclophosphamide and doxorubicin chemotherapy [26].

These youngsters with cancer will have their own concerns about ED at a very early age which will bother them mentally and physically. We may soon get to see increase in the number of PP surgeries in less than 30-year-old individuals [27].

HIV Status

The dilemma whether HIV increases postoperative infection rates continues to exist without robust data. A meta-analysis of HIV patients receiving orthopaedic implants was published by Kigera et al. and the group noted that the pooled risk ratio of infection in the HIV patients when compared to non-HIV patients was 1.8 (95% confidence interval [CI] 1.3–2.4) [28].

Moran et al. also showed that HIV seropositivity should not preclude PP placement in appropriately selected men. The reoperation rates in HIV cohort were similar to non-HIV cohort [29].

In contrast to above findings, in a cross-sectional analysis from Premier Perspective Database of 13 years period, Li et al. noted that HIV-positive status was predictive for PP removals due to infectious causes [30]. There could be association between immune dysregulation and the likelihood of PP removal.

There is contrasting evidence about the outcomes in HIV-positive patients. Our suggestion would be to counsel about the additional risk of PP infection in HIV positive individuals when CD4 T-cell counts <300 [31].

Solid Organ Transplantation (SOT)

It is estimated that the prevalence of ED in patients with a liver, renal and heart transplant is 40–86%, 54–66% and 71–78%, respectively [32].

Higher risk of prosthetic infection due to long-term immunosuppression is the worrisome factor in SOT recipients.

A retrospective study was done by Sun et al. which involved 26 SOT-IPP and 26 age-matched IPP recipients without SOT. Transplants included the heart [3], liver [2], kidney only [16] and kidney and pancreas [4]. The study reported no significant difference in PP infection rates (4% vs 0%, $P = 1.00$) and reoperation rates (11.5% vs 11.5%, $P = 1.00$) when comparing patients with SOT with non-SOT controls [33].

The non-infective concerns in these SOT recipients are that the placement of reservoir may be difficult due to adhesions and fibrosis of the previous pelvic surgical planes.

A 2020 systematic review also opined the same and highlighted that the SOT patients who have received a PP may benefit from the presence of an urologist during any subsequent intra-abdominal surgery to decrease the risk of intraoperative or perioperative complication of the existent PP. [34]

The classical teaching few decades back was to prefer PP without reservoir and hence to avoid three-piece IPP in SOT patients [35].

With improvements in surgical expertise and increase in high-volume centres, it is no longer the same. Recent papers have reported no differences in IPP reoperation rates between two-piece and three-piece IPP models [33, 34].

A submuscular (ectopic) placement of the reservoir to avoid visceral or bladder injury may be considered in pelvic grafts [36].

Although the criteria of Barry [37] published in 2007 on the treatment of ED in renal transplant recipients have been generally accepted, they need to be analysed in detail.

Barry [37] proposed the following recommendations for PP surgery in kidney transplant recipients:

- Stable graft function for at least 6 months
- Low doses of maintenance immunosuppressants
- PP with low probability of device malfunction

- No intra-abdominal components to avoid confusion of the reservoir with the bladder in the event of subsequent kidney transplantation
- Minimal tissue dissection
- No skin or urinary tract infections
- Use of prophylactic antibacterials (parenteral, intraurethral and topical)
- Postoperative broad spectrum oral antibacterials for 1–2 weeks

Although most of the above recommendations have an obvious reason either to avoid infections or abnormal scarring in high-risk patients, the decision to use two-piece or malleable PP to avoid implantation of the intra-abdominal reservoir is based on an analysis of the results of 46 transplant recipients, of which 4 had malfunction of the prosthesis (this was not a side effect related to the fact of being a kidney transplant recipient) and the other 4 had injury of the PP in subsequent surgeries [35]. These complications cannot be due the location of the reservoir but of the surgeons' skills and experience.

Neurological Impairment

Reports from 1980s have showed increased incidence of PP infection in spinal cord injury (SCI) patients in view of recurrent urinary tract infection resulting due to long-term urinary stasis or indwelling urinary catheters [38, 39].

Zermann et al. recommended IPP in neurologically impaired patients because of the lower risk of erosion. Malleable PP had 18% risk of erosion in this study, whereas none was seen with three-piece IPP [40].

Malleable PP, despite its drawbacks of being difficult to conceal and unattractive, has the advantage of being economical in patients who have resting tremors or limited hand movements. Kim et al. obtained different data from SCI patients: of the 48 patients who received malleable PP in SCI, erosion occurred in 2 patients (4.2%) and 2 patients required PP removal due to infection [41].

Simultaneous Artificial Urinary Sphincter (AUS) Implantation

Preliminary papers about doing synchronous dual implants (PP + AUS) have showed encouraging results [42–44]. Rolle et al. compared those who underwent synchronous implants (group 1, $n = 15$) with those who underwent two-stage surgery (group 2, $n = 8$). This Italian study noted that the 92% in group 1 and 95% in group 2 experienced "great improvement" ($P > 0.05$) on Patient Global Impression of Improvement. All group 2 patients stated they would have preferred synchronous surgery. No major complications were noted in either group [42].

Steve Wilson described this technique in 2001, but when he was asked in 2018 about the top 5 lessons that he learned from his 45-year practice in the field of prosthetic urology, he said: "The fifth thing I wish I had known: even though I invented the dual implant via 1 incision, I now discourage it. Experience has taught me to do the implants separately" [45]. The main reason to avoid this single incision dual implant is that when something goes wrong, usually all components from both implants must be removed. This could be avoided if dual implants are inserted through scrotal and perineal incisions separately.

Revision Surgery

Patients with the following scenarios need to be counselled thoroughly about the realistic outcomes as the revision surgeries tend to be more difficult than the primary surgery and are associated with increased infection rates:

- Prior surgical intervention for priapism without primacy placement of PP [46]
- Corporal fibrosis following PP removal due to PP infection [47, 48]
- Prolonged use of intracavernosal injection [49]
- Two retroperitoneal reservoirs already in place
- Thinned out glans and PP erosion

Counselling

Patient and Partner Involvement

Cayan et al. noted higher patient satisfaction rates in the IPP group when compared to malleable PP group (99.2% vs 90.3%). The partner dissatisfaction rates were higher in malleable than IPP group (11.2% with malleable PP, 3.8% with two-piece IPP and 3.3% with three-piece IPP) [50].

Hence involving the partner in preoperative discussions may help ease the matters in postoperative phase as well [51].

Trost et al. defined a simple mnemonic: "CURSED patient" which stands for Compulsive, Unrealistic, Revision, Surgeon Shopping, Entitled, Denial and Psychiatric. Psychological issues with most difficult IPP patients include obsessive/compulsive tendencies, unrealistic expectations, those undergoing revision surgery, those seeking multiple surgical opinions, feelings of entitlement, patients in denial of their prior erectile/sexual function and current disease status or those with other psychiatric disorders [52].

Timed intelligent management of such patients will help improve outcomes and prevent unnecessary law suits.

Pre- and postoperative psychosexual counselling by qualified psychologists may improve postoperative sexual activity and erotic function for both patients and partners following PP surgery [53, 54].

In a patient suspected to have "CURSED" traits, the psychosexual counselling in PP patients should address the following aspects to have a psychologically sound patient at the end of the procedure: the impact of diagnosis, body image issues, fears relating to the surgical procedure and its outcome, the risk of excessive expectations and consequent disillusionment, relationship issues and communication problems [55].

Consent Form

Having a valid informed signed consent form is the first step to medicolegally ensure that one has explained about the positive and negative outcomes of the PP surgery.

Detailed consent forms for PP surgery can be accessed from SMSNA [56] and a document published by Kovac et al. [57]

Device Selection

The majority of high-volume prosthetic urologists would consider a three-piece IPP as the first preference in PP surgery in a virgin uncomplicated case considering the pros and cons of a three-piece IPP.

A three-piece IPP consists of a pair of corporal cylinders, scrotal pump and abdomino-pelvic reservoir. A two-piece IPP (AMS Ambicor™) consists of a pair of corporal cylinders and a scrotal pump. During prosthesis recycling, the pump transfers the solution from small reservoirs located at the proximal end of each cylinder, into each cylinder shaft, thereby causing an erection [58].

The Following Are the List of Currently Available PP Models of Two Major Companies

Boston Scientific (Marlborough, MA, USA)

- Three-piece IPP: AMS 700™ CX (Controlled Expansion) (Fig. 1.1), AMS 700™ LGX (Length Girth Expansion), AMS 700™ CXR (Controlled Expansion Restricted)
- Two-piece IPP: AMS Ambicor™ (Fig. 1.2)
- Malleable: Tactra™ (launched in 2019) (Fig. 1.3)

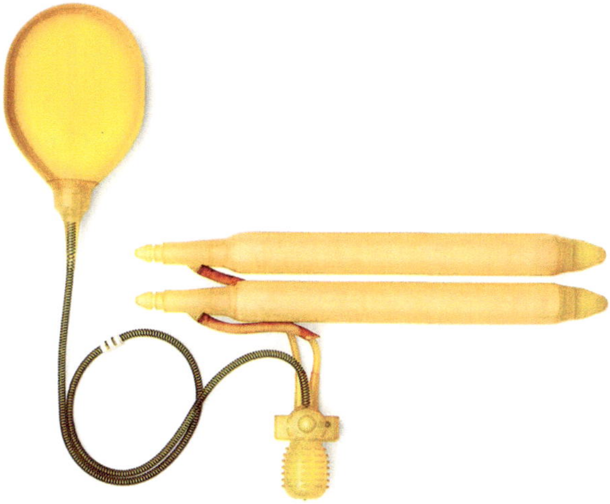

Fig. 1.1 AMS 700CX

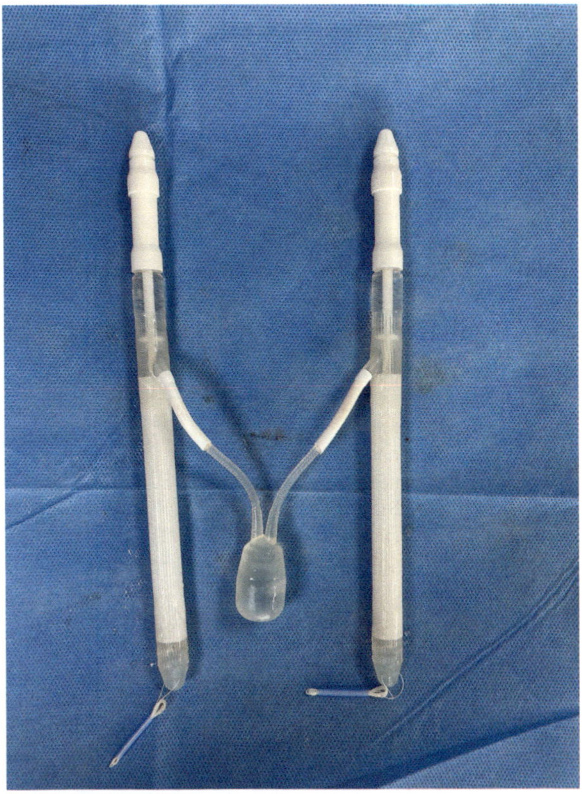

Fig. 1.2 AMS Ambicor

Coloplast (Minneapolis, MN, USA)

- Three-piece IPP: Titan® Touch, Titan® Touch Narrow Base (Fig. 1.4)
- Malleable: Genesis® (Fig. 1.5)

A preliminary study published in 2013 by Chung et al. showed that the AMS 700™ CX and Coloplast Titan® achieved similar clinical outcomes and patient satisfaction rates in Peyronie's disease treatment and modelling procedure [59].

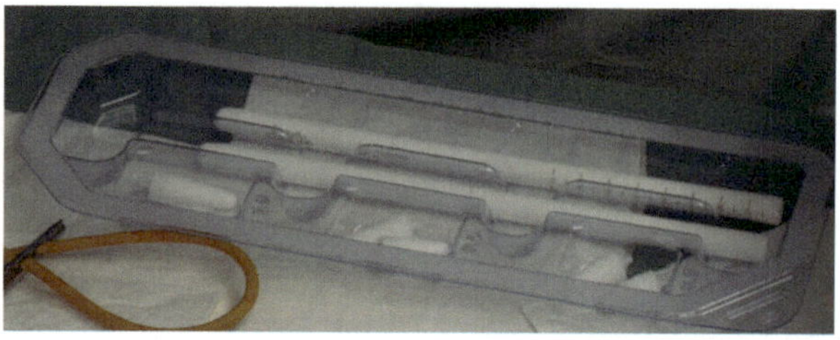

Fig. 1.3 Tactra

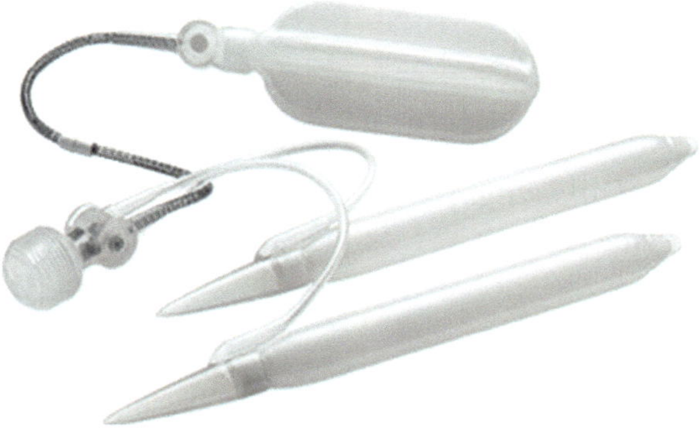

Fig. 1.4 Titan Touch

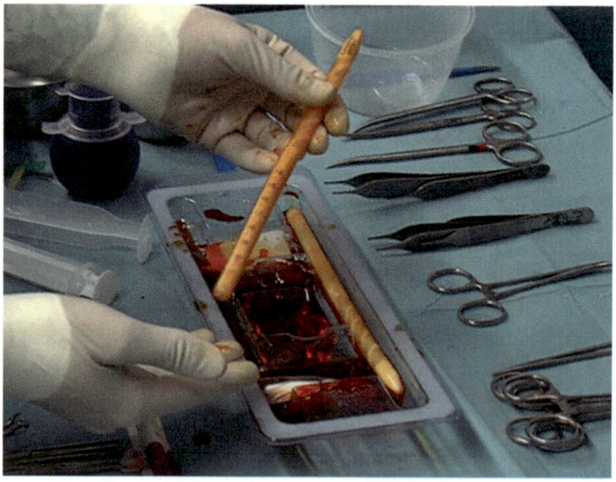

Fig. 1.5 Genesis

Approach

The three-piece IPP models are different for penoscrotal (PS) and infrapubic (IP) approaches. The ones used for PS approach will have shorter scrotal pump tubing length compared to the IP models.

AMS Ambicor™ two-piece IPP has only PS option. Malleable PP doesn't differ based on the approach.

Reservoirs

- Boston Scientific: Spherical and Conceal™
- Coloplast: Cloverleaf™ with lockout valve

The new reservoir designs such as Conceal™ flat reservoir from Boston Scientific and Cloverleaf™ from Coloplast are specially designed for ectopic placement of reservoir (between fascia transversalis and abdominal muscles).

More details about the reservoirs and surgical approaches will be dealt in the upcoming chapters.

The Following Are Some of the Tips in Choosing the Right Device (PP) in Specific Clinical Scenarios

- It is preferable to use AMS 700™ CXR or Titan® Touch Narrow Base in corporal fibrosis and post-radiotherapy cases where corporal dilatation is difficult [60].
- AMS 700™ CX and Titan® Touch which have high-pressure cylinders are preferred for manual modelling in Peyronie's disease [61].
- AMS 700™ LGX is not ideal for penile straightening in scarred corporal bodies, because the lengthening property of these cylinders does not allow for the development of sufficient axial rigidity [62].
- Although few studies [63, 64] claim that AMS 700™ LGX preserves the penile length to some extent, the same has not been observed in a recent study where Wallen et al. observed increase in stretched penile length in only six (23.1%) patients [65].
- Both AMS 700™ and Titan® have antibacterial properties. AMS 700™ has InhibiZone® which is an antibiotic coating impregnated with rifampin and minocycline, whereas Coloplast Titan is coated with polyvinylpyrrolidone (PVP), a hydrophilic substance that retains the antibiotic when dipped in any antibiotic solution. It is difficult to specify which PP offers least infection rates as PP infection depends on so many preoperative, intra-operative and postoperative factors. Dhabuwala et al. noted infection rates of 4.4%, 1.3% and 0% for

Titan® PP coated with vancomycin/gentamycin, InhibiZone-impregnated AMS 700™ PP and Titan® PP coated with rifampin/gentamicin solution, respectively [66].

- In a biomechanical cadaveric pilot study conducted by Wallen et al., the AMS 700™ CX showed the best rigidity in the shortest phallus (with three-point flexure testing) and the Titan® showed slightly better rigidity in the longest phallus and the phallus with mild Peyronie's disease [67].
- Two-piece IPP is best suited in kidney transplant recipients [37].
- Malleable PP are preferred (i) as a "bridge-course" or salvage therapy to prevent complete corporal fibrosis in PP infection or priapism to help easy placement of IPP later; [68] (ii) in those having manual dexterity issues (significant hand tremors) which may hamper handling of scrotal pump; (iii) in patients with Peyronie's disease who require lengthening techniques in which it is important to keep the penis in traction as long as possible in order to maintain the gained length; and (iv) in those unable to afford for IPP, which is mostly the case in many countries where insurance companies do not cover PP surgeries [69].

Table 1.1 summarises the patient and device selection factors that should be considered preoperatively to achieve better results.

Table 1.1 Preoperative decision-making factors

Patient factors	HbA1c less than 8.5
	Urine culture
	Screen for any obvious active infection: groin
	Psychosexual counselling in "CURSED patients"
	Written informed detailed consent
	Involve partner in discussions wherever possible
	Stop antiplatelets 1 week prior to surgery
	Quit smoking at least 4 weeks prior to surgery
	Body mass index <30, preferably
	Previous surgeries (urethral, penile, scrotal, pelvic)
	Low-dose immunosuppression protocols in transplant recipients, if feasible
Device factors	AMS 700™ CXR or Titan® Touch Narrow Base: in severe corporal fibrosis
	AMS 700™ CX and Titan® Touch: for manual modelling in Peyronie's disease
	Avoid doing synchronous dual implants through single incision (in early phase of your career)
	Malleable PP: patients with manual dexterity issues or as bridge-course option in priapism and infection
	Very large phallus: Titan® Touch
	Ectopic reservoir placement: use Conceal™ or Cloverleaf™

References

1. Sunaryo PL, Colaco M, Terlecki R. Penile prostheses and the litigious patient: a legal database review. J Sex Med. 2014;11(10):2589–94.
2. Sørensen LT. Wound healing and infection in surgery. The clinical impact of smoking and smoking cessation: a systematic review and meta-analysis. Arch Surg. 2012;147(4):373–83.
3. Toyoda Y, Fu RH, Li L, Otterburn DM, Rohde CH. Smoking as an independent risk factor for postoperative complications in plastic surgical procedures: a propensity score-matched analysis of 36,454 patients from the NSQIP database from 2005 to 2014. Plast Reconstr Surg. 2018;141(1):226–36.
4. Quan H, Ouyang L, Zhou H, Ouyang Y, Xiao H. The effect of preoperative smoking cessation and smoking dose on postoperative complications following radical gastrectomy for gastric cancer: a retrospective study of 2469 patients. World J Surg Oncol. 2019;17(1):61.
5. Lipsky MJ, Onyeji I, Golan R, Munarriz R, Kashanian JA, Stember DS, Stahl PJ. Diabetes is a risk factor for inflatable penile prosthesis infection: analysis of a large statewide database. Sex Med. 2019;7(1):35–40.
6. Le NN, Rose MB, Levinson H, Klitzman B. Implant healing in experimental animal models of diabetes. J Diabetes Sci Technol. 2011;5(3):605–18.
7. Gefen A, Chen J, Elad D. Stresses in the normal and diabetic human penis following implantation of an inflatable prosthesis. Med Biol Eng Comput. 1999;37(5):625–31.
8. Habous M, Tal R, Tealab A, Soliman T, Nassar M, Mekawi Z, Mahmoud S, Abdelwahab O, Elkhouly M, Kamr H, Remeah A, Binsaleh S, Ralph D, Mulhall J. Defining a glycated haemoglobin (HbA1c) level that predicts increased risk of penile implant infection. BJU Int. 2018;121(2):293–300.
9. Chung E. Penile prosthesis implant in the special populations: diabetics, neurogenic conditions, fibrotic cases, concurrent urinary continence surgery, and salvage implants. Asian J Androl. 2020;22(1):39–44.
10. Hebert KJ, Kohler TS. Penile prosthesis infection: myths and realities. World J Mens Health. 2019;37(3):276–87.
11. Esposito K, Giugliano F, Di Palo C, et al. Effect of lifestyle changes on erectile dysfunction in obese men: a randomized controlled trial. JAMA. 2004;291(24):2978–84.
12. Doyle SL, Lysaght J, Reynolds JV. Obesity and post-operative complications in patients undergoing non-bariatric surgery. Obes Rev. 2010;11(12):875–86.
13. Akin-Olugbade O, Parker M, Guhring P, Mulhall J. Determinants of patient satisfaction following penile prosthesis surgery. J Sex Med. 2006;3(4):743–8.
14. Gross MS. Penile prosthesis infection. AUA Update Ser. 37(11):109–15.
15. Gross MS, Phillips EA, Carrasquillo RJ, Thornton A, Greenfield JM, Levine LA, Alukal JP, Conners WP 3rd, Glina S, Tanrikut C, Honig SC, Becher EF, Bennett NE, Wang R, Perito PE, Stahl PJ, RossellóGayá M, RossellóBarbará M, Cedeno JD, Gheiler EL, Kalejaiye O, Ralph DJ, Köhler TS, Stember DS, Carrion RE, Maria PP, Brant WO, Bickell MW, Garber BB, Pineda M, Burnett AL 2nd, Eid JF, Henry GD, Munarriz RM. Multicenter investigation of the micro-organisms involved in penile prosthesis infection: an analysis of the efficacy of the AUA and EAU guidelines for penile prosthesis prophylaxis. J Sex Med. 2017;14(3):455–63.
16. Mulcahy JJ. Long-term experience with salvage of infected penile implants. J Urol. 2000;163(2):481–2.
17. Weinstein HJ. The relation between the nasal-staphylococcal-carrier state and the incidence of postoperative complications. N Engl J Med. 1959;260:1303–8.

18. von Eiff C, Becker K, Machka K, Stammer H, Peters G. Nasal carriage as a source of Staphylococcus aureus bacteremia. N Engl J Med. 2001;344:11–6.
19. Bode LG, Kluytmans JA, Wertheim HF, Bogaers D, Vandenbroucke-Grauls CM, Roosendaal R, Troelstra A, Box AT, Voss A, van der Tweel I, van Belkum A, Verbrugh HA, Vos MC. Preventing surgical-site infections in nasal carriers of Staphylococcus aureus. N Engl J Med. 2010 Jan 7;362(1):9–17.
20. Kavoussi NL, Siegel JA, Viers BR, Pagliara TJ, Hofer MD, Cordon BH, Shakir N, Scott JM, Morey AF. Preoperative urine culture results correlate poorly with bacteriology of urologic prosthetic device infections. J Sex Med. 2017;14(1):163–8.
21. Kavoussi NL, Viers BR, Pagilara TJ, et al. Are urine cultures necessary prior to urologic prosthetic surgery? Sex Med Rev. 2018;6(1):157–61.
22. Katz DJ, Stember DS, Nelson CJ, Mulhall JP. Perioperative prevention of penile prosthesis infection: practice patterns among surgeons of SMSNA and ISSM. J Sex Med. 2012;9:1705–14.
23. Levine LA, Becher E, Bella A, Brant W, Kohler T, Martinez-Salamanca JI, et al. Penile prosthesis surgery: current recommendations from the international consultation on sexual medicine. J Sex Med. 2016;13(4):489–518.
24. Shabsigh R, Perelman MA, Laumann EO, Lockhart DC. Drivers and barriers to seeking treatment for erectile dysfunction: a comparison of six countries. BJU Int. 2004;94(7):1055–65.
25. Chung E, Solomon M, DeYoung L, Brock GB. Clinical outcomes and patient satisfaction rates among elderly male aged ≥75 years with inflatable penile prosthesis implant for medically refractory erectile dysfunction. World J Urol. 2014;32(1):173–7.
26. Biewenga E, Aisen C, Nguyen T, Gabrielson A, Kim N, Goldstein I. Erectile dysfunction in an adolescent with non-Hodgkin lymphoma following chemotherapy with agents known to induce cardiac fibrosis/myocardial necrosis: a case report and literature review. J Sex Med. 2019;16:S1–S143.
27. Weckx F, Van Renterghem K. Penile implant surgery for conservative therapy resistant erectile dysfunction in a 19y-old. Urol Case Rep. 2020;31:101161. https://doi.org/10.1016/j.eucr.2020.101161.
28. Kigera JW, Straetemans M, Vuhaka SK, Nagel IM, Naddumba EK, Boer K. Is there an increased risk of post-operative surgical site infection after orthopaedic surgery in HIV patients? A systematic review and meta-analysis. PLoS One. 2012;7(8):e42254.
29. Moran G, Asafu-Adjei D, Li G, Lipsky M, Stember D, Stahl PJ. Implant selection patterns and reoperation rates amongst HIV positive and negative patients that underwent penile prosthesis surgery. J Sex Med. 2018;15:S1–S93.
30. Li K, Brandes ER, Chang SL, Leow JJ, Chung BI, Wang Y, Eswara JR. Trends in penile prosthesis implantation and analysis of predictive factors for removal. World J Urol. 2019;37(4):639–46.
31. Guild GN, Moore TJ, Barnes W, Hermann C. CD4 count is associated with postoperative infection in patients with orthopaedic trauma who are HIV positive. Clin Orthop Relat Res. 2012;470:1507–12.
32. Payne K, Popat S, Lipshultz LI, Thirumavalavan N. The prevalence and treatment of erectile dysfunction in male solid organ transplant recipients. Sex Med Rev. 2019:S2050-0521(19)30102-7. https://doi.org/10.1016/j.sxmr.2019.10.002. Epub ahead of print
33. Sun AY, Babbar P, Gill BC, Angermeier KW, Montague DK. Penile prosthesis in solid organ transplant recipients-a matched cohort study. Urology. 2018;117:86–8.
34. Dick B, Greenberg JW, Polchert M, Natale C, Hellstrom WJG, Raheem OA. A systematic review of penile prosthesis surgery in organ transplant recipients [published online ahead of print, 2020 Jul 5]. Sex Med Rev. 2020:S2050-0521(20)30049-4.
35. Cuellar DC, Sklar GN. Penile prosthesis in the organ transplant recipient. Urology. 2001;57(1):138–41.
36. Morey AF, Cefalu CA, Hudak SJ. High submuscular placement of urologic prosthetic balloons and reservoirs via transscrotal approach. J Sex Med. 2013;10:603–10.
37. Barry JM. Treating erectile dysfunction in renal transplant patients. Drugs. 2007;67:975–83.

38. Collins KP, Hackler RH. Complications of penile prostheses in the spinal cord injury population. J Urol. 1988;140:984–5.
39. Diokno AC, Sonda LP. Compatibility of genitourinary prostheses and intermittent self-catheterization. J Urol. 1981;125:659–60.
40. Zermann D-H, Kutzenberger J, Sauerwein D, et al. Penile prosthetic surgery in neurologically impaired patients: long-term followup. J Urol. 2006;175:1041–4.
41. Kim YD, Yang SO, Lee JK, Jung TY, Shim HB. Usefulness of a malleable penile prosthesis in patients with a spinal cord injury. Int J Urol. 2008;15(10):919–23.
42. Rolle L, Ceruti C, Sedigh O, et al. Surgical implantation of artificial urinary device and penile prosthesis through transscrotal incision for post-prostatectomy urinary incontinence and erectile dysfunction: synchronous or delayed procedure? Urology. 2012;80:1046–50.
43. Moncada I. Dual implant in patients with incontinence and erectile dysfunction. J Sex Med. 2006;3(2):367–70.
44. Kendirci M, Gupta S, Shaw K, Morey A, Jones L, Hakim L, Hellstrom WJ. Synchronous prosthetic implantation through a transscrotal incision: an outcome analysis. J Urol. 2006;175(6):2218–22.
45. Wilson S. The top 5 surgical things that I wish I had known earlier in my career: lessons learned from a career of prosthetic urology. J Sex Med. 2018;15(6):809–12.
46. Yücel ÖB, Pazır Y, Kadıoğlu A. Penile prosthesis implantation in priapism. Sex Med Rev. 2018;6(2):310–8.
47. Martínez-Salamanca JI, Mueller A, Moncada I, Carballido J, Mulhall JP. Penile prosthesis surgery in patients with corporal fibrosis: a state of the art review. J Sex Med. 2011;8(7):1880–9.
48. Wilson SK. Reimplantation of inflatable penile prosthesis into scarred corporeal bodies. Int J Impot Res. 2003;15(Suppl. 5):S125–8.
49. Larsen EH, Gasser TC, Bruskewitz RC. Fibrosis of corpus cavernosum after intracavernous injection of phentolamine/papaverine. J Urol. 1987;137:292–3.
50. Çayan S, Aşcı R, Efesoy O, et al. Comparison of long-term results and couples' satisfaction with penile implant types and brands: lessons learned from 883 patients with erectile dysfunction who underwent penile prosthesis implantation. J Sex Med. 2019;16:1092–9.
51. Osmonov D, Christopher AN, Blecher GA, et al. Clinical Recommendations from the European Society for Sexual Medicine Exploring Partner Expectations, Satisfaction in Male and Phalloplasty Cohorts, the Impact of Penile Length, Girth and Implant Type, Reservoir Placement, and the Influence of Comorbidities and Social Circumstances. J Sex Med. 2020;17:210–37.
52. Trost LW, Baum N, Hellstrom WJG. Managing the difficult penile prosthesis patient. J Sex Med. 2013;10:893–907.
53. Ulloa EW, Silberbogen AK, Brown K. Preoperative psychosocial evaluation of penile prosthesis candidates. Am J Mens Health. 2008;2(1):68–75.
54. Pisano F, Falcone M, Abbona A, Oderda M, Soria F, Peraldo F, Marson F, Barale M, Fiorito C, Gurioli A, Frea B, Gontero P. The importance of psychosexual counselling in the re-establishment of organic and erotic functions after penile prosthesis implantation. Int J Impot Res. 2015;27(5):197–200.
55. Vittori-Longhi E, Franco G, Colombo F. Psychosexual counseling in andrological surgery. Cham: Springer; 2019.
56. Penile prosthesis information form, 2008. Available online: http://www.smsna.org/V1/images/SMSNAIPP-policy-ws.pdf.
57. Kovac JR. Informed consent for penile prosthesis surgery. Transl Androl Urol. 2017;6(Suppl 5):S881–2.
58. Chung E. Penile prosthesis implant: scientific advances and technological innovations over the last four decades. Transl Androl Urol. 2017;6(1):37–45.
59. Chung E, Solomon M, DeYoung L, Brock GB. Comparison between AMS 700™ CX and Coloplast™ Titan inflatable penile prosthesis for Peyronie's disease treatment and remodeling: clinical outcomes and patient satisfaction. J Sex Med. 2013;10(11):2855–60.

60. Wilson SK, Delk JR, Mulcahy JJ, Cleves M, Salem EA. Upsizing of inflatable penile implant cylinders in patients with corporal fibrosis. J Sex Med. 2006;3(4):736–42.
61. Wilson SK, Cleves MA, Delk JR 2nd. Ultrex cylinders: problems with uncontrolled lengthening (the S-shaped deformity). J Urol. 1996;155(1):135–7.
62. Mulcahy JJ, Wilson SK. Current use of penile implants in erectile dysfunction. Curr Urol Rep. 2006;7(6):485–9.
63. Negro CL, Paradiso M, Rocca A, Bardari F. Implantation of AMS 700 LGX penile prosthesis preserves penile length without the need for penile lengthening procedures. Asian J Androl. 2016;18:114–7.
64. Barboglio Romo P, Chikkatur HP, Beldona S, Yi Y, Bruns TM, et al. Comparative evaluation of physical characteristics of different inflatable penile prostheses. Scand J Urol. 2017;51:420–5.
65. Wallen JJ, Madiraju SK, Wang R, Henry GD. Implementation of length expanding inflatable penile prosthesis is not sufficient to prevent postsurgical penile shortening. Asian J Androl. 2019;21:98–100.
66. Dhabuwala C, Sheth S, Zamzow B. Infection rates of rifampin/gentamicin-coated Titan Coloplast penile implants. Comparison with Inhibizone-impregnated AMS penile implants. J Sex Med. 2011;8(1):315–20.
67. Wallen JJ, Barrera EV, Ge L, et al. Biomechanical comparison of inflatable penile implants: a cadaveric pilot study. J Sex Med. 2018;15:1034–40.
68. Ralph DJ, Garaffa G, Muneer A, Freeman A, Rees R, Christopher AN, Minhas S. The immediate insertion of a penile prosthesis for acute ischaemic priapism. Eur Urol. 2009;56(6):1033–8.
69. Habous M, Tealab A, Farag M, Soliman T, Williamson B, Mahmoud S, Elserafy A, Mekawi Z, Remeah A, Nassar M, Laban O, Abdelwahab O, Binsaleh S, Giona S, Ralph D, Mulhall J. Malleable penile implant is an effective therapeutic option in men with Peyronie's disease and erectile dysfunction. Sex Med. 2018;6(1):24–9.

Chapter 2
Critical Analysis of Maneuvers to Reduce Infection in Penile Implant Surgery

Karina Evelyn Sidabutar, Jared J. Wallen, and Gerard D. Henry

Introduction

Erectile dysfunction (ED) has been defined as the inability to have and/or sustain an erection sufficient for intercourse [1]. Conditions commonly associated with ED include diabetes mellitus, hypertension, hyperlipidemia, coronary artery disease, obesity, and prostate cancer treatment [2]. While most of those entities are markers of cardiovascular risk, not all have been associated with increased risk of infection with surgical implants [3].

Prosthetic devices are a well-established form of treatment for medically refractory erectile dysfunction. Postoperative infection is the most feared complication of genitourinary prosthetic surgery. In the USA today, most experts report the incidence of infection during the initial implant is only 1–3%, but traditional replacement/revision surgery has had a 10–18% risk [4–6].

Multiple product enhancements during the last 25 years have resulted in markedly decreased mechanical failure rates. In fact, most authorities now believe the devices are more often revised for non-mechanical failure factors such as infection and cylinder issues than mechanical reasons [4–6]. Despite these mechanical improvements, infection has remained a significant complication in prosthetic surgery.

K. E. Sidabutar
Regional Urology, Jakarta, Indonesia

J. J. Wallen
YOU & WEE Urologic Surgery and Wellness, Sarasota, FL, USA

G. D. Henry (✉)
WK Advanced Urology, Bossier City, Louisiana, USA

E. P. Miranda, J. P. Mulhall (eds.), *Penile Implant Surgery*,
https://doi.org/10.1007/978-3-030-82363-4_2

Greater understanding of the mechanisms underlying infection has led to markedly decreased infection rates [7]. However, infection continues to affect a considerable percentage of cases; especially for lower-volume implanters. Current thought is that device infection begins with the contamination of the implant with microorganisms during implantation [8]. Bacteria can attach to the implant surfaces, secreting adhesion molecules and proteins that start to form a biofilm matrix. This structure provides protection by blunting the host immune response and lowering antibiotic effects via decreased penetration [9]. Older research have shown that skin flora bacteria are the most commonly cultured organisms at the time of explant or salvage [10, 11]. However, with the spread of antibiotics, bacterial resistance patterns have changed as was shown by Carrion et al. [12]. Moreover, newer identification techniques, such as DNA sequencing, will be changing the landscape as to what microorganisms are actually causing the implant infections.

Indeed, infection prevention can be a key area for improving outcomes for penile prostheses. More than 20 influential issues have been observed, such as diabetes, immunosuppression, spinal cord injury, reconstruction, revision, concomitant surgeries, preoperative and postoperative antibiotic use, preoperative bathing, surgical site hair removal, adherence to protocol, surgical technique, surgical drain placement/compressive dressings, and skin prepping [13].

Although infection rates are less than 3% in most primary implantation papers today, we may be able to impact modifiable risk factors as discussed above, especially for replacement surgery and at less experienced implant centers. Factors believed to increase replacement IPP infection rates are as follows: decreased host resistance factors, impaired antibiotic penetration of the area due to the capsule surrounding the components, activation of biofilm, and decreased wound healing related to scar formation. For IPP replacement surgery, it appears that performing a revision washout reduces infection rates, and thus it is recommended by the AUA guidelines panel. While infections occur in a higher percentage of patients having revision surgeries than primary surgeries, revision washout is one of the causes for decreased infection rates after inflatable penile prosthesis (IPP) replacement surgery over time [14].

Risk Factors Clearly Associated with Penile Prosthesis Infection

A systematic review and meta-analysis found that diabetes mellitus and immunosuppression were associated with an increased risk for device infection [15]. This review evaluated 15 studies that investigated the relationship between **diabetes mellitus** and penile prosthesis infection, with a total of 35,570 patients: 8033 patients had diabetes mellitus and 27,537 did not. Among these patients, penile device infection was 3% versus 1.44%, respectively. There was a significant association between diabetes mellitus and risk of infection: OR 2.48 (95% CI 1.38 to

4.47) I2 = 71% [15]. *Critical point* – while there is agreement that diabetes mellitus increases infection rates, currently, in prosthetic urology, there is no "magical" hemoglobin A1C level or glucose value that is widely accepted as a breakpoint to not proceeding with the implantation. Immunosuppression was another risk factor that clearly revealed increase infection rates. Three studies were found with a total of 1496 patients. Rates of infection were 31% versus 1.7%, for patients with immunosuppression vs. without immunosuppression, respectively. There was a significant association between immunosuppression and risk of infection: OR 20.99 (95% CI 0.71 to 622.45) I2 = 90% [15].

Two studies investigated the relationship between **obesity** and penile prosthesis infection. Garber et al. [16] presented their series of obese patients who underwent a subcutaneous reservoir of the penile implant with a 12.5% infection rate. Pineda et al. [17] found that 11 of 44 patients (25%) with obesity (body mass index >30 kg/m^2) had a surgical complication or failure to cure, as compared with 5 of 80 non-obese patients (6%; $P < 0.01$). *Critical point* – while these are small single-center studies, metabolic syndrome and other medical conditions associated with many morbidly obese patients may cause higher complication rates. For example, the only patient that the corresponding author has had expire postoperative IPP implantation had a BMI of 48 kg/m^2 and had a fatal pulmonary embolism postop day 3.

Multiple studies in the medical literature have indicated an increased risk of infection when reoperations (revisions) are performed on genitourinary prostheses [4–6, 18, 19]. This increased incidence of infection associated with reoperation has been postulated to be due to decreased host resistance factors, impaired antibiotic penetration of the area because of the capsule surrounding the components, activation of the biofilm, and decreased wound healing related to scar formation. The organism most often found responsible for the infection in reoperation is *S. epidermidis* [18]. This bacterium is also the most common cause of infection during the original implantation, accounting for 35% to 80% of all positive cultures [19]. As alluded to the above, the infectious agent are changing. Nevertheless, revision/replacement surgery is strongly associated with higher infection rates.

Biofilm, Complete Implant Removal, and Culture Sensitivity

Most authorities believe genitourinary prosthetic infection is caused by contamination of the implant at the time of implantation. Studies suggest that preoperative nasal swab cultures of certain staphylococcus species are significantly correlated with postoperative surgical site wound infections [20]. Hematogenous late infections do occur, but rarely [21]. After adherence to the implant, many staphylococcus species produce a protective mucin coat or biofilm [22]. Bacteria present within the biofilm may survive at a decreased metabolic rate chronically and without the patient realizing bacteria are present in the implant spaces. Occasionally bacteria are released from the biofilm in a "planktonic" fashion and may cause symptoms

[22]. Antibiotics or the body's defense mechanisms can kill these planktonic bacteria. Those organisms present within the biofilm are protected and cannot be eradicated except by removal of the implant and lavage of the implant spaces. The majority of clinically uninfected genitourinary prostheses have organisms growing in the implant space at reoperation [10]. A study by Silverstein et al. also shows that bacterial biofilm exists on most inflatable penile prosthesis at revision surgery done for noninfectious reasons. Host mechanisms to control infection may lead to homeostatic balance that enables biofilms to exist on surface of the prostheses without clinical infection (Fig. 2.1). A critical threshold of biofilm extent may exist beyond which clinical infection may occur, but which we currently cannot measure [23]. *Critical point* – bacterial biofilm occurs on almost everything implanted in the body.

In 1996 Brant et al. reported salvage success with overt clinical IPP infections [24]. Their method, since successfully repeated by others, involves removing the infected device, using sequential lavage with antiseptic solutions to sterilize the implant space and immediately re-implantation with a completely new sterile device. Mulcahy's famous salvage rescue protocol described using four antiseptic solutions, that is, (1) 50% peroxide/50% normal saline (NS), (2) 50% povidone-iodine/50% NS, (3) 1 g cefazolin and 40 mg tobramycin sulfate in 1 l NS, and (4) 500 mg vancomycin and 80 mg gentamicin sulfate in 1 l NS. The lavage protocol began with 50% peroxide, then 50% povidone-iodine, then the cefazolin/tobramycin mixture, and then the vancomycin/gentamicin mixture, followed by the same solutions in reverse order (cefazolin/tobramycin mixture, 50% povidone-iodine and 50% peroxide) with the final lavage solution, a combination of the two antibiotic mixtures together. One Asepto syringe full of each solution used in the protocol was irrigated into the different implant spaces. For example, a three-piece penile prosthesis had the two cylinder spaces, the pump space and the reservoir space flushed with all solutions. A large rubber catheter was placed in the reservoir space to assist in the lavage of that area [14]. Only after the complete implant has been removed and the entire capsular space has been thoroughly irrigated is the new implant placed. *We believe* the success of this technique in eradicating infection is *predicated more so on the mechanical removal of the bacteria and the biofilm by the lavage of the solution than the chemical killing of the antiseptics in the solution.*

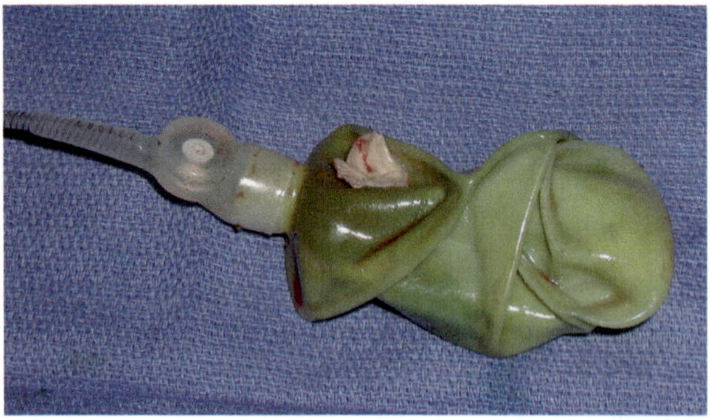

Fig. 2.1 Example of gross biofilm production on reservoir. (Photo courtesy of Gerard Henry)

After components are removed, then a formal salvage rescue washout is performed. If the components are not removed, biofilm would be left behind which might explain the higher rate of infection in any/all revisions [10]. Henry et al. evaluated infection rates and overall device rate, comparing single component exchange and complete replacement of IPP at the time of revision surgery for noninfectious reasons. The results trended toward better outcomes with complete replacement patients. Complete penile prosthesis removal and replacement may have lower infection and higher survival rates. A causal factor may be bacteria on the retained components [25].

Reservoir removal should not be construed as the standard of care in clinically uninfected cases. If reservoir removal proves difficult and there is no evidence of gross infection on the pump and cylinders, the original reservoir can be retained, but a new reservoir is utilized in a different position. A recent study showed no added incidence of subsequent infection in a large series of retained reservoirs [26]. Moreover, *we now believe* that the salvage rescue irrigating solutions made famous by Dr. Mulcahy are not the best protocol; for example, betadine and hydrogen peroxide appear to hurt wound healing. To our current knowledge, the *best irrigating solution appears to be a dilute antiseptic normal saline solution.* A future research study comparing irrigating solutions would require such an enormous number of patients that it would be impractical.

S. epidermidis has been shown to be the most common organism found at removal of a penile prosthesis for infection [10, 27, 28] (Fig. 2.2). Moreover, Licht et al. found that 40% of uninfected penile prostheses and 36% of artificial urinary sphincters had low colony counts of *S. epidermidis* [18]. Of the patients with positive culture, three later became infected, and higher colony counts of the organism were found at explantation. A subsequent prosthetic infection did not develop in any

Organism Cultured	Absolute # (% of total)
S. Epidermidis	25 (39%)
S. Lugdunensis	14 (22%)
S. Capitis	3 (5)
S. Haemolyticus	3 (5)
Strep Mitis	3 (5)
MRSA	2 (3)
S. Auricularis	2 (3)
Propionibacterium	3 (5)
Other	9 (14)

Fig. 2.2 Isolates cultured from clinically uninfected penile prosthesis [10]

patients with penile prosthesis with a negative culture at reoperation. Therefore, ensuring that the replacement implant has a sterile environment in which to be placed at revision/replacement may decrease the rate of prostheses reoperation infection. Even better, using an irrigation protocol with antiseptic solutions at replacement combined with inserting an antibiotic-coated prosthesis could help ensure a sterile environment for the new implant while the antibiotic elution could address bacterial contamination in the subsequent surgery [10].

Henry et al. found that most of these organisms are sensitive to the combination of rifampin and minocycline, which is now available as a coating on penile prostheses [10]. These sensitivity results are almost identical to those found on colonization of catheters with staphylococcus strains [29]. Another study suggested that coating silicone strips "with antibiotics, particularly rifampin/minocycline, can reduce the incidence of graft colonization in contaminated wounds in rats, even in the absence of systemic antibiotics." [30] The presence of rifampin/minocycline eluting into the implant space might have prevented these isolates from colonizing on or near the prostheses. Unexpectedly those revisions due to mechanical failure with positive cultures had significantly worse revision-free duration than those with negative cultures (log rank test p 0.0198). The reason for this finding is unclear [10].

Quick Preoperative Considerations

Alcohol-Based Skin Preparations Since the pathogens found on the patient's skin appear to be the major source of surgical site infection, an optimal preoperative skin preparation may decrease device infection. A prospective, multicenter, randomized clinical trial compared chlorhexidine-alcohol and PVI for surgical site antisepsis. Patients who had their skin prepped with chlorhexidine-alcohol had less surgical site infections than those prepped with PVI (9.5% vs. 16.1%; $P = 0.004$) [31]. In the systematic review and meta-analysis conducted by Lee and colleagues [32], chlorhexidine-based agents were found to decrease the risk of surgical site infections considerably, with an adjusted risk ratio of 0.64, and to decrease positivity of skin culture results (adjusted risk ratio, 0.44) when compared to iodine antisepsis [32, 33]. In 2011, Kava et al. reported a similar result in IPP placement [34]. A total of 117 primary and 72 revision penile implant procedures were analyzed. The first 106 patients had in infection rate of 7.5%. In the last 83 patients, an adjuvant alcohol-based skin prep applied lowered the risk of infection to 1.2% (1 out of 83 patients vs. 8 of the first 106) [8].

Perioperative Prophylactic Antibiotics The new guidelines for antibiotic selection from the American Urological Association (AUA) and European Association of Urology (EAU) have broadened perioperative prophylaxis to encompass the bacteria expected to cause infection [35, 36]. In a recent study, Gross et al. observed and compared the results of retrospective analysis of culture results and profile of antibiotic resistance with the AUA and EAU guidelines [12]. The AUA suggests an aminoglycoside (or aztreonam in patients with renal compromise) in combination with a first- or second-generation cephalosporin or vancomycin. The combination of an aminoglycoside (or aztreonam) and vancomycin showed the highest efficacy, killing 86% of the bacteria cultured in their series. Nonetheless, this combination had weak anaerobic coverage (25%) and did not have fungal coverage. The EAU recommends a second- or third-generation cephalosporin or a penicillin agent with anti-penicillinase. Ampicillin-sulbactam was the most efficient single anti-penicillinase agent in the EAU guidelines and eliminated 72% of the cultured microbes in their series. Anaerobic coverage was 100%, but the Gram-positive and Gram-negative coverage decreased to 72% and 73%, respectively. Also, it did not cover *Candida* species and was not used by their surgeons [12]. These findings of increased fungal infections has led the authors and several other prosthetic urologists to add, *although not stated in the guidelines*, an antifungal agent such as fluconazole preoperatively.

Revision Washout

Salvage rescue by vigorously washing out the implant space with an antibiotic irrigation protocol has been shown to be effective in cases of infected IPPs [24]. Only after the complete implant has been removed and the entire capsular space has been thoroughly irrigated is the new implant placed as discussed above. Revision washout, which is similar antibiotic irrigation protocol, decreases subsequent infection in cases of clinically uninfected IPPs [14]. Perhaps the increased infection rate seen in revision prosthetic surgeries is due to activation of preexisting biofilm. Therefore, we have adopted a policy of removing all components in the surgical exposure of an implant together with foreign material such as polytetrafluoroethylene at prosthesis replacement. The authors acknowledge that in clinically uninfected cases, the reservoir can be left behind in most patients; nevertheless, if the implant is grossly infected or eroded, all components should be removed unless extenuating situations exist. Salvage rescue and revision washout decreases subsequent infections, *most experts believe*, by mechanically cleansing the implant spaces. A decreased bacterial presence in implant spaces after salvage rescue and revision washouts is the basis of the clinical practice [37].

Abouassaly et al. reported decreased infection rates with revision washout using only a copious amount of one type of antibiotic solution instead of the several smaller amounts in the original salvage rescue protocol [38]. It is possible that some irrigants used in the original salvage rescue protocol, i.e., hydrogen peroxide, cause tissue irritation or poor wound healing, making patients more susceptible to infection [37]. A study by Henry et al. found only 2.9% of patients who underwent removal of the IPP with irrigation of the implant spaces with antiseptic solutions and replacement with a three-piece penile prosthesis infection developed within 6–33 months of observation, compared to 11.6% of patients who did not undergo antiseptic irrigation that had infection [14] (Fig. 2.3).

Washout	Number Infections (%) Yes	No	Total #
Yes	4 (2.9)	136 (97.1)	140
No	5 (11.6)	38 (88.4)	43
Total	9 (4.9)	174 (95.1)	183
Fisher's Exact P = 0.034			

Fig. 2.3 Revision penile prosthesis surgery infection rates in patients who did vs. did not undergo revision washout [14]

Another study by the same group demonstrates that in 45% of the revision cases for noninfectious reason, there were culture-positive bacteria on the implant space capsule tissue, which were isolated upon entering the pump space. However, after revision washout, the rate of culture-positive bacteria was decreased by almost half to 25%, indicating a decrease in the number of bacteria present on the implant capsule after surgical lavage of the implant space (Fig. 2.4). It also reduced number of patients with multiple isolates after the washout. A decreased bacterial presence appears to be the basis for the revision washout and the salvage rescue success in decreasing subsequent infection rates. Of note, residual antibiotic fluid used during revision washout could be a contributing factor in the lower culture-positive bacteria rate on the implant space capsule tissue after washout. However, a 25% rate is still quite high, in that prosthetic surgeons are placing a foreign body (the IPP) against a thick capsule of tissue that has live bacteria on it. This indicates that perhaps revision washout should be more aggressive to try to decrease bacterial contamination even more. The patient should receive adequate systemic antibiotics before revision surgery and several applications of the antiseptic lavage washout should be utilized [37]. Indeed, this is consistent with an earlier study by Montague et al. demonstrating that one irrigating solution done with mechanical washout was as good as the four-solution protocol, and revision surgery done in this manner does not carry an increased risk of infection [39].

However, little evaluation of this practice has been performed, and there is wide variation between surgeons and sites regarding the type of irrigant utilized (with or without single or combination antimicrobials). There is also a trend toward irrigant type determined by hospital surgical committees. To date, there is little agreement whether to cease irrigation when the IPP is introduced into the penis (this may or may not be a factor for antibiotic impregnated devices) or continue until the end of the procedure. The lack of uniformity across strategies thought to decrease infection rates for penile prosthesis insertion is of concern [40]. Simply replacing a defective prosthesis with an antibiotic-coated IPP without the revision washout did not alter the higher traditional revision infection rates [14]. Most importantly, there was a significant impact of revision washout, 4% of cases which incorporated washout developed infection or impending extrusion/erosion, as compared with 25% of

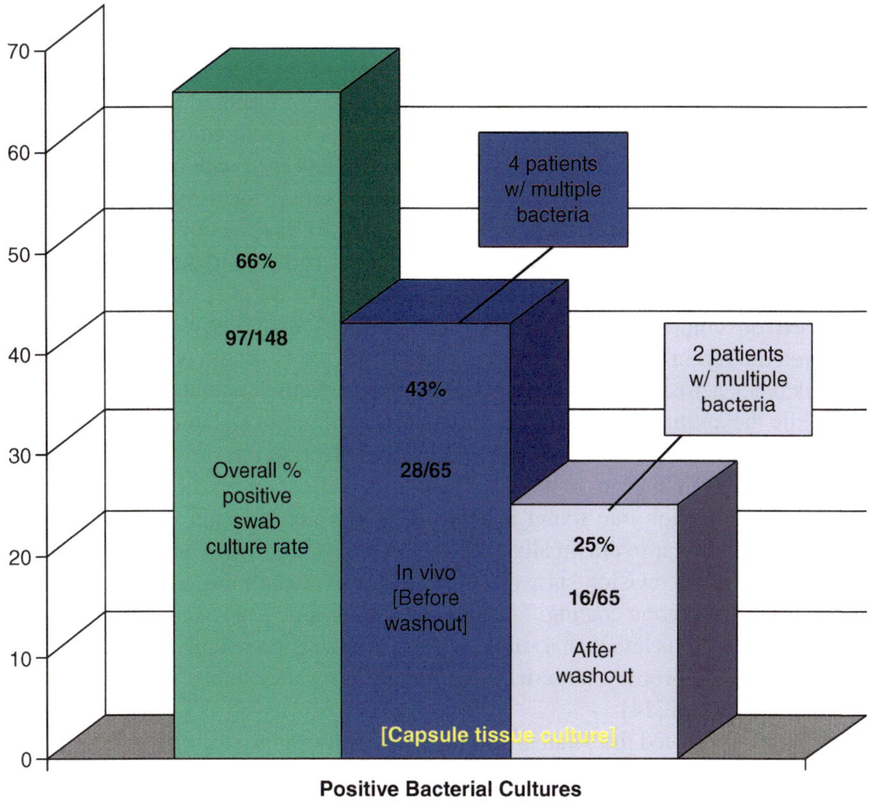

Fig. 2.4 Percent of positive bacterial cultures at IPP revision surgery for noninfectious reasons [37]

cases in which a washout procedure was not performed in another study [41]. A long-term follow-up paper of that series needs to be published. *Critical point* – while there is no uniformity in revision washout, removing the device and a normal saline-based lavage of the implant spaces appears to have real benefit in reducing infection rates and is considered standard of care by most experts.

Antibiotic-Coated Implant

The incidence of primary implantation of an IPP was traditionally 2–5% prior to infection retardant coating and lowered to about 1–2% with infection retardant coatings (IRC) on the IPP [42–44]. However, these IRC prostheses are much less effective in this reduction in revision/replacement infection rates without the addition of a revision washout [14].

The InhibiZone antibiotic coating of the 700 penile prosthesis, a combination of rifampin and minocycline, impregnated into the external silicone surfaces of IPPs has been shown to decrease infection rates for primary implantation surgeries [42, 45]. The antibiotics disperse in vivo, creating a zone of bacterial growth inhibition [45]. In a 2004 study of 700 series prostheses, Carson reported on 2261 men with the InhibiZone-coated IPP and a control group of 1944 men with uncoated prostheses. Infection incidence was 0.28% in the treated group and 1.59% in the control group ($P = 0.0034$) after 60 days, and 0.68% and 1.61%, respectively ($P = 0.0047$), after 180 days. InhibiZone conferred an 82.4% lower infection rate than the control group after 60 days and a 57.8% lower rate after 180 days [42]. However, this data is based on company data, and there are feelings that high-volume customers received the InhibiZone-coated IPPs earlier and therefore would probably have better outcomes across the board compared to lower-volume implanters.

While the antibiotic coating (a combination of rifampin and minocycline) on the outside of 700 IPPs has been shown to decrease infection rates for primary implantation surgeries, it appears to have a less dramatic effect on revision cases [14, 42]. The 11.6% infection rate found in this study in which revision washout was not performed is similar to classically published results (Fig. 2.5). The established biofilm found during revision surgery could be too overwhelming a bacterial colony count for the antibiotic coating. The amount of antibiotic used to coat the outside of the 700 series IPP is less than a single oral pill, which is potentially enough to lower infection rates in primary surgeries but not enough for the established biofilm found in secondary cases [14].

Mentor introduced the Titan in 2002, a hydrophilic substance that reduces bacterial adherence and absorbs and diffuses antibiotics in which the implant is immersed intraoperatively (Fig. 2.6). The Titan IPP offers the advantage that the surgeon chooses the preferred antibiotic for each individual [45]. In 2004, Wolter and Hellstrom published a study comparing 1-year infection rates from the Titan IPP to Mentor's previous alpha-1 prostheses. Data from 2357 patients with the Titan IPP were compared with data from 482 patients with uncoated prostheses. The infection rates were 1.06% (25/2357) for the Titan IPP and 2.07% (10/482) for the alpha-1 noncoated prosthesis ($P = 0.033$) [43]. Similar concerns as with the above Carson paper about this being company data and preferred implanters getting the Titan coating first are valid. The exciting aspect of the Titan coating is the ability to "dip"

Revision Washout	Presentation (mos)	Diabetes	Revision No.	Isolate Cultured	Tetracycline/Rifampin Sensitive
Yes	Erosion + swelling (3)	No	1	S. epidermidis	Sensitive/sensitive
Yes	Adherence + pus (1)	No	1	Citrobacter freudii, Enterococcus faecalis	Sensitive/not available, resistant/sensitive
Yes	Erythema + swelling (2)	No	1	S. epidermidis, Escherichia coli	Sensitive/sensitive, resistant, not available
Yes	Erosion + pus (4)	No	1	Neg	
No	Erythema + pus (4)	No	2	Light yeast	Not available
No	Erosion + pus (15)	Yes	1	Not cultured/removed	
No	Erosion + pus (4)	Yes	1	Light yeast	Not available
No	Overt exudate (1)	No	3	Streptococcus agalactiae	Resistant/resistant
No	Overt exudate (1)	No	4	E. faecalis	Resistant/resistant

Fig. 2.5 Isolates cultured from infected penile prostheses at reoperation [14]

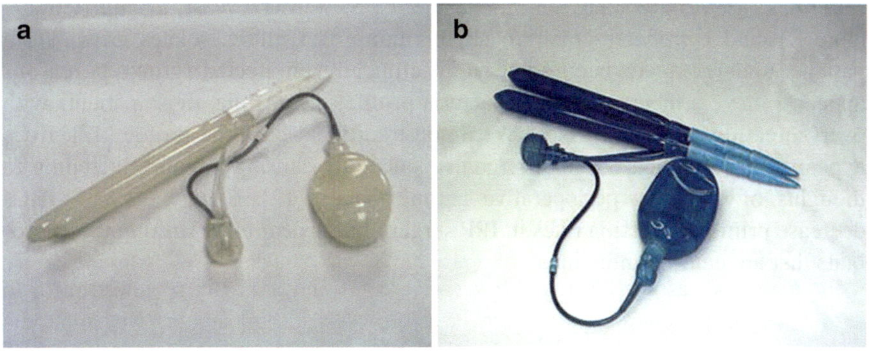

Fig. 2.6 The Titan inflatable penile prosthesis (IPP) demonstrating the absorption properties of its hydrophilic coat. (**a**) Plain hydrophilic coated implant that has not been dipped into a solution, (**b**) Blue dye dipped hydrophilic coated penile prosthesis. (Courtesy of Coloplast Corporation, Minneapolis, MN, USA) [45]

it into a possible future substance that will *not* allow bacteria attachment, the first step in the infection pathway.

Today, virtually all three-piece IPPs placed in the USA have IRCs, InhibiZone on the 700 series and hydrophilic coating on the Titan series. These IRC penile prostheses appear to have made an impact on the microorganisms found on IPPs. An older multicenter center study showed that during revision surgery for noninfected IPPs, culture-positive bacteria had been found in 54 of 77 (70%) patients with noncoated IPP [10]. A similar number, 12 of 20 (60%), of patients with coated IPPs showed positive cultures. Of the 54 noncoated patients, 49 (90%) had positive culture for *Staphylococcus* genus, while 10 (83%) of the 12 patients with coated IPP had a cultured isolate of the *Staphylococcus* genus. Three (5.5%) of the 54 noncoated patients grew more than 1 culture isolate versus none (0%) of the 12 coated IPP patients having more than 1 isolate cultured. Thus, positive cultures and visible bacterial biofilm have been shown to be present on clinically uninfected IPPs at the time of revision surgery in the majority of patients whether or not the IPP is coated with infection retardant coating [46].

A multicenter study evaluated culture isolates from patients with known IRC IPPs to evaluate the bacterial profile [47]. Only patients who already had infection retardant-coated penile prostheses placed and grew out positive culture isolates were included in the study. Patients were further broken down into two groups: clinically uninfected revision/replacement (group 1: 40 patients) and overtly infected undergoing salvage rescue or removal (group 2: 17 patients). In addition, sensitivities to the combination of tetracycline and rifampin were evaluated (sensitive sens; resistant R). A total of 38 isolates were cultured out in these patients with 25 from group 1 and 13 from group 2; some patients grew out more than 1 isolate. Culture-positive isolates from the clinically uninfected revisions (group 1) were 16 *S. epidermidis* (all sens), 3 *S. lugdunensis* (all sens), *Enterococcus faecalis* (intermediate sens), *Klebsiella pneumoniae* (sens), yeast, *Micrococcus* species, Gram rods, and *Peptostreptococcus* species. Culture-positive isolates from overtly infected patients (group 2) were 4 *S. epidermidis* (all sens), 2 MRSA (sens), 2

Enterococcus faecalis (sens), *S. haemolyticus*, S. warneri, yeast, *E. coli* (tetracycline R), and *Citrobacter freundii* (R to rifampin). Culture isolates grown from patients undergoing revision surgery for clinically uninfected (group 1) reasons appear to have a more traditional bacteria profile; meanwhile, those patients with overt infections (group 2) may have a non-traditional bacterial profile [47]. IRCs appear to have shifted the microorganisms actually causing infections, leading to thoughts of changing perioperative antimicrobials [12]. *Critical point* – IRCs decrease primary infection rates in IPP surgery but appear to be shifting the microbials that are causing infections.

Prevention of Hematoma Formation

Techniques to reduce hematoma formation will also decrease nutrient sources available to microorganisms [48, 49]. Large hematomas can cause dark "currant jelly" appearing drainage, which can act like a petri dish for bacteria to grow in. In the past, some prominent prosthetic surgeons advocated for immediate surgical evacuation of large scrotal hematomas to try to avoid high infection rates. The vast majority of prosthetic urologists would agree avoidance of scrotal hematomas is a good idea to prevent infections.

Suction Drain

There is controversy on whether or not to place a drain. In order to avoid postoperative hematoma, Sadeghi-Nejad and colleagues conducted a multi-institutional study on the efficacy of closed suction drainage of the scrotum in IPP surgery. They studied 425 patients and observed a 3.3% infection rate and 0.7% hematoma rate during an 18-month follow-up period. The authors concluded that short-term, closed suction drainage decreased the rate of hematoma formation following penile implant without increasing the risk of infection [49].

In spite of the data presented in that paper, there is still a concern that a drain placed near an implant might increase rates of infection and some may prefer alternative methods of hematoma prevention rather than a closed suction drain. Since the major source of scrotal hematoma could be corporal bleeding, another approach consists of closing the corporotomy with a running water-tight suture after cylinder placement. Arguments against this method include longer operative times to perform the suturing and suturing risks of inadvertent cylinder puncture. Another technique is to place a hemostatic agent along the corporal incision to aid in decrease of post-surgical scrotal hematoma. Alternatively, a newer method to prevent hematomas may be advanced dressings such as a "mummy wrap" variations.

Wilson et al. initially sought to identify methods to decrease scrotal hematoma formation following penile prosthesis surgery. Men were separated into three groups, pressure dressing alone, pressure dressing with drain, and pressure dressing with drain as well as implant inflation. Decreased rate of hematoma was only seen with the combination of all three methods [50].

Further evaluating the potential increase of infection caused by drains, Wallen et al. recently analyzed drain tubing cultures in over 100 IPP procedures. Both distal and proximal (1 cm below skin level) tubing segments were sent for standard culture after 48–72-h placement time following surgery. All distal drain tips were negative for growth and only one proximal section had growth. No cases were noted to be infected on follow-up. As a side note, hematoma formation was not seen in any patient at the time of drain removal [51]. *Critical point* – the jury is still out on the effectiveness and possible increase in infection rates associated with drain usage in IPP implantation; this issue can and has generated heated debates.

Mummy Wrap

Since the insurance reimbursements rules are changing, there is a tendency/hospital administration pressure to do most prosthetic urology as truly outpatient (same-day) surgeries. The use of a drain or complicated "spider web" tape dressing pushes the physician to use an overnight stay in the hospital. The Henry Mummy Wrap™ uses a non-sticky dressing, e.g., a Kerlix™ (Covidien, Dublin Ireland) 4-inch dressing roll. Starting at the top of the penis, the dressing is wrapped loosely, gradually wrapping around the shaft (Fig. 2.7). After the shaft of the penis has been encircled, the dressing is spun around the base of the entire genitalia – lifting the testicles, the pump, and the scrotum, superiorly, in a "broccoli stalk" shaping maneuver [48].

The dressing is then additionally wrapped a few times compressing the already present bandage. The key element is getting the dressing beneath both testicles (the "broccoli stalk"), with the pump positioned in the desired long-term location. Obese patients or those with a small, tight scrotum may need additional circumferential wraps around the base of the whole genitalia to ensure that the testicles and pump are pushed forward into the "cast." The soft cast that develops at the end of this wrap procedure resembles an orthopedic ankle cast. After the dressing is placed, a soft cloth surgical tape, such as Medipore™ (3M, St. Paul, MN), is applied around the soft cast, with minimal tape adhering to the patient's skin. The Foley catheter can be left in until the dressing is removed, with the tubing taped to the patient's abdominal wall to alleviate tension on the Foley catheter, as patients may have difficulty voiding with the dressing in position. Without expansion of the scrotum, there should be minimal to no hematoma while the dressing is in place. One should always leave the glans exposed and avoid aggressive compressive dressing circumferentially around the penis. While controversial, patients on active blood thinner can be done and the mummy wrap left in place for 2 days.

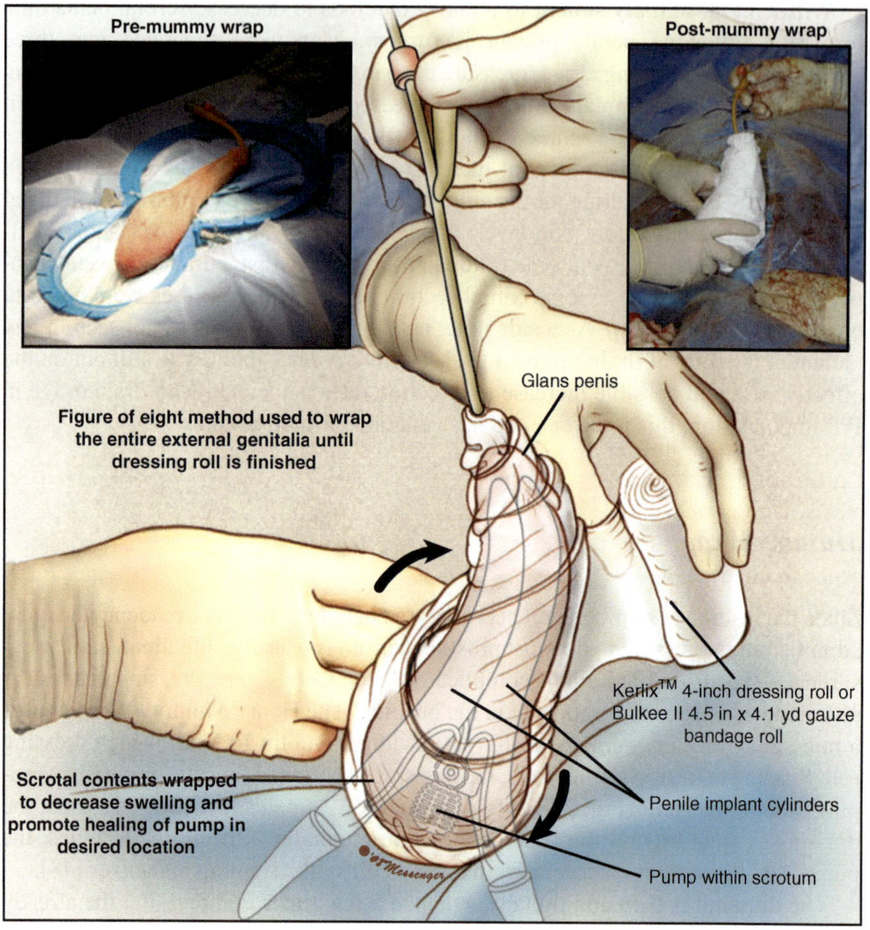

Fig. 2.7 Mummy wrap. A "figure of eight" type of method is used to wrap the entire external genitalia until the dressing roll is finished. The soft cast that develops at the end of the wrap procedure resembles an orthopedic extremity ankle cast. After the dressing is placed, a soft cloth surgical tape, such as Medipore (3M, St. Paul, MN, USA), is applied around the soft cast, with minimal tape adherent to the patient's skin. A Foley catheter can be left in place as long as the wrap is on, as some patients can have difficulty voiding with the soft cast. Typically, the dressing is removed the next day. For patients on anticoagulant therapy, or for other reasons, the wrap may be left on for 2 days. As there is no tape on the patient and no drain, removing the dressing is remarkably easy. If the inflatable penile prosthesis was left inflated, it is now very easy and much less painful to deflate, as there is essentially no swelling and the pump is easily palpated. Without expansion of the scrotum, there should be no hematoma while the dressing is in place [48]

Minimization of Device Skin Contact ("No Touch")

The "no touch" technique consists of decreasing skin contact with the prosthetic material [52]. By changing gloves and surgical tools after opening the skin, subcutaneous tissue, and dartos to the level of Buck's fascia, and usage of a special drape to completely isolate the surgical field from the skin, Eid and Wilson in 2012 showed a decrease in infection rate from 2% with the standard technique and coated devices to only 0.46% with the no touch technique. There were no difference in the 700 and Titan IPP infection rates and no difference between virgin and revision operation infection rates [53].

In a recent study by Weinberg et al., 200 men were operated with a modified "no touch" technique and "mummy wrap" dressing. Using a subcoronal incision and complete penile degloving to place the IPP, the researchers observed that three men developed infections (1.5%). It is important to observe that 74% of patients had diabetes, 24% had Peyronie's plaque plication, and 22% had Peyronie's relaxing incisions to correct penile curvature [54]. The original "no touch" can be burdensome and dangerously slows the procedure so most prosthetic surgeons have their own modified technique that minimizes skin contact. The author *advocates* for *a modified no touch technique and mummy wrap dressing* to reduce IPP infection rates despite limited data supporting the combination of these techniques.

Strict Operative Sterile Technique

Even with sterile procedures, every surgical incision is potentially contaminated with bacteria. Commonly these are bacteria from the patient's own endogenous flora; yet a strict sterile operative technique should be maintained [55]. Notwithstanding the importance of hand scrubbing, and appropriate use of sterile gloves and gowns, other perioperative measures including hair removal, perioperative patient warming, and optimization of the operating room environment should be a priority and is outside the scope of this chapter. Perioperative hypothermia, however, is associated with a significant increase in surgical site infection risk, and the patient should be warmed during surgery; meanwhile the actual room is cooler with low humidity being ideal [33]. The lowest risk of surgical site infection (SSI) has always been associated with not removing hair. If hair needs to be removed because of interference with the procedure, then it should be done immediately before the surgery. While clipping has been shown to be better than shaving for cardiac bypass grafting, it can be difficult and abrasive to clip the scrotum [56].

However, Grober et al. showed "that preoperative hair removal on the scrotal skin using a razor results in less skin trauma and improved overall shave quality with no apparent increased risk of SSIs." [57].

The use of double gloves may offer additional benefit. In a recent study Makama et al. encouraged the use of double gloves [58]. After analyzing total of 1536 gloves, a perforation rate of 15.2% was observed in single gloves and 14.4% in double gloves. However, the number of through and through puncture from outer to the inner gloves was only 1.17%. Thus, the double glove technique offered a protection for 98.83% of cases of outer glove perforation. Double gloving appears to be more and more the standard of care for the patient, staff, and doctors.

Future Research, Ideas, and Advancements

Planktonic (free floating) bacteria are different from bacteria in a biofilm as discussed above. Biofilm bacteria can and do alter their local environment, distinguishing themselves even further from planktonic ones. Bacteria in a biofilm can sustain slow growth rates and remain inactive for long periods. Since conventional laboratory bacterial cultures were developed to identify planktonic bacteria, they are often unable to identify bacteria present in a biofilm, thus increasing the likelihood of failure when culturing biofilm for an implanted device [37]. Moreover, there is a long-standing worry that "wimpy skin organisms" contaminate cultures: for example, Staphylococcus epidermis is the most common bacteria found [37].

Taking into account these difficulties, there is an increase in the use of clinical molecular microbiological methods to investigate the microbiota of chronic and now acute infections. Molecular testing is more sensitive than culturing, which results in markedly different results being reported to clinicians. When comparing molecular and culture testing, the culture-free 16S ribosomal DNA sequencing and its relative abundance score can help clinicians decide the best course of treatment by displaying the bacteria more common in a sample and therefore more likely to be responsible for the infection. The *corresponding author believes* that DNA sequencing with its "relative abundance" data will rewrite causative microbiomes that are actually causing the infections of IPPs.

The slow growth speeds of the biofilm offer protection against immune defenses and many antimicrobial agents, such as antibiotics and biocides. The bacteria deep into the biofilm can withstand antibiotic concentrations 1000–1500 times higher than the concentrations that kill same species freely floating (planktonic) bacteria [22]. Thus, biofilms are particularly hard to prevent and even harder to destroy once they are formed, increasing the risk of persistent/chronic infection [22, 59]. Molecular testing delivers fast results even in the setting of a negative culture and will detect dormant bacteria. Additionally, biofilm pathogens are evaluated against resistance genes, more than a standard culture's susceptibility testing. Clinical molecular microbiological methods are now considered the gold standard in other medical specialties such as wound care.

Other ideas for future research in decreasing implant infections should include different types of surface/shielding of the surface of the implant – for example, a surface that does not allow attachment of the bacteria on a scanning microscopy level. It has been reported the European Union is soon to require a large clinical study of InhibiZone in order to keep using it after 2021, and this may be not feasible to the company. Therefore, expanded research of IPP surface design may be imminent. In addition, as we learn more about the actual causative agents of IPP infections, InhibiZone maybe the wrong coating anyway.

While discussed and presented at several meetings including those of the Sexual Medicine Society of North America (SMSNA) and the AUA, the authors were discouraged to write up "observation of local clinical penile prostheses infections instead of immediate salvage rescue/removal" in cases of draining clear fluid from the postoperative incision in patients with no systemic symptoms [60, 61]. The point of when to observe the patient versus surgical readmission of a patient for implant removal versus salvage rescue remains indeterminate and controversial. The *authors believe* it is time to move forward with defining these issues with research. In addition, despite it being mandatory to irrigate infected wounds, there is only one paper found in PubMed that compared tissue cultures before and after any type of surgical washout in our field of surgery and there should be more.

References

1. Zegers-Hochschild F, Adamson GD, Dyer S, Racowsky C, De Mouzon J, Sokol R, et al. The international glossary on infertility and fertility care, 2017. Fertil Steril. 2017;108(3):393–406.
2. Rew KT, Heidelbaugh JJ. Erectile dysfunction. Am Fam Physician. 2016;94(10):820–7.
3. Billups KL, Bank AJ, Padma-Nathan H, Katz S, Williams R. Erectile dysfunction is a marker for cardiovascular disease: results of the Minority Health Institute Expert Advisory Panel. J Sex Med. 2005;2(1):40-50-52.
4. Wilson SK, Delk JR II. Inflatable penile implant infection: predisposing factors and treatment suggestion. J Urol. 1995;153:659.
5. Lotan Y, Roehrnborn CG, Mcconnel JD, Hendin BN. Factors influencing the outcomes of penile prosthesis surgery at a teaching institution. Urology. 2003;62:918.
6. Jarow JP. Risk factors for penile prosthetic infection. J Urol. 1996;156:402.
7. Darouiche RO, Bella AJ, Boone TB, Brock G, Broderick GA, Burnett AL, et al. North American consensus document on infection of penile prostheses. Urology. 2013;82(4):937–42.
8. Dawn LE, Henry GD, Tan GK, Wilson SK. Biofilm and infectious agents present at the time of penile prosthesis revision surgery: times are a changing. Sex Med Rev. 2017;5(2):236–43.
9. Wilson SK, Costerton JW. Biofilm and penile prosthesis infections in the era of coated implants: a review. J Sex Med. 2012;9(1):44–53.
10. Henry GD, Wilson SK, Delk JR II, Carson CC, Silverstein A, Cleves MA, Donatucci CF. Penile prosthesis cultures during revision surgery: a Multicenter study. J Urol. 2004;172:153–6.
11. Mulcahy JJ, Kramer A, Brant WO, Parker JL, Perito PE, Myers JB, et al. Current management of penile implant infections, device reliability, and optimizing cosmetic outcome. Curr Urol Rep. 2014;15(6):413.
12. Gross MS, Phillips EA, Carrasquillo RJ, Thornton A, Greenfield JM, Levine LA, et al. Multicenter investigation of the micro-organisms involved in penile prosthesis infection: an

analysis of the efficacy of the Aua and Eau guidelines for penile prosthesis prophylaxis. J Sex Med. 2017;14(3):455–63.
13. Pineda M, Burnett AL. Penile prosthesis infections-a review of risk factors, prevention, and treatment. Sex Med Rev. 2016;4(4):389–98.
14. Henry GD, Wilson SK, Delk JR 2nd, Carson CC, Wiygul J, Tornehl C, et al. Revision washout decreases penile prosthesis infection in revision surgery: a Multicenter study. J Urol. 2005;173(1):89–92.
15. Carvajal A, Benavides J, García-Perdomo HA, et al. Risk factors associated with penile prosthesis infection: systematic review and meta-analysis. Int J Impot Res. 2020; https://doi.org/10.1038/s41443-020-0232-x.
16. Garber BB, Bickell M. Subcutaneous placement of inflatable penile prosthesis reservoirs. Urology. 2016;88:93–6.
17. Pineda M, Burnett AL. Distinguishing failure to cure from complication after penile prosthesis implantation. J Sex Med. 2017;14(5):731–7.
18. Licht MR, Montague DK, Angermeier KW, Lakin MM. Cultures from genitourinary prostheses at reoperation: questioning the role of Staphylococcus epidermidis in periprosthetic infection. J Urol. 1995;154:387.
19. Blum MD. Infections of genitourinary prostheses. Infect Dis Clin N Am. 1989;3:259.
20. Casewell MW. The nose: an underestimated source of Staphylococcus aureus causing wound infection. J Hosp Infect. 1998;40:S3.
21. Carson CC, Robertson CN. Late hematogenous infection of penile prosthesis. J Urol. 1988;139:50.
22. Stewart PS, Costerton JW. Antibiotic resistance of Bacteria in biofilms. Lancet. 2001;358:135.
23. Silverstein AD, Henry GD, Evans B, Pasmore M, Simmons CJ, Donatucci CF. Biofilm formation on clinically noninfected penile prosthesis. J Urol. 2006;176:1008–11.
24. Brant MD, Ludlow JK, Mulcahy JJ. The prosthesis salvage operation: immediate replacement of the infected penile prosthesis. J Urol. 1996;155:155.
25. Henry GD, Wilson SK, Donatucci CF, Delk JR II, Lentz A, Mcnamara E, Cleves M, Jennerman C, Carson CC. Single component exchange during penile prosthesis revision appears to have higher infection rates and lower overall device survival rates than complete component replacement: a multicenter analysis. J Urol. 2012;187(4s)
26. Rajpurkar AD, Bianco FJ, Terlecki R, Dhabuwala CB. Fate of the retained reservoir after replacement of a three-piece penile implant. J Urol. 2003;Suppl. 169:326., Abstract 1266.
27. Montague DK. Periprosthetic infections. J Urol. 1987;138:68.
28. Thomalla JV, Thompson ST, Rowland RG, Mulcahy JJ. Infectious complications of penile prosthetic implants. J Urol. 1987;138:65.
29. Raad I, Darouiche R, Hachem R, Mansourt M, Bodey GP. The broad-spectrum activity and efficacy of catheters coated with minocycline and rifampin. J Infect Dis. 1996;173:418.
30. Li H, Fairfax MR, Dubocq F, Darouiche RO, Rajpurkar A, Thompson M, et al. Antibacterial activity of antibiotic coated silicone grafts. J Urol. 1998;160:1910.
31. Darouiche RO, Wall MJ Jr, Itani KM, Otterson MF, Webb AL, Carrick MM, et al. Chlorhexidine-alcohol versus povidone-iodine for surgical-site antisepsis. N Engl J Med. 2010;362(1):18–26. https://doi.org/10.1056/NEJMoa0810988.
32. Lee I, Agarwal RK, Lee BY, Fishman NO, Umscheid CA. Systematic review and cost analysis comparing use of chlorhexidine with use of iodine for preoperative skin antisepsis to prevent surgical site infection. Infect Control Hosp Epidemiol. 2010;31(12):1219–29. https://doi.org/10.1086/657134.
33. Young PY, Khadaroo RG. Surgical site infections. Surg Clin North Am. 2014;94(6):1245–64. https://doi.org/10.1016/j.suc.2014.08.008.
34. Kava BR, Kanagarajah P, Ayyathurai R. Contemporary revision penile prosthesis surgery is not associated with a high risk of implant colonization or infection: a single-surgeon series. J Sex Med. 2011;8(5):1540–6. https://doi.org/10.1111/j.1743-6109.2011.02222.x.

35. Wolf JS Jr, Bennett CJ, Dmochowski RR, Hollenbeck BK, Pearle MS, Schaeffer AJ, et al. Best practice policy statement on urologic surgery antimicrobial prophylaxis. J Urol. 2008;179(4):1379–90. https://doi.org/10.1016/j.juro.2008.01.068.
36. Bonkat G, Pickard R, Bartoletti R, Bruyère F, Geerlings SE, Wagenlehner F, et al.. EAU guidelines on urological infections. European Association of Urology; 2017.
37. Henry GD, Carson CC, Wilson SK, Wiygul J, Tornehl C, Cleves MA, Simmons CJ, Donatucci CF. Revision washout decreases implant capsule tissue culture positivity: a Multicenter study. J Urol. 2008;179:186–90.
38. Abouassaly R, Angermeier KW, Montague DK. Risk of infection with an antibiotic coated prosthesis at device replacement for mechanical failure. J Urol. 2006;176:2471.
39. Montague DK, Angermeier KW, Lakin MM. Penile prosthesis infections. Int J Impot Res. 2001;13:326–8.
40. Bella AJ, Christine BS, Henry G, Kramer AC, Rhee E, Khera M, Brant WO, Bennett NE, Karpman E, Jones LA, Carrion R. Review of 1103 inflatable penile prosthetic surgeries performed in 2009 demonstrates almost complete variability for irrigation and antibiotic practice amongst eleven high-volume reconstructive surgeons. J Urol. 2011;185(4s)
41. Henry GD, Donatucci CF, Conners W, Greenfield JM, Carson CC, Wilson SK, Delk J, Lentz AC, Cleves MA, Jennermann CJ, Kramer AC. An outcomes analysis of over 200 revision surgeries for penile prosthesis implantation: a multicenter study. J Sex Med. 2012;9:309–15.
42. Carson CC. Efficacy of antibiotic impregnation of inflatable penile prostheses in decreasing infection in original implants. J Urol. 2004;171:1611–4.
43. Wolter CE, Hellstrom WJ. The hydrophilic-coated inflatable penile prosthesis: 1-year experience. J Sex Med. 2004;1:221.
44. Wilson SK, Zumbe J, Henry GD, Salem EA, Delk JR, Cleves MA. Infection reduction using antibiotic coated inflatable penile prosthesis. Urology. 2007;70:337–40.
45. Gerard D, Henry MD. Historical review of penile prosthesis design and surgical techniques: part 1 of a three-part review series on penile prosthetic surgery. J Sex Med. 2009;6:675–81.
46. Henry GD, Wilson SK, Carson CC III, Greenfield J, Lentz AC, Connors W, Rampersaud EN, Bella AJ, Donatucci CF. Infection retardant coated versus non-coated penile prosthesis cultures during revision surgery: a multicenter study. J Urol. 2009;181(4, Supplement)
47. Henry G, Carson C, Delk J II, Mckim S, Mcnamara E, Cleves M, Simmons C, Bella A, Donatucci C. Positive culture growths from infection retardant-coated penile prostheses at the time of revision/savlage surgery: a multicenter study. J Urol. 2011;185(4s)
48. Henry GD. Surgical techniques: the Henry Mummy Wrap™ and the Henry Finger Sweep™ surgical techniques. J Sex Med. 2009;6(3):619–22. https://doi.org/10.1111/j.1743-6109.2008.01200.x.
49. Sadeghi-Nejad H, Ilbeigi P, Wilson SK, Delk JR, Siegel A, Seftel AD, et al. Multi-institutional outcome study on the efficacy of closed-suction drainage of the scrotum in three-piece inflatable penile prosthesis surgery. Int J Impot Res. 2005;17(6):535–8. https://doi.org/10.1038/sj.ijir.3901354.
50. Wilson SK, Delk JL. Hematoma formation following penile prosthesis implantation: to drain or not to drain. J Urol. 1996;55(634A)
51. Wallen J, Beilan J, Emtage J, Bickell M, Martinez D, Carrion R, et al. 062 "Just the Tip" closed suction drain cultures after implantation of penile prosthesis. J Sex Med. 2016;13(5) https://doi.org/10.1016/j.jsxm.2016.02.065.
52. Eid JF. No-touch technique. J Sex Med. 2011;8(1):5–8. https://doi.org/10.1111/j.1743-6109.2010.02137.x.
53. Eid JF, Wilson SK, Cleves M, Salem EA. Coated implants and "no touch" surgical technique decreases risk of infection in inflatable penile prosthesis implantation to 0.46%. Urology. 2012;79(6):1310–5. https://doi.org/10.1016/j.urology.2011.11.076.

54. Weinberg AC, Pagano MJ, Deibert CM, Valenzuela RJ. Sub-coronal inflatable penile prosthesis placement with modified no-touch technique: a step-by-step approach with outcomes. J Sex Med. 2016;13(2):270–6. https://doi.org/10.1016/j.jsxm.2015.12.016.
55. Tacconelli E, Muller NF, Lemmen S, Mutters NT, Hagel S, Meyer E. Infection risk in sterile operative procedures. Dtsch Arztebl Int. 2016;113(16):271–8. https://doi.org/10.3238/arztebl.2016.0271.
56. Graf K, Sohr D, Haverich A, Kuhn C, Gastmeier P, Chaberny IF. Decrease of deep sternal surgical site infection rates after cardiac surgery by a comprehensive infection control program. Interact Cardiovasc Thorac Surg. 2009;9(2):282–6. https://doi.org/10.1510/icvts.2009.205286.
57. Grober ED, Domes T, Fanipour M, Copp JE. Preoperative hair removal on the male genitalia: clippers vs. razors. J Sex Med. 2013;10(2):589–94. https://doi.org/10.1111/j.1743-6109.2012.02904.x.
58. Makama JG, Okeme IM, Makama EJ, Ameh EA. Glove perforation rate in surgery: a randomized, controlled study to evaluate the efficacy of double gloving. Surg Infect. 2016;17(4):436–42. https://doi.org/10.1089/sur.2015.165.
59. Lewis K. Riddle of biofilm resistance. Antimicrob Agents Chemother. 2001;45(4):999–1007. https://doi.org/10.1128/AAC.45.4.999-1007.2001.
60. Henry G, Price G, Pryor M, Greenfield J, Jones L, Perito P, et al. Observation of local clinical penile prostheses infections instead of immediate salvage rescue/removal: ten center study with surprising results. Abstract #92. Proceedings of the 20(th) Annual Fall Scientific Meeting of the Sexual Medicine Society of North America, Miami Beach, USA, November 20-23, 2014. J Sex Med. 2015;12(Suppl 2):101–83. https://doi.org/10.1111/jsm.12808.
61. Henry G, Price G, Pryor M, Greenfield J, Jones L, Perito P, et al. Pd20-04 observation of local clinical penile prostheses infections instead of immediate salvage rescue / removal: multicenter study with surprising results. J Urol. 2014;191(4S) https://doi.org/10.1016/j.juro.2014.02.1694.

Chapter 3
Strategies for Optimal Pain Control in the Penile Implant Patient

Bruno C. G. Nascimento, Eduardo P. Miranda, and John P. Mulhall

Introduction

According to the International Association for the Study of Pain, pain is defined as "an unpleasant sensory and emotional experience associated with actual or potential tissue damage" and usually involves patient apprehension with their body integrity [1, 2]. The importance of its recognition and appropriate treatment is currently well recognized, which led to development of fellowship training programs focused on the study and management of pain [3].

In the field of surgical specialties, the importance of pain management is remarkable. It has been shown that inappropriate postoperative pain control delays functional recovery, increases risk of complications, and increases the risk of persistent pain, ultimately decreasing patients quality of life [4]. Most of these concepts are derived from extensive studies in orthopedic and thoracic surgery, in which pain control has direct impact on functional recovery.

B. C. G. Nascimento (✉)
Sexual & Reproductive Medicine Program, Urology Service, Memorial Sloan Kettering Cancer Center, New York, NY, USA

Sexual Medicine Group, Division of Urology, Hospital das Clinicas – University of Sao Paulo Medical School, Sao Paulo, Brazil

E. P. Miranda
Sexual & Reproductive Medicine Program, Urology Service, Memorial Sloan Kettering Cancer Center, New York, NY, USA

Division of Urology, Federal University of Ceara, Fortaleza, Brazil

J. P. Mulhall
Sexual & Reproductive Medicine Program, Urology Service, Memorial Sloan Kettering Cancer Center, New York, NY, USA

E. P. Miranda, J. P. Mulhall (eds.), *Penile Implant Surgery*,
https://doi.org/10.1007/978-3-030-82363-4_3

Therefore, it is important to acknowledge the relative lack of published evidence regarding the adequate evaluation and management of pain in the urologic field. In a PubMed literature search conducted on May 6, 2020, while the terms "hip replacement surgery" and "pain management" retrieved 917 results, only 39 publications were identified for the terms "penile implant surgery" and "pain management." Still, the presence of post-op pain in penile implant (PI) surgery has been reported in 2–5% of patients and is linked to patient dissatisfaction [5, 6].

Considering this scenario, the high prevalence of ED and the steady increase in PI surgeries worldwide, reaching more than 60,000 cases between 2005 and 2012, improvements in the quality of care and pain management are warranted [7]. In addition to that, the attempt to perform PI surgery in an outpatient setting and the epidemic of opioid abuse have been progressively increasing the awareness of the necessity of an optimal pain management following PI surgery. The aim of this chapter is to perform a comprehensive review of this topic and discuss multimodal pain management strategies, while providing recommendations for an optimal approach to PI perioperative pain.

Literature Challenges

A common challenge in surgical literature is the absence of trials to evaluate the effect of a single drug on a given specific outcome. This is the case for studies evaluating strategies to reduce PI infection, in which many prospective studies have tested a combination of interventions or the implementation of checklists, but not the efficacy of each measure alone [8, 9]. Nevertheless, these studies are valuable as they provide combined evidence to reduce infection rates, which was the scientific question in the first place. A similar scenario is found in the assessment of pain control after PI. Moreover, given the paucity of high-quality evidence in this subject, studies presented in urological meetings but not published in peer-reviewed journals, lessons learned from anesthesiology and other surgical areas were taken in consideration for the structured discussion that follows.

Preoperative Strategies

Education and Patient History

First of all, there are data showing that patient understanding of the surgery, realistic expectation toward the pain, and knowledge of available tools for pain reduction have a positive effect on pain control, and these measures are recommended by the guidelines from the American Pain Society [10]. In fact, these relatively simple and low-cost interventions are associated with reduced length of stay after surgery and decreased pre-op anxiety in orthopedic [11] and cardiothoracic surgery [12, 13]. In addition, preoperative education was able to reduce post-op opioid use in two recent studies on knee and shoulder surgeries [14, 15].

Another simple but still important preoperative measure brought by the American Pain Society guidelines is to be aware of history of psychiatric comorbidities, substance abuse, and/or opioid chronic use. Ideally, a consultation with pain specialist should be available for those patients with high risk of inadequate pain control [10].

Pre-op Medication: Acetaminophen, NSAID/COX-2, and Gabapentin/Pregabalin

Still in the preoperative setting, several agents can be used in an attempt to desensitize pain receptors. In a randomized placebo-controlled trial evaluating the need for opioid use after subpectoral breast augmentation, Parsa and colleagues [16] showed in 695 patients that the administration of 400 mg of celecoxib 30 min before surgery significantly reduced the need for post-op opioid use (6.1 vs. 10.3 hydrocodone tablets in the first 48 h, $p < 0.001$). Later, the same group published a second analysis comparing the preoperative use of either celecoxib 400 mg alone or in combination with gabapentin 1200 mg. In this second study, the authors showed a significant reduction in pain scores, and the need for opioid use dropped from around 80% in the celecoxib alone group, to less than 5% in the combination group [17].

Animal studies had already suggested a possible synergic effect with the administration of anticonvulsants (gabapentin, pregabalin) and COX inhibitors (naproxen) [18], and its preoperative use is mentioned in the recommendations 16 and 17 of the American Pain Society guideline [10]. Finally, the association of pre-op acetaminophen, gabapentin, and NSAID have been tested in PI surgery settings as part of a more complex multimodal protocol with interesting results [19, 20] and will be discussed later in this chapter.

Intraoperative Strategies

Local Anesthesia

The anatomy of penile and scrotal sensory pathways and the focal nature of PI surgeries allow different regional block anesthetic strategies. The afferent fibers located in the penile skin, glans, and urethra converge in the dorsal penile nerve, while in the superficial perineal nerve innervate the scrotum and small branches can innervate the ventral aspect of the penis. Both join the pudendal nerve and reach the spinal cord at the level of S2-S4. This pathway can be successfully targeted with local anesthetics by different approaches [21, 22].

A combination of several regional blockage and anesthetic agents have been reported in PI surgery. In studies evaluating the tolerability of PI surgery using mainly local anesthesia, a combination of penile ring block (PRB), dorsal nerve

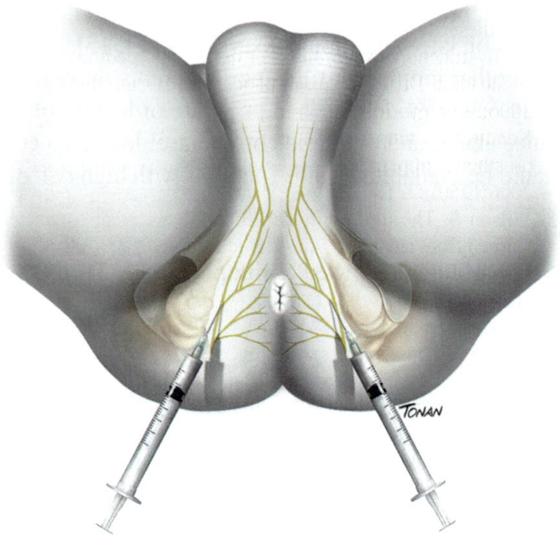

Fig. 3.1 Pudendal block representation. (Credit: medical illustrations Rodrigo Tonan)

penile block (DNPB), intracorporeal anesthesia, and pudendal block (PB), illustrated in Fig. 3.1, is seen [23–26]. In one of the first reports, Kaufman et al. [23] described a 2-year successful experience with PI surgery with pudendal and intracorporeal anesthesia using lidocaine. In his article from 1982, Kaufmann cautiously described and illustrated both techniques and reported over 100 cases, mostly malleable implants, without the need of supplement local or general anesthesia. For the intracorporeal anesthesia, authors applied a tourniquet at the base of the penis, to decrease concerns with systemic effects of lidocaine in the elderly. Recently, however, Taniguchi and colleagues [27] showed in 56 patients that intraoperative intracavernosal administration of liposomal bupivacaine without a tourniquet does not affect systemic hemodynamics.

Despite those studies increasing the body of evidence of local anesthesia effectiveness and safety, the evaluation of postoperative pain control was not the goal. On the other hand, Raynor et al. investigated the beneficial effect of local anesthesia in post-op pain control in a randomized placebo (saline injection) control trial in 30 patients, using de DNPB technique [22]. The authors demonstrated that pain immediately and 4 h postoperatively was lower in patients receiving DNPB with 1% lidocaine and 0.5% bupivacaine than those in the saline group (VAS 2.5 vs. 5.3, $P = 0.009$ at 0 h; VAS 2.8 vs. 5.1, $P = 0.011$ at 4 h). In their study, no peri- or early post-op complication was seen in either group [22].

Similarly, in a prospective study with 131 patients, Xie and colleagues [28] compared the level of post-op pain between those receiving either no block or DNPB with PRB using bupivacaine or ropivacaine. Pain score using VAS was assessed 2 h post-op and every day for the first 7 days. The authors showed that both drugs reduced pain significantly in the first 48 h as compared to the control group, being greater in the no block group but statistically similar from day 2 through 7 [28].

Also, the development of novel longer-lasting agents such as liposomal bupivacaine fostered new studies. In this form of presentation, a multivesicular structure filled with bupivacaine is injected, which enables a gradual release of the agent for up to 96 h and has an expected duration of local anesthesia around 3 days [26, 29]. In 2016, Cota and colleagues [26] reported its use in 13 patients performing IPP. In this study, the authors administered liposomal bupivacaine diluted in saline to form a 20 cc suspension and administered in several sites: peri-incisional, testicular cord, intracorporeally, in the reservoir space, and in the area of expected pump location. When comparing to patients that did not receive it, the authors showed similar overall pain scores but with a reduction in narcotics used by 3.2 times. Of note, the study followed patients for the first 23 h only, and in the control group there were patients receiving regular bupivacaine blockage [26].

Similarly, King et al. [30] reported their experience with DNPB with liposomal bupivacaine in 28 patients, and, in comparison to the traditional DNPB with ropivacaine or bupivacaine, patients receiving liposomal bupivacaine demanded significant less narcotics pills in the following 4 weeks (8.2 vs. 24.1, $p < 0.0001$) postoperatively.

Overall, the utility of local blockage in post-op pain control is still limited by the small number of studies evaluating its efficacy and the short duration of action of the available agents. For early pain control, however, its use seems to be beneficial and also appears to reduce the use of opioids without adding morbidity.

Surgical Technique

The association of different surgical techniques and pain is still a matter of debate [31, 32] Although it seems intuitive that the penoscrotal approach tends to be more painful when early device cycling is desired, no specific study has ever evaluated the prevalence or magnitude of such discomfort.

Also, another surgical aspect that could potentially influence post-op pain control is corporeal dilation. On that matter, Moncada and colleagues [33] showed in a randomized study with 100 patients undergoing primary implantation of inflatable penile prosthesis a significant reduction in post-op pain on those who were in the group of no corporeal dilation (VAS 1 vs. 2 in postoperative day 1, 5, and 7, $p < 0.01$). In this study, the authors also reported similar surgical complication rates in those who performed cavernous tissue sparing technique, which involved the absence of corporeal dilation with Hegar dilators [33].

Alternative Approaches

Different analgesic approaches have already been reported, although these strategies have been less popular in the field of urologic surgery, namely, acupuncture and the use of local anesthetic in the PI intraoperative soaking solution [34, 35].

Hsu and colleagues evaluated the applicability of acupuncture as an adjuvant technique for a variety of penile surgeries, including PI. Although the authors did not report a structured comparison, they reported their experience with almost 1500 cases of penile surgeries combining local blockage and acupuncture targeting acupoints of Hegu (LI4), Shou San Li (LI10), Quchi (LI11), and either Waiguan (TE5) or Neiguan (PC6). In this study, the authors advocate that the use of acupuncture in combination to traditional nerve blockage seems to be beneficial, but present little objective data [34].

In regard to the inclusion of local anesthetic in soaking solutions, Chung et al. [35] presented a randomized study with 40 patients using an IPP with hydrophilic layer, which permits diluted agents to be fixated. Comparing patients in whom standard soaking solution was applied to those using 0.75% ropivacaine and 0.5% marcaine, there was a significant decrease in both VAS scores and the need for analgesic medication in the group using diluted anesthetic solution. Using the same principle but comparing it to the standard combination of DNPB and PRB, Brennan and colleagues [36] showed no difference in VAS at the recovery room or follow-up appointments, with similar time to start device activation. These results, therefore, would signal for an efficacy of adding local anesthetic in the soaking solution of hydrophilic IPPs, maybe comparable in terms of post-op pain control to its delivery through the traditional nerve block. Of importance, a second study with in vitro data showed that the addition of bupivacaine in the soaking solution does not impact the antimicrobial properties of the penile implants – InhibiZone on the AMS700 (Boston Scientific, Marlborough, MA) and the antibiotic-soaked Titan (Coloplast Corporation, Minneapolis, MN) [37].

Postoperative Strategies

Finally, postoperative prescription is surely a key factor for pain control. First, as described and recommended from anesthesiology guidelines, doctors should always adjust and respond to the level of pain presenting at any given stage, regardless of the strategy chosen initially [10].

From those same guidelines, it can be said that both acetaminophen and NSAIDs should be used if not contraindicated and are proven to decrease post-op pain and opioid use [10]. In fact, Weimberg et al. [38] reported that the use of NSAIDs alone in post-op pain management may be sufficient for a majority of patients undergoing PI surgery. In their study, patients underwent an IPP through subcoronal approach and combined penile block (PRB + pudendal) with a combination of anesthetic agents (0.5% ropivacaine, 1.0% lidocaine, sodium bicarbonate (2 cc), and dexamethasone 4 mg). In this series, only nine patients (16%) required narcotics prescription on post-op day 2, and none on post-op days 7–10 [38].

Nevertheless, opioid-based analgesia after PI surgery may be required and should be used if needed. As a general rule, the use of oral and short acting opioids is preferred for acute postoperative pain [10]. Another important drug that can be used postoperatively is gabapentin or pregabalin, but these are usually part of a multimodal analgesia protocol with a structured pre-defined analgesic strategy combining several drugs and encompassing pre-op, intra-op, and post-op strategies.

Multimodal Analgesia

The American Pain Society guidelines on the management of postoperative pain define multimodal analgesia (MMA) as "the use of a variety of analgesic medications and techniques that target different mechanisms of action in the peripheral and/or central nervous system (which might also be combined with nonpharmacological interventions) might have additive or synergistic effects and more effective pain relief compared with single-modality interventions." [10]

Probably the most complex and well-conducted study about MMA in penile implants is from Tong and colleagues, published in 2018 [19]. In a retrospective but matched control analysis, the results of post-op pain (VAS) and opioid use (TME, total morphine equivalents) at the post-anesthesia recovery unit (PACU), post-op day 0 (POD0), and post-op day 1 (POD1) were compared in two different groups – opioid-based regimen and MMA. The MMA group received a complex regimen including most of the possible discussed drugs and techniques so far and included:

Pre-op

- 975 mg acetaminophen
- 300 mg gabapentin
- 7.5 or 15 mg of meloxicam

Intra-op

- General anesthesia
- Dorsal penile nerve and pudendal block prior to incision – using 20 ml of a 50/50% mixture of 1% lidocaine and 0.5% bupivacaine without epinephrine for each blockage (40 ml total)

Post-op

- 975 mg acetaminophen every 6 h
- 300 mg gabapentin every 8 h
- 7.5 or 15 mg of meloxicam daily
- If moderate pain – oxycodone 5 mg, no more than every 4 h
- If severe pain – morphine 2 mg, no more than every 2 h

Discharge Prescription

30-day regimen of in-hospital pain regimen + oxycodone 5 mg every 4 h as needed

This complex multimodal pain management efficacy was compared to patients in the "traditional" opioid-based (OB) regimen, in which there was no drug utilization preoperatively, no local injection during surgery and postoperatively they were allowed to receive acetaminophen/oxycodone (650/10 mg) every 4 h and morphine 2 mg every 2 h as needed. Patients in the OB group were discharged with

Table 3.1 Comparison of postoperative course between treatment groups

	OB (n = 38)	MMA (n = 19)	p-value
Operative time (min) mean ± SD	93.6 ± 53.6	87.6 ± 26.8	0.33
PACU			
VAS mean ± SD	2.97 ± 3.23	0.84 ± 1.95	0.01
TME (mg) mean ± SD	4.32 ± 5.55	1.26 ± 2.33	0.03
POD0			
VAS mean ± SD	4.73 ± 2.56	2.62 ± 2.3	0.003
TME (mg) mean ± SD	13.8 ± 10.5	4.08 ± 5.00	<0.001
POD1			
VAS mean ± SD	4.0 ± 2.3	2.26 ± 2.76	0.01
TME (mg) mean ± SD	25.1 ± 22.3	5.05 ± 7.16	<0.001
No narcotics prescribed at discharge (mean ± SD)	51.3 ± 14.8	12.7 ± 2.6	<0.001
No of patients requiring prescription refills (n/%)	18 / 37 (49%)	2 / 19 (11%)	0.007

Adapted from Tong et al. [19]
OB opioid-based, *MMA* multimodal analgesic, *PACU* post-anesthesia recovery unit, *POD* postoperative day, *TME* total morphine equivalents, *VAS* visual analogue scale

acetaminophen/oxycodone (650/10 mg) every 4 h as needed for pain control. Despite the limited number of patients in the study (38 patients in OB and 19 MMA groups, respectively), the MMA group reported less pain and required less opioid at all three time points assessed (PACU, POD0, and POD1) as shown in Table 3.1. Of interest, results remained significant in subgroup analysis evaluating the penoscrotal approach and surgeries with longer duration (>90 min). Also, the authors showed a remarkable reduction in the amount of pills received by discharged patients in the MMA group (12.7 vs. 51.3 pill, $p < 0.001$) and in the refill requests outside the hospital (11% vs. 49%).

It is important to highlight, however, that it is very difficult to predict the isolated effect of each specific drug, a common challenge in studies with such methodology [39]. It could also be argued that the outcome of number of pills at discharge has an inherent bias, as a result of its retrospective design. Nevertheless, the requirement of less narcotic refills postoperatively points toward a better pain control in the MMA group [40].

Another recent study has also supported these findings. Lucas et al. evaluated 203 patients comparing MMA protocol vs. matched cohort post-IPP implantation in a multicenter study. These authors have utilized a very similar MMA protocol to Tong et al. In their analysis, VAS and opioid used in PACU, POD0, POD1, and immediate post-discharge were evaluated. Results showed a significant reduction in pain and opioid use in all PACU (median 0 vs. 2, $p = 0.001$), POD0 (median 3 vs. 4, $p = 0.001$), and POD1 (median 3 vs. 4.3, $p = 0.04$). In addition, MMA patients required significantly less narcotics (in PACU, POD0, and POD1), less opioid pills at discharge (20 vs. 30 tablets, $p < 0.001$), and a smaller proportion required narcotic refills (10.7% vs. 28%, $p = 0.001$) [20].

Finally, it is very important to recognize the importance of communicating and adopting strategies from other surgical specialties, such as anesthesiology, orthopedics, and general surgery, among others [40]. While we are still starting this discussion in the setting of PI surgery, MMA has already been the gold standard in many other procedures, likely due to a more painful nature of such surgeries which might have urged for more effective alternatives earlier.

Limitations

As mentioned before, the literature exploring optimization of pain control following PI surgery is still scarce, with multiple limitations: short follow-up, no data on patient satisfaction, and functional outcomes, among others. Although current designs should suffice to evaluate short-term pain control and the achievement of a significant decrease in opioid use, it is not possible to evaluate long-term consequences of prolonged pain such as delayed or diminished IPP use, increased difficulties to start cycling, penile length loss, decreased confidence for engaging on intercourse, and overall IPP satisfaction. Also, there is a significant amount of studies in this area that were presented in society meetings but were never published in peer-reviewed journals, limiting the dissemination of these data. Finally, it is known that the costs associated with MMA protocols are not insignificant; however, this merit was not discussed as it was beyond the scope of this chapter.

Summary

Pain is a relevant aspect in the process of PI surgery as it might be linked to patient dissatisfaction [5, 6]. Optimization of pain control is important to improve outcomes and minimize potential complications. Although no clear recommendations based on high-quality evidence can be made, there are strategies available that could be included in routine care, which include:

- Appropriate preoperative *patient education*
- *Involve pain specialist* if patient with risk factor for difficult management (history of substance/opioid abuse or psychiatric illness)
- *Multimodal analgesia is preferable* over opioid based. Multimodal protocol include:
  - *Pre-op acetaminophen, NSAID, and gabapentin.*
  - Intra-op *local blockage* – combined blockage (DNPB + PRB or pudendal block). Longer-lasting agents are desirable, if available.
  - *Post-op around the clock acetaminophen, NSAID, and gabapentin.*
  - At discharge, *prefer oral and short-acting opioid agent*, per demand use.

- Intraoperative possible strategies to be used:
  - Avoid corporal dilation if safe (first PI surgery and no fibrosis).
  - Intracavernosal injection of local anesthetics or adding local anesthetics in the soaking solution for PI with hydrophilic layer.

Conclusions

There are several strategies to optimize pain control on PI surgery. Multimodal analgesia appears to reduce post-op pain and the amount of opioid at discharge, with possible consequences in patient satisfaction and reduction in opioid abuse. Prospective studies with longer follow-up time and evaluation of functional outcomes such as patient satisfaction are needed.

References

1. Treede RD. The International Association for the Study of Pain definition of pain: as valid in 2018 as in 1979, but in need of regularly updated footnotes. Pain Rep. 2018;3:e643.
2. Cohen M, Quintner J, van Rysewyk S. Reconsidering the International Association for the Study of Pain definition of pain. Pain Rep. 2018;3:e634.
3. Hochberg U, Perez J, Borod M. New frontier: cancer pain management clinical fellowship. Support Care Cancer. 2018;26:2453–7.
4. Kehlet H, Jensen TS, Woolf CJ. Persistent postsurgical pain: risk factors and prevention. Lancet. 2006;367:1618–25.
5. Trost LW, Baum N, Hellstrom WJ. Managing the difficult penile prosthesis patient. J Sex Med. 2013;10:893–906; quiz 07
6. Judith C, Hagedorn NO, Lundy S, Miest T, Voelzke BB. Inflatable penile prosthesis failure and complications: review of a national database. J Urol. 2015;193:e43–4.
7. Baas W, O'Connor B, Welliver C, et al. Worldwide trends in penile implantation surgery: data from over 63,000 implants. Transl Androl Urol. 2020;9:31–7.
8. Katz BF, Gaunay GS, Barazani Y, et al. Use of a preoperative checklist reduces risk of penile prosthesis infection. J Urol. 2014;192:130–5.
9. Pineda M, Burnett AL. Penile prosthesis infections-a review of risk factors, prevention, and treatment. Sex Med Rev. 2016;4:389–98.
10. Chou R, Gordon DB, de Leon-Casasola OA, et al. Management of postoperative pain: a clinical practice guideline from the American Pain Society, the American Society of Regional Anesthesia and Pain Medicine, and the American Society of Anesthesiologists' Committee on Regional Anesthesia, Executive Committee, and Administrative Council. J Pain. 2016;17:131–57.
11. Crowe J, Henderson J. Pre-arthroplasty rehabilitation is effective in reducing hospital stay. Can J Occup Ther. 2003;70:88–96.
12. Arthur HM, Daniels C, McKelvie R, Hirsh J, Rush B. Effect of a preoperative intervention on preoperative and postoperative outcomes in low-risk patients awaiting elective coronary artery bypass graft surgery. A randomized, controlled trial. Ann Intern Med. 2000;133:253–62.

13. Anderson EA. Preoperative preparation for cardiac surgery facilitates recovery, reduces psychological distress, and reduces the incidence of acute postoperative hypertension. J Consult Clin Psychol. 1987;55:513–20.
14. Syed UAM, Aleem AW, Wowkanech C, et al. Neer Award 2018: the effect of preoperative education on opioid consumption in patients undergoing arthroscopic rotator cuff repair: a prospective, randomized clinical trial. J Shoulder Elb Surg. 2018;27:962–7.
15. Andelman SM, Bu D, Debellis N, et al. Preoperative patient education may decrease postoperative opioid use after meniscectomy. Arthrosc Sports Med Rehabil. 2020;2:e33–8.
16. Parsa AA, Soon CW, Parsa FD. The use of celecoxib for reduction of pain after subpectoral breast augmentation. Aesthet Plast Surg. 2005;29:441–4; discussion 45
17. Parsa AA, Sprouse-Blum AS, Jackowe DJ, Lee M, Oyama J, Parsa FD. Combined preoperative use of celecoxib and gabapentin in the management of postoperative pain. Aesthet Plast Surg. 2009;33:98–103.
18. Hurley RW, Chatterjea D, Rose Feng M, Taylor CP, Hammond DL. Gabapentin and pregabalin can interact synergistically with naproxen to produce antihyperalgesia. Anesthesiology. 2002;97:1263–73.
19. Tong CMC, Lucas J, Shah A, Foote C, Simhan J. Novel multi-modal analgesia protocol significantly decreases opioid requirements in inflatable penile prosthesis patients. J Sex Med. 2018;15:1187–94.
20. Lucas J, Gross M, Yafi F, et al. A multi-institutional assessment of multimodal analgesia in penile implant recipients demonstrates dramatic reduction in pain scores and narcotic usage. J Sex Med. 2020;17:518–25.
21. Kinter KJ, Newton BW. Anatomy, abdomen and pelvis, pudendal nerve. Treasure Island: StatPearls; 2020.
22. Raynor MC, Smith A, Vyas SN, Selph JP, Carson CC 3rd. Dorsal penile nerve block prior to inflatable penile prosthesis placement: a randomized, placebo-controlled trial. J Sex Med. 2012;9:2975–9.
23. Kaufman JJ. Penile prosthetic surgery under local anesthesia. J Urol. 1982;128:1190–1.
24. Dos Reis JM, Glina S, Da Silva MF, Furlan V. Penile prosthesis surgery with the patient under local regional anesthesia. J Urol. 1993;150:1179–81.
25. Ghanem H, Fouad G. Penile prosthesis surgery under local penile block anesthesia via the infrapubic space. Int J Androl. 2000;23:357–9.
26. Cotta BH, Welliver C, Brahmamdam A, Bednarchik CL, Dynda D, Kohler TS. Long-acting liposomal bupivacaine decreases inpatient narcotic requirements in men undergoing penile prosthesis implantation. Turk J Urol. 2016;42:230–4.
27. Taniguchi H, Mulhall JP. Intraoperative intracavernosal liposomal bupivacaine (exparel) injection does not affect systemic hemodynamics. J Sex Med. 2020;17:526–30.
28. Xie D, Nicholson M, Azaiza M, et al. Effect of operative local anesthesia on postoperative pain outcomes of inflatable penile prosthesis: prospective comparison of two medications. Int J Impot Res. 2018;30:93–6.
29. Chahar P, Cummings KC 3rd. Liposomal bupivacaine: a review of a new bupivacaine formulation. J Pain Res. 2012;5:257–64.
30. Sherita King JG, Goldstein I. MP48-10 use of dorsal nerve block with bupivacaine liposome injectable suspension (exparel) for pain management following three-piece penile prosthesis surgery. J Urol. 2016;195:e639–e39.
31. Reinstatler L, Shee K, Gross MS. Pain management in penile prosthetic surgery: a review of the literature. Sex Med Rev. 2018;6:162–9.
32. Ellis JL, Higgins AM, Simhan J. Pain management strategies in penile implantation. Asian J Androl. 2020;22:34–8.
33. Moncada I, Martinez-Salamanca JI, Jara J, Cabello R, Moralejo M, Hernandez C. Inflatable penile prosthesis implantation without corporeal dilation: a cavernous tissue sparing technique. J Urol. 2010;183:1123–6.

34. Hsu GL, Zaid UX, Hsieh CH, Huang SJ. Acupuncture assisted local anesthesia for penile surgeries. Transl Androl Urol. 2013;2:291–300.
35. Chung E. 059 Local anaesthesia eluting property of Coloplast Titan penile prosthesis hydrophilic coating: an in-vitro drug elution profile and a randomised double-blind clinical outcome study. J Sex Med. 2018;15(Supplement 3)
36. Mea B. 038 Analgesic implant soaks with ropivacaine are as effective as perioperative penile blocks. J Sex Med. 2019;16:S18.
37. Lokeshwar SD, Horodyski L, Lahorewala SS, et al. The effect of bupivacaine on the efficacy of antibiotic coating on penile implants in preventing infection. Sex Med. 2019;7:337–44.
38. Aea W. 142 Preoperative local anesthetic block reduces the need for narcotic medications following penile prosthesis surgery. J Sex Med. 2016;13:S66–7.
39. Kovac JR. Editorial commentary on "Novel multimodal analgesia protocol significantly decreases opioid requirements in inflatable penile prosthesis patients". J Sex Med. 2018;15:1366–7.
40. Carmen Tong CM, Lucas J, Shah A, Foote C, Simhan J. Author reply to editorial comment on "Novel multimodal analgesia protocol significantly decreases opioid requirements in inflatable penile prosthesis patients". J Sex Med. 2018;15:1364–5.

Chapter 4
Perioperative Management of Antithrombotic Therapy in Penile Implant Surgery

Kevin J. Hebert, David Y. Yang, and Tobias S. Köhler

Introduction

Increased patient awareness and earlier consideration of surgical management for erectile dysfunction (ED) has led to a more medically diverse patient population undergoing inflatable penile prosthesis (IPP) surgery. Risk factors for ED including hypertension, stroke, hyperlipidemia, smoking, and diabetes are associated with multiple cardiopulmonary conditions [1]. This extensive overlap of comorbidities as well as increasing patient age has resulted in an increasingly complex patient population seeking IPP surgery. While many aspects of IPP surgical management are debated, the management and evaluation of one patient population is particularly controversial: the patient on antithrombotic therapy.

In our surgical practice, over 50% of patients electing for IPP surgery are also on an antithrombotic medication (anticoagulation and/or antiplatelet therapy). Due to the risk of acute hemorrhage and delayed scrotal hematoma formation, the traditional perioperative dogma suggests discontinuation of antithrombotic therapy (AT) at the time of IPP surgery. However, increasing awareness of the potential morbidity of discontinuation of AT has led to reconsideration of this practice. In this chapter, we aim to review the appropriate evaluation and perioperative management of a patient on antithrombotic therapy who wishes to undergo IPP surgery.

K. J. Hebert · D. Y. Yang · T. S. Köhler (✉)
Mayo Clinic, Rochester, MN, USA
e-mail: kohler.tobias@mayo.edu

E. P. Miranda, J. P. Mulhall (eds.), *Penile Implant Surgery*,
https://doi.org/10.1007/978-3-030-82363-4_4

Periprocedural Evaluation

The initial evaluation for patients considering IPP surgery should start with a thorough history and physical exam. This includes a detailed review of comorbidities, current AT, and prior abdominal/pelvic surgery. Specifically, providers must ascertain the indications for specific AT as well as the duration of usage and whether these medications have been previously discontinued for surgery. Understanding of the planned duration of antithrombotic therapy is also important as many medications are not continued lifelong. Thus, a safer period to undergo IPP surgery may be present in the future. Perioperative management of AT relies on surgeons having a thorough understanding of the pharmacokinetics of antiplatelets and oral anticoagulants.

AT is divided into antiplatelet and anticoagulation therapy. Broadly, antiplatelet therapy (Table 4.1) affects platelet function, while oral anticoagulants (Table 4.2) impact the clotting cascade. Antiplatelet therapy includes irreversible cyclooxygenase inhibitors (aspirin) and ADP receptor inhibitors (clopidogrel, prasugrel, and ticagrelor).

Table 4.1 Common antiplatelet pharmacokinetics

Antiplatelet	Mechanism of action	Antithrombotic effect	Half-life	Onset	Metabolized	Antithrombotic duration
Aspirin	Irreversible COX-1 inhibitor	Impairs platelet aggregation, reduces thrombin generation, enhances fibrinolysis	2–3 hr	3–4 hr (enteric coated)	Hepatic	10 days (lifespan of platelet)
ADP receptor inhibitor	Inhibition of ADP receptor	Reduces platelet aggregation				
Clopidogrel (Plavix)	Active metabolite irreversibly blocks P2Y12	Reduces platelet aggregation	6 hr	24 hr (75 mg)	Hepatic	~5–10 days
Prasugrel (Effient)	Active metabolite irreversibly blocks P2Y12	Reduces platelet aggregation	7 hr	<30 min (60 mg)	Hepatic	~5–10 days
Ticagrelor (Brilinta)	Reversibly blocks P2Y12	Reduces platelet aggregation	7 hr	30 min (180 mg)	Hepatic	3 days

Key: *ADP* adenosine diphosphate, *COX* cyclooxygenase, *hr* hour, mg milligram

Table 4.2 Common oral anticoagulant pharmacokinetics

Oral anticoagulant	Mechanism of action	Antithrombotic effect	Half-life	Onset	Metabolized	Antithrombotic duration
Warfarin	Competitively inhibits vitamin K-dependent coagulation factors	Reduces prothrombin	40 hr (variable)	5–7 days	Hepatic	2–5 days
Dabigatran	Reversible, direct thrombin inhibitor	Prevents thrombin-mediated effects	12–17 hr	0.5–1 hr	Hepatic	24 hr
Direct factor Xa inhibitor						
Apixaban (Eliquis)	Selective, reversible inhibition of Xa	Prevents thrombin generation	12 hr	3–4 hr	Hepatic	2–3 days
Rivaroxaban (Xarelto)	Selective, reversible inhibition of Xa	Prevents thrombin generation	5–9 hr	2–4 hr	Hepatic	2–3 days

Key: *hr* hours

Antiplatelet Therapy

Aspirin

Indications/Prevalence

Aspirin (acetylsalicylic acid) is a nonsteroidal anti-inflammatory drug (NSAID) with broad indications and applications. The role of aspirin use for primary prevention is under debate [2]; however, the high prevalence of this medication is indisputable with as many as 30 million patients in the United States over the age 40 admitting to its use for primary prevention alone in 2017 [3]. Additionally, near one-quarter of patients over the age of 40 use aspirin without a physician recommendation due to perceived cardiovascular benefit [3].

Use for secondary prevention is also common in the setting of prior history of acute coronary syndromes (myocardial infarction and unstable angina), acute occlusive stroke, chronic coronary syndrome, revascularization following cardiac stent or coronary artery bypass graft surgery, peripheral arterial disease, or carotid artery disease. These populations likely benefit most from continuation of aspirin during the perioperative IPP surgery period.

Mechanism of Action

Aspirin exerts its antithrombotic effects through three main mechanisms via irreversible inhibitor of cyclooxygenase-1 (COX-1): (1) impaired platelet aggregation, (2) thrombin generation reduction, and (3) enhanced fibrinolysis.

Perioperative Management of Aspirin

Continuation of aspirin during IPP surgery should be carefully reviewed prior to surgery as this patient population may be at highest risk for postoperative hematoma formation. We suspect this is related to the high use of aspirin in the general population for inappropriate primary prevention in the absence of cardiovascular risk factors. Thus, all patients on aspirin should be evaluated preoperatively by their primary care provider to assess if a true indication for aspirin use is present. Patients on aspirin for primary prevention or if taken without a physician's recommendation should discontinue aspirin prior to IPP surgery as the perioperative benefit is unlikely to outweigh the risk of bleeding. Patients on aspirin for secondary prevention (81 mg or 325 mg) are commonly continued on aspirin through the perioperative period by our team following shared decision-making discussion with the patient.

ADP Receptor Inhibitors (Clopidogrel, Prasugrel, Ticagrelor)

Indications/Prevalence

Primary indications for ADP receptor inhibitors include prior history of acute coronary syndrome, percutaneous coronary intervention (PCI), and ischemic stroke. Commonly, ADP receptor inhibitors are used in conjunction with aspirin which forms the basis of dual-antiplatelet therapy. Limited data is available on the number of patients in the United States on ADP receptor inhibitors; however clopidogrel (Plavix) is the most commonly prescribed ADP receptor inhibitor in the United States.

Antithrombotic Mechanism of Action

ADP receptor inhibitors block the function of $P2Y_{12}$ receptor which under normal conditions is activated by ADP. Inhibition of the $P2Y_{12}$ receptor affects glycoprotein IIb/IIIa receptors which increases thromboxane production and inhibits platelet aggregation. ADP receptor inhibitors are generally perceived as irreversible, lasting the lifespan of the platelet, and thus return of platelet function is dependent on platelet production. Prasugrel (Effient) is a third-generation ADP receptor inhibitor which differs in metabolism compared to clopidogrel and results in more stable antiplatelet effects and quicker onset of action. Ticagrelor (Brilinta) represents a new-generation ADP receptor inhibitor which utilizes an ADP analogue leading to rapid onset of action but differs from clopidogrel and ticagrelor in that it is reversible.

Perioperative Management of ADP Receptor Inhibitors

Presurgical evaluation by cardiology, vascular medicine, or neurology is paramount to assess risk of ADP receptor inhibitor discontinuation at the time of IPP surgery. Continuation of dual-antiplatelet therapy is also considered if perioperative risk warrants continuation. Following risk assessment, we again hold a shared decision-making discussion with the patient to determine a perioperative plan. We routinely continue both clopidogrel and dual-antiplatelet therapy if the patient understands the small increase of postoperative hematoma. Owing to the higher prevalence of clopidogrel, these authors have limited experience with continuing prasugrel and ticagrelor during the perioperative period and are unable to include these medications in this discussion.

Anticoagulation Therapy

Anticoagulation therapy represents classes of medications that affect the intrinsic or extrinsic pathway of the coagulation cascade including vitamin K antagonists (warfarin), direct thrombin inhibitor (Pradaxa), and direct factor Xa inhibitors (rivaroxaban and apixaban).

Warfarin

Indications/Prevalence

Indications for warfarin therapy include prior cardiac valve surgery, atrial fibrillation, myocardial infarction with ventricular thrombus, venous thromboembolism, and antiphospholipid syndrome. Management of warfarin is often directed by vascular medicine, thrombophilia clinics, or cardiology. Most commonly, warfarin is used for risk reduction in patients with a history of atrial fibrillation. Over the past decade, increasing use of direct-acting oral anticoagulants (DOAC) compared to warfarin has been noted [4].

Mechanism of Action

Warfarin blocks vitamin K epoxide reductase which prevents development of the active forms of vitamin K-dependent clotting factors (II, VII, IX, and X). Warfarin therapy includes frequent adjustments based on a narrow international normalized ratio (INR) range depending on indication. This range typically is either 2.0–3.0 or 2.5–3.5. Warfarin therapy is highly dependent on P450 system metabolization and vitamin K consumption which can lead to wide fluctuation of INR levels and variable risk of hemorrhage.

Perioperative Management of Warfarin

Due to variable degree of bleeding risk with warfarin therapy, patients on warfarin require careful risk assessment and perioperative monitoring. As with any antithrombotic medication, patients on warfarin should be assessed by the prescribing provider to evaluate perioperative risk of cardiovascular events. Modifiable risk factors should be optimized. Patients at low risk for perioperative events including those on warfarin for paroxysmal atrial fibrillation should consider discontinuation at time of IPP surgery. If patient is on short-term warfarin therapy, IPP surgery should be delayed until warfarin is no longer necessary. Patients on lifelong warfarin who are at high risk for perioperative events as determined by vascular medicine or cardiology should consider continuation of warfarin through the perioperative period after a thorough surgeon directed shared decision-making discussion. In this population, we avoid retropubic reservoir placement in this population due to the risk of pelvic hematoma formation. Patients should understand that a point of care INR is absolutely necessary the day of surgery and that surgery should be canceled if any evidence of supratherapeutic INR is present. In fact, these authors target the lower half of a patient's INR range to decrease bleeding risk. Lastly, consideration can be given to malleable prosthesis in this population as risk of bleeding is mostly related to the scrotal dissection and reservoir placement.

Direct Thrombin Inhibitor (Dabigatran)

Indications/Prevalence

Dabigatran is FDA approved for use in prevention of embolic events in patients with non-valvular atrial fibrillation. It is also used for venous thromboembolism and ischemic heart disease. In 2017, dabigatran prescriptions represented 12.3% of all oral anticoagulants used for non-valvular atrial fibrillation, while warfarin and direct factor Xa inhibitors represented 45% and 42%, respectively [5].

Mechanism of Action

Dabigatran is a prodrug that undergoes hepatic conversion into a reversible direct thrombin inhibitor which prevents thrombin-mediated activation of coagulation factors and possibly enhances fibrinolysis. Half-life is 12–17 h in patients with normal renal function. Maximum anticoagulation occurs within 2–3 h of the first dose.

Perioperative Management of Dabigatran

Consultation with cardiology or vascular medicine is necessary in the IPP perioperative period. As with other oral anticoagulants, dabigatran should be held if possible. These authors have no experience with concurrent dabigatran use at the time of IPP surgery and thus recommend careful multispecialty discussion including regarding continuation of this medication during IPP surgery. As more patients transition away from warfarin therapy for oral anticoagulation, we expect perioperative management of dabigatran to become more common.

Direct Factor Xa Inhibitors (Apixaban, Rivaroxaban)

Indications/Prevalence

Direct factor Xa inhibitors are used for stroke prevention in atrial fibrillation, ischemic heart disease, and treatment of venous thromboembolism. Apixaban and rivaroxaban are used more commonly in treatment of atrial fibrillation 21.0% and 21.6%, respectively. [5].

Mechanism of Action

Direct factor Xa inhibitors selectively inhibit factor Xa which blocks propagation phase of the coagulation cascade. As a result, thrombin generation is decreased.

Perioperative Management of Direct Factor Xa Inhibitors

Apixaban and rivaroxaban are common oral anticoagulants encountered by a prosthetic surgeon in the perioperative period. As with any antithrombotic, referral to the prescribing provider should occur to allow a perioperative risk assessment to be performed. If temporary discontinuation is considered low risk, factor Xa inhibitors should be held. If the patient is considered high risk for discontinuation and is on lifelong therapy, continuation of factor Xa inhibitors should be considered after appropriate counseling. In our experience with apixaban and rivaroxaban, no increased risk of hematoma formation has occurred in non-revision IPP surgery. We prefer ectopic reservoir placement in this patient population due to the risk of pelvic hematoma with retropubic reservoir placement.

Perioperative management of antithrombotic therapy must involve a multidisciplinary evaluation to perform a perioperative risk assessment of discontinuation of antithrombotic therapy. Broad continuation of AT should not be performed, but rather continuation of AT should occur after a through risk assessment and shared decision-making with the patient. Bridging therapy can also be considered although its utility during elective surgery has been questioned [6]. We routinely refer patients with a history of cerebral vascular accidents on antiplatelet therapy to neurology to perform a risk assessment. Patients with cardiovascular indications for AT including cardiac stents, atrial fibrillation, prosthetic or mechanical valves, and vascular grafts should be evaluated by cardiology and or vascular medicine. Prior history of venous thromboembolism should include a preoperative Caprini Score calculation and evaluation by vascular medicine [7]. Interestingly, in our institutional experience, the risk of postoperative hematoma increases in the setting of continuation of aspirin 81 mg taken for preventative measures or anticoagulation taken in the setting of revision IPP surgery. However, no increased hematoma risk was seen in patients on AT for a cardiovascular indication (CVA, MI, s/p CABG/Stent, AF, VTE, etc.). Furthermore, when postoperative hematomas have occurred, it has only resulted in delayed device activation. No patients have required scrotal drainage, exploration, or surgical intervention.

After multidisciplinary evaluation, patients should revisit with the prosthetic surgeon to discuss the risks and benefits of AT continuation or discontinuation at time of IPP surgery. If risk assessment favors discontinuation of antithrombotic therapy, we make perioperative recommendations based on the AskMayoExpert perioperative antithrombotic management calculator (Table 4.3).

Table 4.3 Antithrombotic duration, perioperative dosing, and reversal agents

Oral antithrombotic	Antithrombotic duration	Creatinine clearance	Last dose	Reversal agent(s)
Aspirin	10 days		8 days prior	Platelets
ADP receptor inhibitor				
Clopidogrel (Plavix)	5–10 days		6 days prior	Platelets
Prasugrel (Effient)	5–10 days		8 days prior	Platelets
Ticagrelor (Brilinta)	3 days		6 days prior	Platelets
Warfarin	2–5 days		6 days prior	Vitamin K, PCC (Kcentra), FFP
Dabigatran (Pradaxa)	24 hr	≥ 50 mL/Min	6 days prior	Idarucizumab
		30–49 mL/Min	7 days prior	
Direct factor Xa inhibitor				
Apixaban (Eliquis)	2–3 days	≥ 50 mL/Min	3 days prior	Andexxa, Kcentra
		30–49 mL/Min	4 days prior	
Rivaroxaban (Xarelto)	2–3 days	≥ 50 mL/Min	4 days prior	Andexxa, Kcentra
		30–49 mL/Min	5 days prior	

Last dose is "x" days prior to surgical date. Antithrombotic dosing was determined based on a high bleeding risk with IPP surgery. This table is meant to service as a guide and should not replace clinical decision-making. Surgeons should have a low index for referral to vascular medicine or anticoagulation services to direct perioperative antithrombotic management. Key: *PCC* prothrombin complex concentrate, *FFP* fresh frozen plasma, *mL* milliliter, *Min* minute

Perioperative Management

When continuing anticoagulation in the perioperative setting, the implanter must consider additional steps during surgery to reduce the risk of hematoma and other bleeding complications. Within this section, we describe our surgical technique for IPP placement in patients on AT.

In our experience, we perform our IPPs through a penoscrotal approach which allows direct pump placement and control of any scrotal vessels.

Corporotomy closure is often surgeon specific (tying preplaced sutures vs running closure). However, we prefer tying preplaced sutures to avoid risk to the implant device. The key, especially when operating on anticoagulation, is to create a watertight closure to entrap any bleeding that may come from the corpora. This is further controlled by leaving the device 60% inflated at the end of the case to provide intra-corporeal tamponade. We counsel our patients that the device is left partially inflated until their activation visit.

During reservoir placement, we recommend utilizing a high-submuscular reservoir placement. In this setting, we avoid the space of Retzius at all costs as there are unnamed pelvic vessels, beyond the iliacs, that can be injured and are difficult to control. While everyone is aware of and concerned about the "bleeding you can hear" associated with iliac injury, small pelvic bleeders that normally will self-resolve can be more dangerous in the AT patient. The space of Retzius can become a large potential space, as seen in traumatic pelvic fractures, and therefore, bleeding within this space can be indolent. Postoperative blood work is rarely utilized in IPP patients. As such, slow pelvic bleeding may not be diagnosed until there are signs and symptoms of anemia. Reservoir placement in the submuscular position avoids creating this potential space and while rare, any significant bleeding should be easier to identify.

Recently, post-surgical drains have become more accepted especially within the high-volume implanter community as there is mounting evidence that there is no increased risk of infection [8]. In patients on AT, a drain is essential. We utilize a ten French Jackson-Pratt drain placed through a dependent scrotal incision that is removed on postoperative day 1 if output is <50 cc over the preceding 8-h shift. In addition to a drain, we also utilize the mummy wrap for the scrotum to provide compression and reduce potential space [9]. This should be kept in place for 48–72 h postoperatively. Scrotal supports in the form of a jock strap or biking shorts are also used. Combined, this should greatly reduce the risk of postoperative hematoma formation.

With depreciating reimbursement and the recent healthcare crisis, the push toward outpatient prosthetic surgery has shown that in most instances, outpatient IPP surgery is safe. We would caution outpatient surgery in the AT patient for the abovementioned reasons. Specifically, an overnight stay allows serial vital measurements, accurate drain outputs, and a postoperative physical exam in a controlled environment.

Lastly, timing for device activation is a double-edged sword. We want our patients to start using their devices as soon as possible, but postoperative pain and swelling can make early activation difficult. With the aforementioned techniques, risk of postoperative hematoma can be reduced. In our experience, we typically have primary IPP patients return at 3–4 weeks for activation visit. In our experience, patients on AT may have a slightly increased risk of not being able to activate early, whether due to pain, swelling that prevents patient manipulation, or true hematoma. In all our patients on AT, they were able to be activated by 6 weeks. As such, we are considering making it standard to wait 6 weeks for activation in our AT patients.

Conclusion

Perioperative antithrombotic management in the IPP surgery population remains a controversial topic due to an absence of literature addressing its management. This has led to surgeon-dependent management often based on anecdotal evidence. As IPP surgery volume increases with the aging patient population in the United States, AT management will continue to be a source of significant perioperative decision-making. Surgeons must consider perioperative risk stratification, multispecialty input, and patient wishes when formulating an IPP perioperative AT management plan. With appropriate risk stratification and perioperative measures (scrotal drain, device inflated, scrotal support, mummy wrap, avoidance of space of Retzius), IPP surgery can be performed with concurrent antithrombotic therapy with minimal risk to the patient. Until large-volume, multicenter, prospectively collected data is available, perioperative antithrombotic therapy will continue to be a source of debate among the prosthetic surgery community (Table 4.4).

Table 4.4 Summary of recommendations for perioperative AT management

Perioperative antithrombotic management
Widespread continuation of antithrombotics during IPP is not advisable
Absence of peer-reviewed data on IPP perioperative antithrombotic management
Preoperative thromboembolic/cardiovascular risk stratification is key
Refer to anticoagulation clinic, cardiology, and vascular medicine for preoperative counseling
Shared decision-making with surgeon, internist, and patient regarding risks and benefits
Aspirin for primary prevention should not be continued
Point of care INR on the day of surgery must be obtained in patients continuing warfarin
Measures to decrease hematoma rate should be employed
If held, antithrombotics should be restarted within 24–48 h

References

1. Nguyen HMT, Gabrielson AT, Hellstrom WJG. Erectile dysfunction in young men-a review of the prevalence and risk factors. Sex Med Rev. 2017;5(4):508–20.
2. Zheng SL, Roddick AJ. Association of aspirin use for primary prevention with cardiovascular events and bleeding events: a systematic review and meta-analysis. JAMA. 2019;321(3):277–87.
3. O'Brien CW, Juraschek SP, Wee CC. Prevalence of aspirin use for primary prevention of cardiovascular disease in the United States: results from the 2017 National Health Interview Survey. Ann Intern Med. 2019;171(8):596–8.
4. Alcusky M, McManus DD, Hume AL, Fisher M, Tjia J, Lapane KL. Changes in anticoagulant utilization among United States nursing home residents with atrial fibrillation from 2011 to 2016. J Am Heart Assoc. 2019;8(9):e012023.
5. Zhu J, Alexander GC, Nazarian S, Segal JB, Wu AW. Trends and variation in oral anticoagulant choice in patients with atrial fibrillation, 2010-2017. Pharmacotherapy. 2018;38(9):907–20.
6. Douketis JD, Spyropoulos AC, Kaatz S, Becker RC, Caprini JA, Dunn AS, et al. Perioperative bridging anticoagulation in patients with atrial fibrillation. N Engl J Med. 2015;373(9):823–33.
7. Caprini JA. Thrombosis risk assessment as a guide to quality patient care. Dis Mon. 2005;51(2-3):70–8.
8. Hebert KJ, Kohler TS. Penile prosthesis infection: myths and realities. World J Mens Health. 2019;37(3):276–87.
9. Henry GD. The Henry mummy wrap and the Henry finger sweep surgical techniques. J Sex Med. 2009;6(3):619–22.

Chapter 5
Management of Residual Curvature in Men with Peyronie's Disease Following Penile Prosthesis Implantation

Eiftu Haile, Petar Bajic, and Laurence A. Levine

Introduction

The name "Peyronie's disease" (PD) is attributed to François de la Peyronie who reported a case series of men with penile deformity in 1743 [1]. Three patients were reported to have a thickening of the shaft of the penis, causing curvature in the shaft during erections. PD remains underreported with autopsy studies revealing a higher prevalence of the disease than self-reported studies [2]. This may be a result of the prevalence of the disease being greater than the rate of bothersome deformity in patients.

Men with Peyronie's disease can also suffer from concomitant erectile dysfunction (ED) [3]. While there has been much debate regarding which of these two conditions leads to the other, it is likely that they may each be a risk factor for the other. A subset of men with both PD and ED require penile prosthesis implantation due to bothersome deformity and/or insufficient erectile response to pharmacotherapy.

Etiology of PD

PD is an acquired fibrotic disorder characterized by "plaque" (scar) formation in the penile tunica albuginea which causes penile deformity [4]. While this disease has been recognized for centuries, the etiology of PD remains incompletely understood.

E. Haile · P. Bajic (✉)
Glickman Urological and Kidney Institute, Cleveland Clinic, Cleveland, OH, USA
e-mail: bajicp@ccf.org

L. A. Levine
Division of Urology, Rush University Medical Center, Chicago, IL, USA

E. P. Miranda, J. P. Mulhall (eds.), *Penile Implant Surgery*,
https://doi.org/10.1007/978-3-030-82363-4_5

PD plaque is presumed to be a result of abnormal or exuberant scar tissue formation in response to (often asymptomatic) trauma, most commonly during sexual intercourse [2]. This microtrauma and resultant inflammation, in susceptible men, results in changes in the collagen composition of the tunica albuginea with excessive collagen deposition, breakdown of the elastin framework, and fibroblast proliferation resulting in the formation of fibrous plaque which creates a segmental limitation in elasticity of the diseased tunica. The diminished elasticity of this scar tissue results in penile deformity in the erect state, the hallmark of the disease. While penile curvature is the most common presentation of Peyronie's disease, various combinations of deformities may be present. Reduced tunical elasticity may result in both length and girth loss. Girth loss, sometimes referred to as "volume loss," may involve the entire penis or only the diseased segment. Segmental girth loss exists on a spectrum ranging from indentation to non-circumferential narrowing to complete hourglass deformity. Patients with more distal narrowing may exhibit distal tapering or a "Bordeaux bottle" appearance (Fig. 5.1).

Risk factors for PD include penile trauma (most commonly with the partner on top), smoking, family or personal history of Dupuytren's contracture, and a family history of PD [5].

Anatomy and Pathophysiology

The tunica albuginea is composed of inner circular and outer longitudinal layers [6]. This fascial structure is formed from a lattice of elastin and collagen arranged around and surrounding the penile corpora cavernosa. PD plaque forms in the tunica albuginea and is anchored to the fibers of the septum dividing the two corporal bodies [2]. In the acute phase of PD, the plaque undergoes structural changes and becomes more fibrotic, and the penile shaft deformity appears which can initially be accompanied by pain. Due to failure of the remodeling process which occurs during normal wound healing, this deformity persists, and there is stabilization of the deformity in the chronic (stable) phase [2].

Surgical Indications for Inflatable Penile Prosthesis (IPP) in PD

Generally speaking, surgical management is indicated in the chronic (stable) phase of PD; this implies that deformity has been stable and without inflammatory pain for 3–6 months, ideally with disease duration of at least 1 year. Deformity should prevent satisfactory sexual intercourse or results in pain for the patient or partner. Surgical intervention is indicated for patients with severe deformity or those desiring the most rapid and reliable results [7, 8]. For patients with PD and medication refractory ED or who are anticipated to have a high likelihood of medication refractory ED after PD surgery, it is recommended that the patient undergo upfront penile

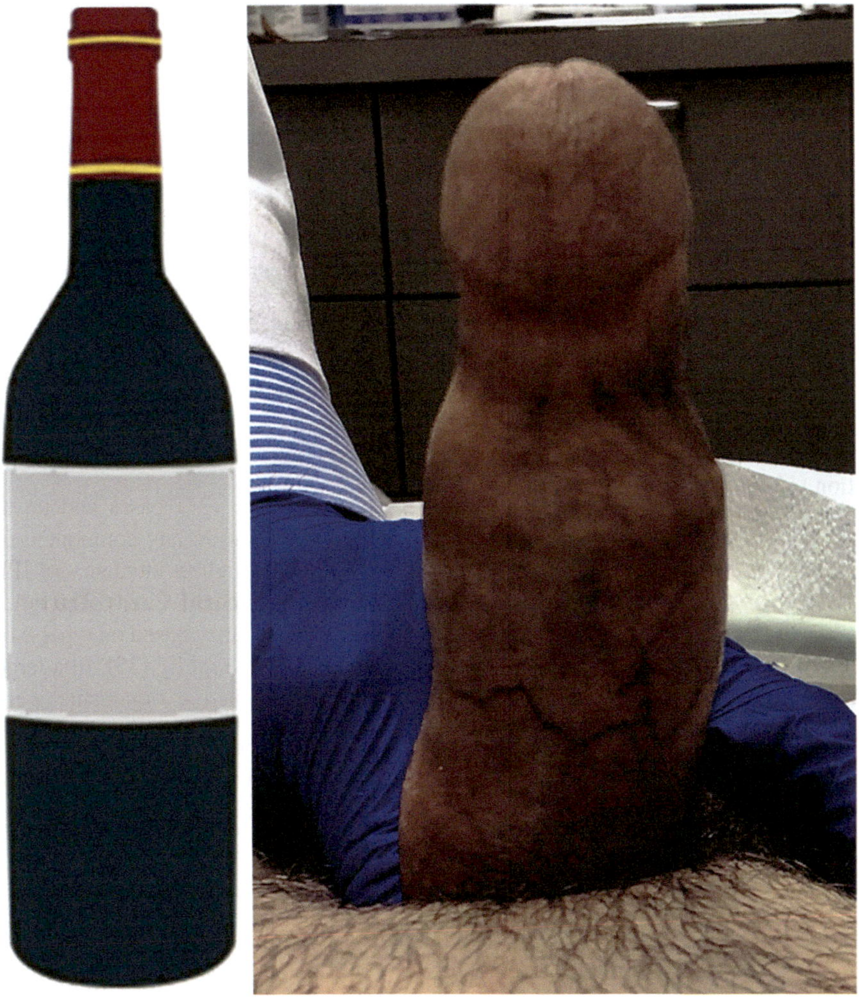

Fig. 5.1 "Bordeaux bottle" appearance of distal penile girth loss due to Peyronie's disease without evidence of curvature

prosthesis implantation with straightening maneuvers (which may include manual modeling, plication or plaque incision, and grafting). The optimal candidates for this approach are those patients with borderline or poor erectile function, diabetes, ventral curvature requiring urethral mobilization, or those desiring reliable erections and minimization of de novo ED risk with surgical correction of their penile deformity. Patients who have PD with mild ED adequately controlled with medications may also elect for penile prosthesis implantation without waiting to fail pharmacologic therapy. Patients in the acute phase of PD who have ED may also benefit from early prosthesis implantation in order to reduce the risk of further penile length loss due to PD. Preoperative counseling must take into consideration the fact that up to 73% of men complain of penile length loss following IPP implantation for PD with concomitant ED [9]. Similarly, patients must be made aware that the revision rate for penile prosthesis in this population has been reported to be 6–13% within 4–5 years [10, 11].

Relative to the malleable penile prosthesis, the inflatable penile prosthesis (IPP) is preferred in patients with PD and ED given the increased likelihood of curvature correction (due to greater rigidity), the concealable nature of the device, ease of use for patients, and arguably higher patient satisfaction rates [10, 12]. For this patient population in particular, IPPs have been shown to correct curvature without additional interventions with success rates ranging from 33% to 90% [8]. However, for patients with residual curvature greater than 30°, adjuvant maneuvers are indicated to correct residual curvature. In this chapter, we detail the various options for ensuring the optimal final result in men with residual curvature after IPP implantation. Our approach to these cases was reported in the first surgical algorithm documenting the sequence of maneuvers to address residual curvature after IPP implantation [13].

Intraoperative Methods for Correction of Residual Curvature

Manual Modeling

The manual modeling technique is an option for patients where residual curvature is minimal (i.e., <30°) after IPP implantation or as an initial attempt to improve curvature in men with more severe deformity [13, 14]. This method was first described in 1994 by Wilson and Delk in a landmark case series from which this technique gained notoriety for its efficiency and noninvasive nature [15]. In this series, manual modeling was performed following cylinder implantation but prior to pump placement. Our practice has been to always perform manual modeling as the initial maneuver regardless of degree of curvature as many deformities may have adequate improvement with modeling alone [13]. Furthermore, partial improvement after modeling may facilitate less invasive adjunctive measures to achieve the desired result.

Technique

Following implantation of the IPP cylinders, but before corporotomy closure, the cylinders are maximally inflated via a surrogate reservoir, and rubber shods are placed on the tubing to minimize pressure on the pump from saline backflow. While grasping the shaft at the level of the distal cylinders with one hand and the proximal shaft with the contralateral hand, applying digital pressure to the corporotomy sites, the cylinders are forcibly bent in the direction opposite the curvature [14, 16]. Care must be taken not to apply downward pressure on the corporal tips as this may encourage distal urethral perforation. This position is held for 60–90 seconds and presumably relies on disruption of the fibrotic plaque. The procedure is repeated until residual curvature is <20–30° [14]. It is possible that multiple rounds of modeling may be required [16]. Wilson and Delk, in their original series, reported an 86% success rate with this technique, while other longer-term studies have quoted a success rate closer to 80% [14, 15].

Complications

Urethral injury is the most feared, albeit rare, complication associated with manual modeling [14]. Wilson and Delk, in comparing patients who had undergone manual modeling to those who had not, reported that 4% of the cohort who underwent the adjunct procedure experienced distal urethral perforation [15]. The complication occurs from inadequate protection of the glans when applying pressure on the cylinders; a distal tip can ultimately be forced through the urethra in the fossa navicularis and emerge through the meatus [16]. This illustrates the importance of placing the hand performing the modeling on the distal shaft of the penis and not the glans [14]. The cylinder that perforates must be removed; however, the contralateral cylinder can be left in place and may provide for satisfactory sexual intercourse [16]. The patient should be treated with urethral catheterization for 7–10 days followed by replacement of the cylinder(s) 6 weeks postoperatively with confirmation of a normal-appearing urethra on cystoscopy [16].

Summary

Manual modeling is favored in the literature due to its high success rates, high patient satisfaction, and minimization of residual curvature to <20° [17]. In 2010, our group published a study of 90 patients with median curvature of 53° who underwent IPP placement with manual modeling and had an 83% patient satisfaction rate [10]. The rest of the cohort underwent adjuvant plaque incision or grafting. Seven of these patients had mechanical failure of their IPP, of whom two underwent distal corporoplasty for impending distal erosion. In a similar work, Chung et al. in 2013 performed a randomized trial of 130 patients to compare manual modeling in patients who received an AMS 700 CX to those receiving a Coloplast Titan over a mean follow-up period of 5 years [11]. 98% of the patients with curvature <60° had complete resolution with manual modeling and the two systems had equal 5-year Kaplan-Meier estimates for mechanical survival.

Plication

When manual modeling does not decrease the degree of curvature to less than 30° or when the degree of residual curvature is such that manual modeling is unlikely to be wholly successful, other adjunct procedures should be considered including plaque incision with or without grafting and plication. Plication entails shortening the convex side of the penis to match the concave side which has been shortened by Peyronie's disease. Patients who have residual severe indentation causing poor cosmesis and/or structural weakness are inappropriate candidates for this procedure.

Technique

Several different techniques for plication have been described. Our preferred approach, the tunica albuginea plication (TAP) procedure (performed via a subcoronal incision), entails partial thickness excision of the outer longitudinal fibers of the tunica albuginea over a 1 cm segment and uses a central 2-0 Tevdek suture (Teleflex Medical; Wayne, PA, USA) in an inverting vertical mattress fashion to perform the plication with a buried knot. This suture is flanked by two 3-0 PDS sutures to provide further support. When this procedure is performed without a penile prosthesis, an artificial erection is created to assess for residual curvature, and the procedure is repeated as many times as necessary to ensure a straight penis. In the setting of a penile prosthesis, we generally avoid plication as incision and grafting tends to result in better preservation of penile length. However, if plication were to be performed, the sutures may be placed before the prosthesis is implanted, as described by Rahman et al. in 2004 and Chung, Scott, and Morey in 2014 [9, 18].

Complications and Considerations

One contemporary series of plication with penile prosthesis implantation was published by the Lue Group at University of California San Francisco [18]. In this series, five men underwent the combination procedure and all had greater than or equal to 90 degree curvature (three ventral, two dorsal). All patients had complete correction of curvature, and at a mean follow-up of 22 months, the authors noted no recurrences. The authors stated that patients reported no complication in regard to the prosthesis. No mention was made of transient or long-term sensory changes or change in stretched penile length.

Another series from Chung et al. reviewed synchronous IPP implantation and plication in 18 patients from a single institution over a 3-year period [9]. Mean preoperative curvature was relatively mild at 39° and no patient had greater than 60° curvature. Curvature was corrected to a mean of <5° using a median of four plication sutures (range 3–6). Of these 18 patients, 15 completed a postoperative satisfaction survey at a mean of 11 months post-op and all noted improvement in their overall condition and penile curvature. A single patient with biplanar deformity noted a minor residual curvature. No patients reported pain with erections. The authors did not report on sensory changes, shortening complaints, or measurements of penile length, and no validated questionnaires were reported.

Plaque Incision or Partial Excision and Grafting (PIG/PEG)

Plaque incision and grafting (PIG) has been our preferred approach for residual curvature after manual modeling or as an initial approach to correct severe deformity following prosthesis implantation. Occasionally, partial plaque excision is required for bothersome palpable calcified plaques or to ensure normal shaft contour after prosthesis implantation. Some authors have described non-grafting approaches, although our preference has been to use TachoSil (Baxter Pharmaceuticals, Deerfield, IL, USA) which does not require suturing. We have also successfully utilized other hemostatic patches including Nu-Knit and Evarrest (Ethicon; Somerville, NJ, USA) [19].

Technique

We begin by implanting the penile prosthesis cylinders by a subcoronal approach. A surrogate reservoir is used to assess curvature, and the cylinders are left mostly inflated. Buck's fascia is incised longitudinally just lateral to the corpus spongiosum on both sides. This is performed along a sufficient length to facilitate elevation of the neurovascular bundle to expose the area of the tunica albuginea to be incised. The bundle is elevated and a double-Y incision is marked at the point of maximum curvature. This incision must cross the midline as all Peyronie's plaques are tethered to the septum of the corpora cavernosa. The prosthesis is deflated to about 50% and the incision is created with electrocautery over the implant on a 30-watt or less coagulation setting. The device is then reinflated and modeling is performed. The incision may be modified as needed to ensure a straight result. The defect is then covered with TachoSil or Evarrest which should also cover a 0.5–1 cm rim of tunica albuginea around the defect. The graft should be sized with the device in the inflated position to correct shaft caliber. Once the graft is applied, the device is deflated and Buck's fascia is closed to provide hemostasis and support for the graft. The remainder of the prosthesis is placed in the standard fashion. At the end of the procedure, the device is left partially inflated (about 50%) for up to 2 weeks to ensure proper healing of the tissues around the implant.

Scratch Technique

While manual modeling and PIG have been the mainstay of surgical PD correction in the setting of a penile prosthesis, other approaches have been proposed in recent years. The scratch technique was first described by Dr. Paul Perito in 2013 [20]. This procedure was developed to lower the risk of distal urethral injury during manual modeling which is as high as 5% [8, 20]. According to Perito et al. the procedure can also be used to improve both curvature and hourglass deformity prior to IPP placement. This procedure is considered investigational as no clinical trials have been performed to compare the efficacy of this technique to other more widely accepted techniques. Furthermore, it remains unclear how longitudinal incisions could correct curvature.

Technique

The procedure begins with identification and marking of the area with the plaque on the penis. An infrapubic incision is made in order to proceed with dilation of the corpora cavernosa. The corporotomy is explored with the insertion of a long nasal speculum. A 12-blade hook scalpel is inserted along the path of the nasal speculum, and longitudinal "scratches" are created in several locations. According to Perito et al., this method facilitates disruption of the plaque in three dimensions (x-, y-, and z-axes). Once this is performed, the IPP is implanted in the usual fashion. If residual curvature $\geq 30°$ is present, then manual modeling is performed.

Postoperative Management

Antonini et al. in 2018 added postoperative vacuum therapy to reduce recurrent curvature and/or inadequate correction of intraoperative curvature. This resulted in over 93% of the patients within the cohort having final curvature $<15°$, although the median follow-up interval was not clearly reported [21].

Length Restoration

Several more involved techniques have been described for penile lengthening at the time of IPP implantation in patients with bothersome length loss due to PD. Notably, surgical techniques to increase penile length require augmentation of the tunica albuginea, particularly on the concave side in men with curvature [22]. Lengthening procedures can be successful in the hands of experienced surgeons but carry with them higher risk of catastrophic complications like glans necrosis. The following are some of the procedures that have been described for this indication:

Sliding Technique

The sliding technique was first described by Rolle et al. in a small case series of three patients with concomitant ED, PD, and penile shortening in 2012 [23]. This procedure relies on a multiplanar incision that allows telescoping of the penis away from the body up to the limit of the dorsal neurovascular bundle and urethra. Two separate grafts are used to cover proximal and distal tunical defects. As is the case with any length restoration procedure, adequate skin is also necessary to ensure coverage of the elongated penile shaft.

Technique

The sliding technique involves exposure of the tunica albuginea via a circumferential subcoronal incision [23]. Buck's fascia is longitudinally incised and the neurovascular bundle is elevated to facilitate maximum elongation. The corpus spongiosum is carefully separated from the corpora to gain access to the ventral surface of the corpora cavernosa. Lateral longitudinal incisions are made bilaterally and a dorsal semicircular incision is made to connect these lateral incisions. This is repeated ventrally and gentle traction is applied to distract the distal and proximal penis to the limit of the neurovascular bundle. The lateral incisions are sutured in their new position. Proximally, dilation of the corpora is performed followed by insertion of the prosthesis cylinders. The staggered edges are then sutured in place with two rectangular grafts (porcine small intestinal submucosa was used in this study). Grafting may be performed prior to placement of the IPP cylinders to prevent damage to the prosthesis.

An update by Rolle et al. in 2016 to the technique proceeds in the same fashion but uses a proximal semi-circumferential incision on the ventral penile shaft at the level of the penoscrotal junction [24]. This prevents the need for a second ventral corporotomy for insertion of the cylinders.

Complications and Considerations

In the initial series, no major intraoperative or postoperative complications were noted. Over the 13 months of follow-up, patients had a median increase in the total IIEF scores from 24 at their preoperative visit to 60 (maximum score of 70) at the 12-month postoperative evaluation. In the second series of 28 patients with penile shortening secondary to PD and concomitant ED with 21 of them receiving IPPs, postoperative complications were reported. One patient on anticoagulant therapy had profuse bleeding requiring transfusion (Clavien-Dindo grade II). Two patients had infection of their prostheses requiring explantation (grade III). Notably, both of these patients were diabetic. Hematoma formation was noted to be common but was managed conservatively in all cases. The rate of prosthesis infection was high overall at 7%. Further prospective analysis of patients and longer-term follow-up will provide more information for this technique's impact over time as long-term complications have yet to be elucidated.

Modified Sliding Technique (MoST)

This technique, first described by Egydio et al. in 2015 is a modification of the Rolle technique in which essentially the same procedure is performed, but without grafting [25]. In this approach, defects in the tunica albuginea are covered by Buck's fascia only.

Technique

The procedure begins with a standard subcoronal degloving approach. Buck's fascia is longitudinally incised lateral to the urethra and the NVB is elevated along the length of the shaft. The urethra is mobilized in a similar fashion. The penis is held on stretch to allow for corporal markings: a semi-circumferential line ventrally 2 cm proximal to the coronal sulcus and a second semi-circumferential marking dorsally 1–2 cm distal from the penoscrotal junction. These lines are then connected by longitudinal lines on the lateral aspects of both corpora. The corporotomies for IPP cylinders placement are then made just proximal to the semicircular incision. This ensures there is a proximal exit for the tubing of the IPP. A proximal dorsal semicircular incision is created to allow for corporal dilation and the corporal bodies are distracted to the limit allowed by the stretch of the NVB. Buck's fascia is closed over the defects without placement of a graft. The remainder of the IPP implantation proceeds in the usual fashion. A dressing is applied to the wound and compression gauze is placed around the penis and scrotum.

Postoperative Management

The implant remains fully inflated for 1–2 h postoperatively to decrease the risk of hematoma formation. It is then deflated to 50% and, on the next day, cycled by the surgeon based on the patient's pain tolerance. The dressing is reapplied and the implant is inflated to >50%. The patient is instructed to cycle the implant daily starting 1 week postoperatively, maintaining the implant at partial inflation with the glans pointing up and then maximally inflating the implant for 1 h in the morning and 1 h in the evening.

Multiple-Slit Technique (MuST)

The multiple-slit technique (MuST) was first described by Egydio et al. in 2018 [26]. In this procedure, multiple small incisions are made rather than a single larger incision. Between July 2013 and January 2016, 138 patients underwent surgical management of their PD with concomitant ED. 35 of these patients underwent IPP placement, while the other 103 had a malleable penile prosthesis placed. Patients received a 2-week course of acetylsalicylic acid *(ASA)* 50 mg starting 2 days before surgery to reduce the risk of glans ischemia.

Technique

The shaft of the penis is degloved to its base and the dartos fascia is everted and sutured to the surgical drape to facilitate a "no-touch" technique. Two longitudinal paraurethral incisions are made into the Buck fascia to facilitate mobilization of the neurovascular bundle (NVB). The distal NVB is then everted over the glans and further mobilized with care given to preserving the fan-shaped laterality of the nerve branches. The semicircular incisions are similar to the MoST technique; however, instead of just two incisions, multiple small tunica defects are made on the concave side of the curvature. The penis is stretched to the maximum elasticity of the NVB or the urethra.

Two additional proximal corporotomies are made in order to proceed with IPP placement in the usual fashion. The multiple tunical defects are then covered with Buck's fascia without additional grafting.

Postoperative Management

The cylinders are kept semi-inflated for 2–3 weeks until the patient can manipulate the scrotal pump. Patients are instructed not to overpump the cylinders to avoid bulging defects. The most common complication was postoperative hematoma (18.8%) which resolved with observation in every case. 2.9% of patients reported partial glans numbness which was self-resolving. 5.1% of patients were anorgasmic for up to 4 months. There was one case of glans necrosis in a patient who underwent malleable prosthesis placement, requiring glans resurfacing and exchange of prosthesis. No infections were noted in this cohort.

Outcomes

The mean reported penile length gain of 3.1 cm (2–5 cm) with all PD cases resulting in subjective straightening. The average IIEF score increased from 22 to 61 at 6 months of follow-up. Other purported benefits of this approach include reducing bulging without the need for grafting (Table 5.1).

Table 5.1 Summarizes all described techniques and contains the most relevant data pertaining their outcomes

Authors	Date	Size of study population	Adjunct technique to IPP placement	Residual curvature pre-intervention	Residual curvature post-intervention	Complications
Wilson and Delk	10/1994	138	Manual modeling	Not quantified	Not quantified	Unsatisfactory straightening requiring adjunct procedures (6%)
						Urethral perforation (3%)
						Infection (3%)
Levine et al.	11/1/2010	90	Manual modeling	53°	Functionally straight (<20°)	Mechanical failure requiring device replacement (7.8%)
						Revision surgery (2.2.%)
						Distal tunica erosion (2.2%)
						Infected device (1.1%)
Lue et al.	6/2004	5	Plication	90°	No recurrent curvature reported	No complications reported at 36 months of follow-up
Chung et al.	6/1/2014	18	Plication	39° (range 30–60°)	<5°	Further manipulation after initial postoperative visit for recurrent curvature (11%)
Levine et al.	7/1/2019	33	Plaque Incision and Grafting (PIG)	75° (hemostatic patches = HP)	>20% in 13% of patients with PA and 17% in patients with HP	Bothersome residual curvature (13% with PA and 6% with HP)
				78° (pericardium allografts = PA)		Revision surgery (12%)
Perito et al.	9/1/2018	145	Scratch technique +12 weeks vacuum pump therapy	Middle third plaques: 65.6+/−10°	Middle third plaques: 9.2+/−2.9°	Significant relapse (>15° curvature, 6.2%)
				Proximal third: 71.8+/−4.5°	Proximal third: 9.5+/−3.1°	Severe scrotal hematoma (4.1%)
				Subcoronal zone: 49.2+/−7.4°	Subcoronal zone: 8.5+/−1.3°	Prosthesis extrusion (2.1%)
						Mechanical failure (1.4%)

Rolle et al.	12/21/2015	28 (7 malleable prosthesis implants, 21 IPPs)	Sliding technique	Dorsal curvature: 39° (25–70°)	No recurrent curvature reported	Profuse bleeding requiring transfusion (3.5%)
				Lateral curvature: 30° (20–60°)		Infection of prosthesis requiring removal (7%)
				Ventral curvature: 41° (25–60)		Penile hematoma (28.5%)
						Penoscrotal hematoma (10.7%)
Egydio et al.	1/28/2015	143 (77 patients, 53.8%, with PD)	Modified "Sliding" Technique (MOST)	Mean deviation of penile axis = 45° (range: 0–100°)	All PD cases resulted in subjective straightening	Hematoma (self-resolving, 24.5%)
						Partial glans numbness (self-resolving, 4.9%)
						Anorgasmia (resolved by 4 months, 10.5%)
Egydio et al.	12/2/2017	138 (103 malleable prosthesis implants, 35 IPPs)	Multiple-Slit Technique (MUST)	Mean deviation of penile axis = 55° (range: 0–90°)	All PD cases resulted in subjective straightening	Hematoma (self-resolving, 18.8%)
						Anorgasmia (resolved by 4 months, 5.1%)
						Partial glans numbness (self-resolving, 2.9%)
						Glans necrosis (0.7%)
Moncada et al.	2/9/2020	92	Structured home modeling (SHM) protocol after IPP placement	Mean preoperative penile curvature = 39.4° +/− 5.7°	≤10° at 6 months of SHM (94.7% of patient population)	Hematoma (non-surgical, 6 patients)
						Pain lasting <6 weeks [4]
						Pump revision for malfunction [1]
						Mechanical failure [1]
						Impending erosion [1]

Postoperative Techniques for Straightening

Home Manual Modeling

A recent study by Moncada et al. in 2020 reviewed a series of 92 patients with PD who underwent IPP implantation [27]. A subset of 76 patients underwent manual modeling and had between 0° and 45° residual curvature. No further straightening maneuvers were undertaken in the operating room, but patients were instructed to perform home modeling for 6 months, starting 4 weeks after penile prosthesis implantation. The mean postoperative residual curvature after modeling was 29.7° (SD 3.2°), and 85.5% of patients who performed home modeling had 10° or less residual curvature at 3-month follow-up. At 6-month follow-up, this rate increased to 94.7%. Subjective patient satisfaction was reported at 92.1% at 6 months. The authors concluded that home modeling may be reasonable in patients with <45° curvature. Further investigation is needed to assess the role of postoperative modeling in a multi-institutional setting.

Penile Traction Therapy and Vacuum Erection Devices

While they are often used in the preoperative setting to maximize penile length at the time of implantation, mechanical therapies for PD have not been described to treat residual curvature in the post-IPP setting. Further studies are needed to determine whether there may be a role for these treatments.

Residual Curvature Algorithm

In summary of the techniques presented, our standardized approach to residual curvature after IPP implantation is presented in Fig. 5.2. Patients with bothersome length loss may also be offered lengthening procedures but require thorough counseling on the risks including glans necrosis.

Conclusions

Peyronie's disease is a relatively common finding among men undergoing penile prosthesis implantation. Efforts should be made to recognize this condition in the preoperative setting whenever possible in order to facilitate detailed counseling on the risks and benefits of various approaches. The penis should be examined for plaque and restricted tunical elasticity during every evaluation for penile prosthesis

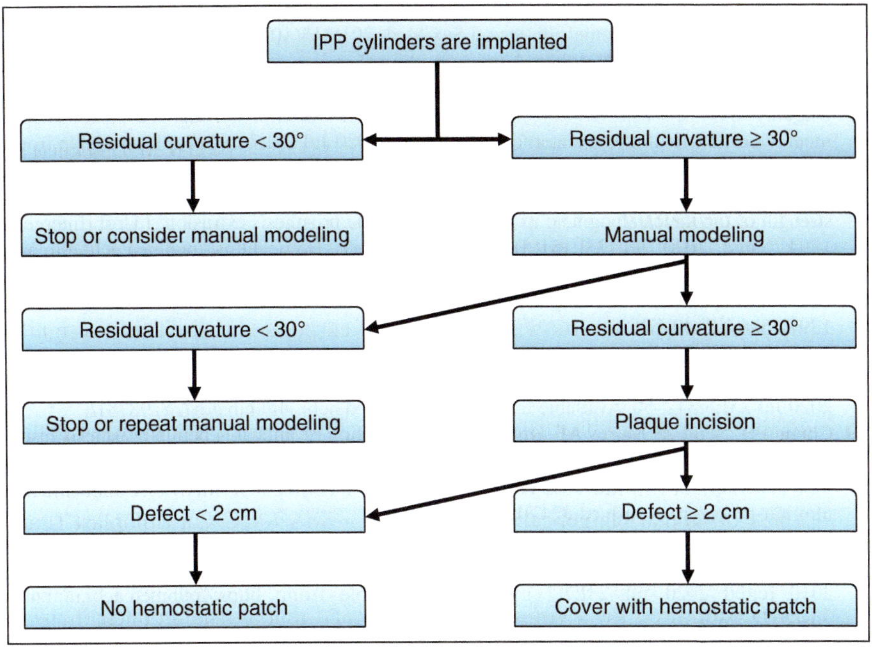

Fig. 5.2 Algorithm for the management of residual curvature after inflatable penile prosthesis (IPP) implantation in men with Peyronie's disease [13]

implantation. Patients who undergo penile duplex ultrasound or intracavernosal injection in the office should be evaluated with a goniometer and assessment of girth so that degree of curvature and character of deformity can be documented. This evaluation is critical to determining which straightening maneuvers may be indicated and allows patients the opportunity to learn about the relative risks and benefits of each approach before choosing a surgical approach. In our practice, manual modeling followed by PIG with TachoSil or Evarrest patching if residual curvature is greater than 30 degrees (or if the patient insists on complete straightening during the preoperative consultation) continues to be our standard approach. Finally, length restoration procedures should be performed with great caution and by centers of excellence in order to minimize the risk of neurovascular injury and glans necrosis.

References

1. Chir F de la P-MAR, 1743Paperpile undefined. Sur quelques obstacles qui s' opposent a l'ejaculation naturelle de la semence.
2. Tsambarlis P, Levine LA. Nonsurgical management of Peyronie's disease. Nat Rev Urol [Internet]. 2019 [cited 2019 Dec 22];16(3):172–86. Available from: http://www.nature.com/articles/s41585-018-0117-7.

3. Terrier JE, Tal R, Nelson CJ, Mulhall JP. Penile sensory changes after plaque incision and grafting surgery for Peyronie's disease. J Sex Med. 2018;15(10):1491–7.
4. Mulcahy JJ. In: Klein EA, editor. A guide to clinical management male sexual function. 2nd ed. Totwa: Humana Press Inc.; 2006.
5. Bilgutay AN, Pastuszak AW. Peyronie's disease: a review of etiology, diagnosis, and management. Curr Sex Health Rep [Internet]. 2015 [cited 2020 Jul 23];7(2):117–31. Available from: https://pubmed.ncbi.nlm.nih.gov/26279643/.
6. Hsu GL, Brock G, Martinez-Pineiro L, Von Heyden B, Lue TF, Tanagho EA. Anatomy and strength of the tunica albuginea: its relevance to penile prosthesis extrusion. J Urol [Internet]. 1994 [cited 2020 Jul 23];151(5):1205–8. Available from: https://pubmed.ncbi.nlm.nih.gov/8158761/.
7. Levine LA, Lenting EL. A surgical algorithm for the treatment of Peyronie's disease. J Urol. 1997;158(6):2149–52.
8. Anaissie J, Yafi FA. A review of surgical strategies for penile prosthesis implantation in patients with Peyronie's disease [Internet]. Transl Androl Urol. AME Publishing Company. 2016 [cited 2020 Jul 23];5:342–50. Available from: https://pubmed.ncbi.nlm.nih.gov/27298781/.
9. Chung PH, Scott JF, Morey AF. High patient satisfaction of inflatable penile prosthesis insertion with synchronous penile plication for erectile dysfunction and Peyronie's disease. J Sex Med [Internet]. 2014 [cited 2020 Jul 28];11(6):1593–8. Available from: https://pubmed-ncbi-nlm-nih-gov.ezproxy.rush.edu/24708140/.
10. Levine LA, Benson J, Hoover C. Inflatable penile prosthesis placement in men with Peyronie's disease and drug-resistant erectile dysfunction: a single-center study. J Sex Med [Internet]. 2010 [cited 2020 Jul 23];7(11):3775–83. Available from: https://pubmed.ncbi.nlm.nih.gov/20722782/.
11. Chung E, Solomon M, Deyoung L, Brock GB. Comparison between AMS 700™ CX and Coloplast™ Titan inflatable penile prosthesis for Peyronie's disease treatment and remodeling: clinical outcomes and patient satisfaction. J Sex Med [Internet]. 2013 [cited 2020 Jul 23];10(11):2855–60. Available from: https://pubmed.ncbi.nlm.nih.gov/23210973/.
12. Montorsi F, Guazzoni G, Bergamaschi F, Rigatti P. Patient-partner satisfaction with semirigid penile prostheses for Peyronie's disease: a 5-year followup study. J Urol [Internet]. 1993 [cited 2020 Jul 28];150(6):1819–21. Available from: https://pubmed-ncbi-nlm-nih-gov.ezproxy.rush.edu/8230513/.
13. Levine LA, Dimitriou RJ. A surgical algorithm for penile prosthesis placement in men with erectile failure and Peyronie's disease. Int J Impot Res [Internet]. 2000 [cited 2020 Jul 28];12(3):147–51. Available from: https://pubmed-ncbi-nlm-nih-gov.ezproxy.rush.edu/11045907/.
14. El-Khatib FM, Huynh LM, Yafi FA. Intraoperative methods for residual curvature correction during penile prosthesis implantation in patients with Peyronie's disease and refractory erectile dysfunction [Internet]. Int J Impot Res. Springer Nature; 2020 [cited 2020 Jul 23];32:43–51. Available from: https://pubmed.ncbi.nlm.nih.gov/31754245/.
15. Wilson SK, Delk JR. A new treatment for Peyronie's disease: modeling the penis over an inflatable penile prosthesis. J Urol [Internet]. 1994 [cited 2020 Jul 23];152(4):1121–3. Available from: https://pubmed.ncbi.nlm.nih.gov/8072079/.
16. Martins FE, Kulkarni SB, Kohler TS, editors. Textbook of male genitourethral reconstruction. 1st ed. Cham: Springer; 2020.
17. Berookhim BM, Karpman E, Carrion R. Adjuvant maneuvers for residual curvature correction during penile prosthesis implantation in men with Peyronie's disease. J Sex Med [Internet]. 2015 [cited 2020 Jul 23];12:449–54. Available from: https://pubmed.ncbi.nlm.nih.gov/26565576/.
18. Rahman NU, Carrion RE, Bochinski D, Lue TF. Combined penile plication surgery and insertion of penile prosthesis for severe penile curvature and erectile dysfunction. J Urol [Internet]. 2004 [cited 2020 Jul 31];171(6 I):2346–9. Available from: https://pubmed-ncbi-nlm-nih-gov.ezproxy.rush.edu/15126818/.

19. Farrell MR, Abdelsayed GA, Ziegelmann MJ, Levine LA. A comparison of hemostatic patches versus pericardium allograft for the treatment of complex Peyronie's disease with penile prosthesis and plaque incision. Urology [Internet]. 2019 [cited 2020 Jul 28];129:113–8. Available from: https://pubmed-ncbi-nlm-nih-gov.ezproxy.rush.edu/30914333/.
20. Perito P, Wilson S. The Peyronie's plaque " scratch": an adjunct to modeling. J Sex Med [Internet]. 2013 [cited 2020 Jul 23];10(5):1194–7. Available from: https://pubmed.ncbi.nlm.nih.gov/23750353/.
21. Antonini G, De Berardinis E, Del Giudice F, Busetto GM, Lauretti S, Fragas R, et al. Inflatable penile prosthesis placement, scratch technique and postoperative vacuum therapy as a combined approach to definitive treatment of Peyronie's disease. J Urol [Internet]. 2018 [cited 2020 Jul 23];200(3):642–7. Available from: https://pubmed.ncbi.nlm.nih.gov/29678456/.
22. Gaffney CD, Pagano MJ, Weinberg AC, Small AC, Kuehas FE, Egydio PH, et al. Lengthening strategies for Peyronie's disease [internet]. Transl Androl Urol. AME Publishing Company. 2016 [cited 2020 Jul 23];5:351–62. Available from: https://pubmed.ncbi.nlm.nih.gov/27298782/.
23. Rolle L, Ceruti C, Timpano M, Sedigh O, Destefanis P, Galletto E, et al. A new, innovative, lengthening surgical procedure for Peyronie's disease by penile prosthesis implantation with double dorsal-ventral patch graft: the "sliding technique." J Sex Med [Internet]. 2012 [cited 2020 Jul 28];9(9):2389–95. Available from: https://pubmed.ncbi.nlm.nih.gov/22429331/
24. Rolle L, Falcone M, Ceruti C, Timpano M, Sedigh O, Ralph DJ, et al. A prospective multicentric international study on the surgical outcomes and patients' satisfaction rates of the "sliding" technique for end-stage Peyronie's disease with severe shortening of the penis and erectile dysfunction. BJU Int [Internet]. 2016 [cited 2020 Jul 23];117(5):814–20. Available from: https://pubmed.ncbi.nlm.nih.gov/26688436/
25. Egydio PH, Kuehhas FE. Penile lengthening and widening without grafting according to a modified "sliding" technique. BJU Int [Internet]. 2015 [cited 2020 Jul 23];116(6):965–72. Available from: https://pubmed.ncbi.nlm.nih.gov/25644141/
26. Egydio PH, Kuehhas FE. The Multiple-Slit Technique (MUST) for penile length and girth restoration. J Sex Med [Internet]. 2018 [cited 2020 Jul 23];15(2):261–9. Available from: https://pubmed.ncbi.nlm.nih.gov/29275049/.
27. Moncada I, Krishnappa P, Ascencios J, Lopez I, Martinez-Salamanca JI. Home modeling after penile prosthesis implantation in the management of residual curvature in Peyronie's disease. Int J Impot Res [Internet]. 2020 [cited 2020 Jul 23]; Available from: https://pubmed.ncbi.nlm.nih.gov/32641777/.

Chapter 6
Considerations on Inflatable Penile Prosthesis Reservoir Placement

Brian Dick, Michael Polchert, Ayman Soubra, and Wayne J. G. Hellstrom

Introduction

When it comes to surgically managing erectile dysfunction, there are numerous different penile implants. The prosthetic options include malleable penile prosthesis and two-piece and three-piece inflatable penile prosthesis (IPP). The three-piece IPP is the most popular among patients, as it most closely mimics the natural flaccid and erect states of the penis. It is composed of three components: two identical inflatable cylinders, which are inserted within either corpus cavernosum, a scrotal pump that is used to inflate and deflate the aforementioned cylinders and a reservoir that stores saline when the device is in the detumesced state. The reservoir is what allows for flaccidity and hence the patient's desire for the three-piece system.

While the prosthetic reservoir confers obvious benefits to the patient, it can provide challenges for the urologist. Regardless of surgical approach, reservoir placement is performed somewhat blindly, placing the patient at potential risk for bladder, bowel, or vascular injury. Postoperatively, the reservoir may become infected, fail mechanically, or erode into surrounding tissue. Lastly, depending on where the reservoir is placed, it can pose an additional challenge if the patient has future abdominal or pelvic surgeries. The experienced urologist considers these factors to ensure optimal reservoir placement. This chapter covers different techniques of reservoir placement for a three-piece IPP and provides the advantages/disadvantages of each.

B. Dick · M. Polchert · A. Soubra · W. J. G. Hellstrom (✉)
Department of Urology, Tulane University School of Medicine, New Orleans, LA, USA
e-mail: bdick@tulane.edu; mpolchert@tulane.edu; asoubra@tulane.edu; whellst@tulane.edu

E. P. Miranda, J. P. Mulhall (eds.), *Penile Implant Surgery*,
https://doi.org/10.1007/978-3-030-82363-4_6

Preoperative Considerations

After it is decided that a patient will undergo placement of a three-piece IPP, the surgeon needs to consider the optimal location to place the reservoir. There are a number of locations to choose from, each offering unique advantages and disadvantages (Table 6.1, Fig. 6.1). A thorough patient history is important in deciding on a location that will result in the best outcome.

The traditional location to place an IPP reservoir is into the space of Retzius (SOR), or prevesical space. This is an extraperitoneal space located posterior to the pubic symphysis and anterior and lateral to the urinary bladder. This was the preferred location for older-generation reservoirs, which lacked lock-out valve features, as it exerted minimal pressure on the reservoir and reduced the risk of auto-inflation [12]. Despite the advent of a lock-out reservoir, surgeons continue to place the reservoir in the SOR because of custom and its imperceptibility to patients. The main disadvantage in choosing this location is the blind insertion of the reservoir, placing the patient at potential risk of bowel, bladder, and vascular injury

Table 6.1 Locations to place IPP reservoir

Location	Advantages	Disadvantages	Considerations
Space of Retzius (SOR) aka prevesical space	Imperceptible to patient	Risk of bowel, bladder, and vascular injury [1–3]	RALP can alter anatomy [2]
		Risk of herniation or erosion into nearby structures [3–5]	Pelvic radiation might pose technical difficulty
Peritoneal	No capsular formation [6]	Risk of damage/ erosion into peritoneal structures [2]	Fell out of use after advent of lock-out valves
	Low risk of auto-inflation		
Epigastrium	No capsular formation	Requires a complex, additional incision	Fell out of use after advent of lock-out valves
	Low risk of bowel or vascular injury		
	Low risk of auto-inflation		
Anterior to transversalis fascia (ATF)	Avoids adhesions and scarring in patients with history of pelvic surgery [7]	Palpable or visible in some patients [8]	Useful in patients with history of pelvic surgery
	Low risk of vascular, bowel, or bladder injury [8]	Groin herniation [8]	
Posterior to transversalis fascia (PTF)	Same advantages as ATF placement but it is less perceptible to patient and less likely to herniate [8]	More difficult placement in patients with history of pelvic surgery [8]	Useful in patients without history of pelvic surgery

Table 6.1 (continued)

Location	Advantages	Disadvantages	Considerations
High submuscular (HSM)	Avoids adhesions and scarring in patients with history of pelvic surgery [9]	Reservoir more difficult to remove [10, 11]	Gaining popularity among some high-volume implanters
	Low risk of vascular, bowel, or bladder injury [9]	Reservoir may be palpable or visibile [12]	
Subcutaneous	Easy intraoperative placement	Patient must have high BMI [13]	If patient loses weight, the reservoir may become more apparent
	Low risk of vascular, bowel, or bladder injury		

RALP robot-assisted laparoscopic prostatectomy

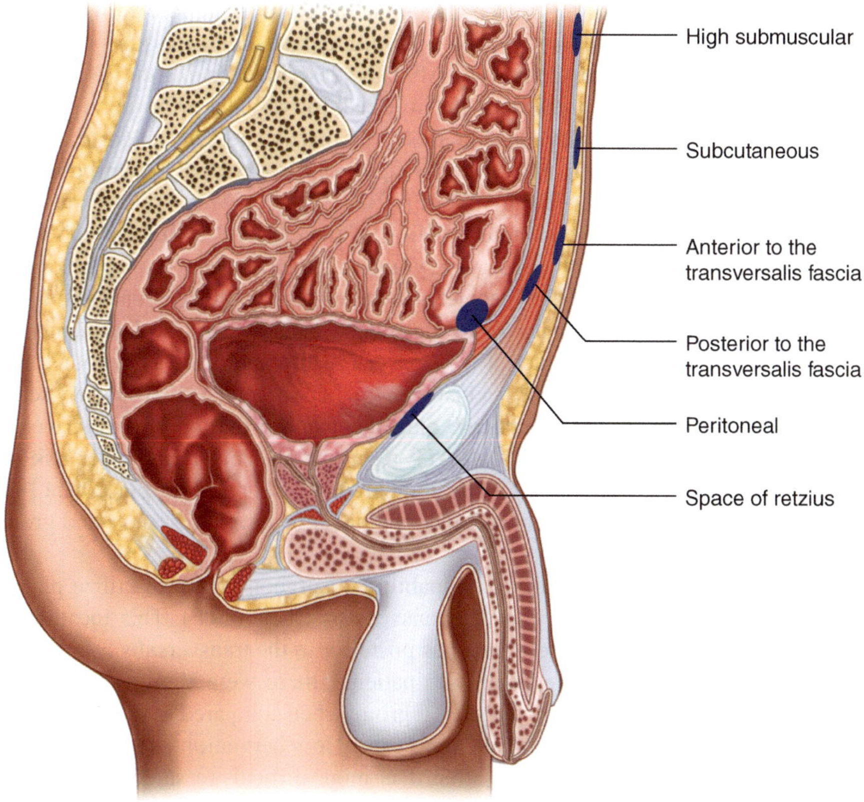

Fig. 6.1 Locations to place inflatable penile prosthesis reservoir. *1* Space of Retzius; *2* peritoneal; *3* posterior to the transversalis fascia; *4* anterior to the transversalis fascia; *5* subcutaneous; *6* high submuscular. Rectus muscles not pictured. All reservoir locations are deep to the rectus muscles except the subcutaneous location

[1–3]. Erosion into nearby structures and herniation, although rare, have also been reported [3–5]. Care must be taken in patients with a history of robot-assisted laparoscopic prostatectomy (RALP), as these patients may have altered anatomy of the SOR, resulting in increased risk of inadvertent intraperitoneal placement of the reservoir [2]. This is especially important given that radical prostatectomy (RP) usually causes medical refractory erectile dysfunction and many IPPs are placed in post-RP patients. This space can also be problematic in patients with prior history of pelvic surgery or pelvic radiation, as adhesions and scar tissue may have altered the anatomy.

Ectopic reservoir placement refers to reservoir placement in a location besides the SOR. The first ectopic location utilized was the peritoneal cavity. Similar to the SOR, the peritoneal cavity exerts little pressure on the reservoir and poses little risk of auto-inflation. An additional benefit of peritoneal reservoir placement is that capsular formation is avoided, eliminating risk of capsule-related mechanical failure [6]. A drawback of this location is that the peritoneal cavity holds many vital organs which may be damaged during device placement or device migration/herniation [2]. Further, this location may also be problematic in patients with a history of pelvic surgery. To avoid these "hostile pelves," Mulcahy described placing the reservoir in the epigastrium [6]. The epigastrium has little risk for vascular or bowel injury but requires the use of a secondary incision. Reservoir placement in the epigastrium and peritoneum fell out of favor when Mentor Corporation (Irvine, CA) introduced a lock-out valve on their reservoir in 1998 [6].

The lock-out valve prevents auto-inflation of the corporal cylinders with fluid when pressure is applied to the reservoir, granting surgeons access to a plethora of new ectopic locations. In 2001, Wilson et al. detailed reservoir placement behind the abdominal musculature but anterior to the transversalis fascia – a placement that would come to be known as anterior to transversalis fascia (ATF)[7]. They found this location was useful in patients with a history of pelvic surgery, as it avoids any scarring or adhesions that may complicate placement in the retroperitoneal space or SOR. More recent studies report that ATF reservoir placement has lower risk of bladder, bowel, or vascular injury when compared to SOR reservoir placement [8]. Disadvantages of ATF placement include a palpable or visible reservoir and groin herniation [8].

In an effort to decrease reservoir palpability, a surgeon may also utilize placement of the reservoir posterior to the transversalis fascia (PTF). This location is similar to ATF; however, the reservoir lies posterior to the transversalis fascia. In a single surgeon series of more than 2600 patients, there were significantly fewer revisions for palpable reservoirs in the PTF group when compared to the ATF group [8]. Additionally, the PTF group had significantly less herniation and device auto-inflation. A disadvantage of PTF is that it is more difficult to safely perform in patients with a history of pelvic surgery or radiation [8].

Both ATF and PTF approaches have been largely superseded by the high submuscular placement (HSM), first described by Morey et al. in 2013. A channel is created between the transversalis fascia and rectus abdominis muscle, and the reservoir is placed as cephalad as possible [9]. Advantages of HSM reservoir placement are that it can be performed in those with a history of pelvic surgery, and the risk of herniation is virtually eliminated due to its high location. Drawbacks of HSM reservoir placement are that it is often more difficult to explant [11]. In fact, a cadaveric study noted that only 1/3 of reservoirs placed in the HSM were found in their intended location [10]. Additionally, patients may see or feel the reservoir, especially if they are slender in build [12]. This issue improves over time as a capsule forms around the reservoir.

If a patient is particularly obese, the surgeon may consider a subcutaneous reservoir placement (SRP). A review of eight patients who received an IPP with SRP reported that none of the patients could palpate or see the reservoir [13]. The average BMI of this cohort of patients was 39. SRP avoids adhesions and scarring from previous surgeries, making it ideal in overweight patients who have undergone multiple previous surgeries. A drawback of this location is that the reservoir may become palpable or visible if the patient undergoes weight loss.

Surgical Technique

Once a location for the reservoir has been decided upon, the implanter must choose which surgical approach will provide the best results for the patient. The SOR (Fig. 6.2) is typically accessed blindly whether the IPP is being placed via a penoscrotal or infrapubic approach. The surgeon inserts a finger through the incision to find the periosteum of the pubic bone and then moves the finger toward the ipsilateral shoulder until it is over the superior edge of the pubic bone. The external inguinal ring can be found here with medial and lateral sweeping just above the pubic bone [14]. Once the external inguinal ring is identified, the reservoir is inserted through the transversalis fascia edge into the SOR. It is recommended to place the patient in Trendelenburg position so that the bowel and bladder contents fall away from the inguinal ring, thus reducing the risk of organ damage. As previously mentioned, a history of pelvic surgery or radiation may make it more difficult to access the SOR. In these more complex patients, Levine and Hoeh recommend entering the SOR sharply with a pair of curved Jorgenson scissors. The scissors are placed curve-side down just over the superior aspect of the pubis, and the handle is lifted causing the curved tips to perforate the transversalis fascia [15]. The space is then opened bluntly or sharply, and using the finger, the surgeon will sweep around to enlarge the space to accommodate the reservoir. This approach has the added benefit of reduced inguinal floor weakness.

The initial surgical steps are identical between ATF and PTF reservoir placement. After emptying the bladder, a finger is used to identify the external inguinal

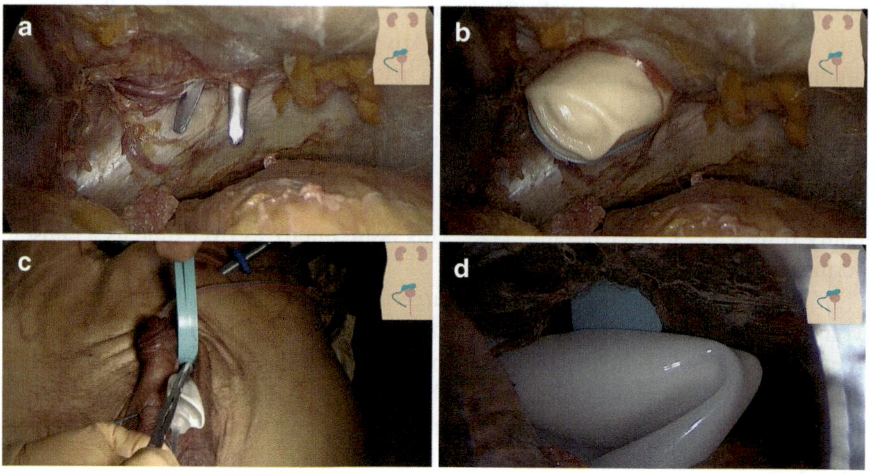

Fig. 6.2 Placement of reservoir in space of Retzius in a cadaver under laparoscopic visualization. (**a**) Space of Retzius is opened by piercing the transversalis fascia, (**b**) space is enlarged by sweeping finger movement, (**c**) reservoir deployed under a s-retractor into the space, (**d**) reservoir filled and well seated in wanted position. (Images obtained, with permission, from Osmonov D. VJPU 2018; 2: 122)

ring. An 80 mm closed nasal speculum can be used and is inserted along the ventral aspect of the finger and into the ring. In a PTF reservoir placement (Fig. 6.3), the speculum handle tip is used to perforate the transversalis fascia in a downward fashion. The handle is then rotated such that the tip is oriented toward the head. The speculum is advanced cephalad to the hilt and the paddles are spread to open a potential space. A deflated reservoir is then inserted. If the device is a Coloplast® (Minneapolis, MN) model, care must be taken to ensure the lock-out mechanism is anterior facing, as nearby structures may interfere with its proper function [8]. In ATF reservoir placement, the speculum is inserted through the external inguinal ring and advanced cephalad, without piercing the transversalis fascia [8].

HSM reservoir placement (Fig. 6.4) is similar to ATF reservoir placement. After the external inguinal ring is identified, a space is fashioned between the transversalis fascia and rectus muscles. A Foerster lung clamp or other similar device is then inserted through the external inguinal ring, and the paddles are spread in the anterior-posterior plane to widen the space. The clamp is advanced cephalad in this manner toward the ipsilateral nipple; the paddle may be spread in the horizontal plane if needed to advance the instrument [9]. A deflated reservoir is inserted as cephalad as possible.

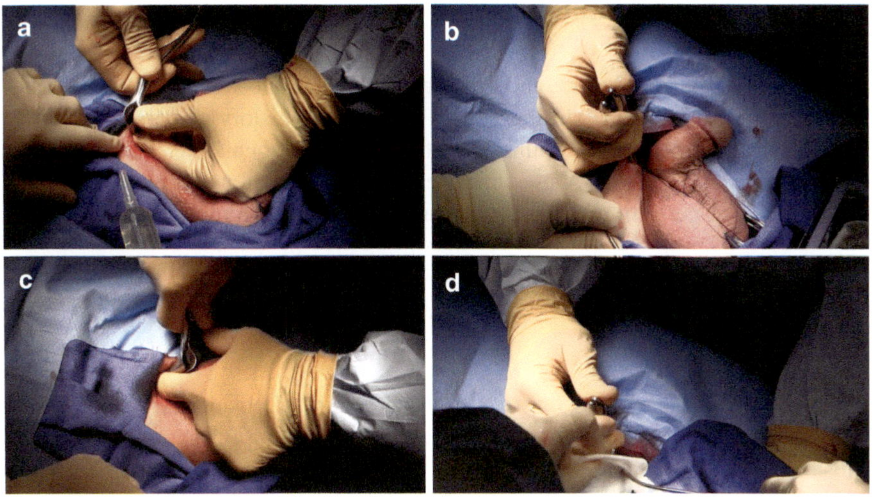

Fig. 6.3 Placement of reservoir in posterior transversalis fascial space during an infrapubic approach to inflatable penile prosthesis placement. (**a**) Transversalis fascia is pierced by pushing on the speculum downward fashion, (**b**) speculum blades are then dropped and pointed cephalad, (**c**) space is developed with sweeping finger movement, (**d**) reservoir advanced into the space with the help of a clamp/suction tip. (Images obtained, with permission, from Perito P. VJPU 2018; 2: 141)

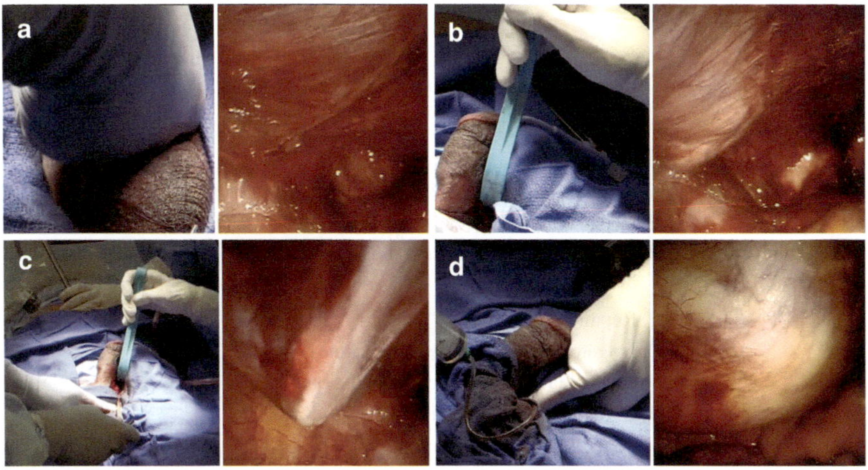

Fig. 6.4 High submuscular placement of reservoir with robotic-assisted laparoscopic visualization at the time of prostatectomy. (**a**) The surgeon identifying external inguinal ring, (**b**) S-shaped retractor placed through the external ring, (**c**) a clamp passed through the ring and pointed cephalad toward the ipsilateral nipple to create the space, (**d**) reservoir filled and well seated outside the peritoneum. (Images obtained, with permission, from Simhan J, Kutikov A, et al. VJPU 2018; 2: 143)

Intraoperative Complications

Intraoperative bladder, bowel, and vascular injuries are most commonly associated with reservoir placement into the SOR. Patients with history of pelvic surgery or radiation are at higher risk. Utilization of ectopic placements, i.e., ATF, PTF, and HSM, reduces the risk of these intraoperative complications. Table 6.2 outlines what actions to perform when encountering intraoperative complications.

Bladder Injury

There are numerous reports throughout the literature of bladder laceration during reservoir placement [8, 11]. This is not surprising, given a full bladder may be as close as 2 cm to the inguinal ring [16]. It is mandatory that the bladder is drained prior to IPP reservoir placement. Patients with a history of pelvic surgery or radiation are at increased risk due to adhesions causing distorted anatomy. If the bladder injury went unnoticed, patients will typically present with irritative voiding, gross hematuria, or IPP infection [11]. Postoperatively, bladder injury can be confirmed with cystoscopy, ultrasound, and computed tomography (CT) scans. Ideally, if the injury is suspected intraoperatively, a confirmatory cystogram or cystoscopy will indicate if the bladder needs to be repaired and the reservoir placed on the contralateral side.

Table 6.2 Intraoperative complications and solutions

Intraoperative complication	Solution
Bladder laceration	1. Confirm injury with intraoperative cystogram or cystoscopy
	2. Repair laceration, relocate reservoir to contralateral side
	3. Use Foley catheter or suprapubic cystostomy and drain until bladder is healed
Bowel laceration	1. Repair laceration[a]
	2. Irrigate copiously with sterile saline
	3. Relocate reservoir to ectopic location
	4. If visible fecal material, abort case
Vascular injury	1. Create adequate exposure to identify the bleed
	2. Apply pressure to site of bleed
	3. Repair or ligate damaged vasculature
	4. If bleeding does not stop, notify anesthesia of the situation, cross and match blood, and immediately consult a general or vascular surgeon

[a]Consult general surgery

Bowel Injury

Bowel injury is uncommon, although cases have been reported [8, 11]. Similar to bladder injury, patients with a history of pelvic surgery or radiation are predisposed to bowel injury. Patients who have undergone RALP are at increased risk of inadvertent, intraperitoneal reservoir insertion which can lead to bowel laceration or erosion [2]. If bowel laceration is noticed intraoperatively, it needs immediate attention, with prosthesis removal or, in certain cases, reservoir relocation to an ectopic location [17]. A general surgeon should always be consulted to aid in the repair, as future litigation may arise [11].

Vascular Injury

Vascular damage or postoperative compression by a reservoir can be minimized through adequate evaluation of any potential risk factors, including unique anatomy and past-surgical history. The vessels at risk of injury during reservoir placement are the internal iliac vein and its branches including the inferior epigastric, external superficial pudendal, and cremasteric vessels [11]. The iliac vessels lie 3 cm from the SOR and may be partially obstructed if the reservoir is not carefully placed. Management of patients with partial venous obstruction involves surgical exploration through a suprapubic approach with relocation of the reservoir to an ectopic position [11]. While it is possible to lacerate these vessels during reservoir placement, it is a more commonly reported issue with reservoir removal [8]. If extensive bleeding is noted during reservoir placement or removal, adequate exposure should be created while applying pressure to the site of the bleed. This may require a second incision to maintain adequate pressure on the hemorrhage while the vessel is ligated or repaired [15]. Ultrasound can be used to diagnose and to confirm return of normal blood flow. If bleeding does not stop, anesthesia should be notified of the situation and a general or vascular surgeon consulted [11].

Postoperative Complications

Postoperative reservoir complications include infection, damage to surrounding structures, herniation, mechanical dysfunction, and patient dissatisfaction. Surgeons should ensure that patients are both made aware and reminded of postoperative instructions to reduce the risk of any preventable complications. Strenuous activities and inadequate rest/healing time can cause serious complications in any IPP surgery. Even in revision surgery, patients should be reminded of precautions, as they may become careless, having previously undergone this operation without difficulty [18]. After intake of pertinent patient history, the physician can use an MRI or other imaging modalities of IPP prosthesis components in both flaccid and inflated states to confidently diagnose IPP reservoir complications [19]. Routine postoperative appointments should be used to glean any mild or potentially more severe symptoms a patient may be experiencing with the new reservoir/implant.

Infection

Infections of primary implants occur in an estimated 1–3% of cases and up to 8–18% of revision procedures [20, 21]. Biofilms may form on any component of IPP implants – including solely on the reservoir [22]. The highest incidence of IPP infection is reported during the first 3–6 months after placement [23, 24]. The timeline of IPP reservoir infection will generally progress in severity based on type(s) of microorganism present; anaerobic infections progress most rapidly [25]. In a large multicenter study of penile implant infections, gram-positive organisms were detected in 73% of cultures, while gram-negative bacteria were noted in 39% [23]. General infection reduction principles are extensively reviewed in the literature and include selection of proper antibiotic IPP coatings [26]/prophylactic treatment, as well as utilization of surgical techniques, i.e., the "no-touch" technique, and the washout for revision cases [27].

Alternative reservoir location placements appear to have similar infection rates as those for SOR localizations. In a large series evaluating ATF and PTF reservoir placements, infection occurred in 6/447 patients (1.24%) with ATF reservoir placement and 21/2239 patients (0.94%) with PTF reservoir placement [28]. In the case of a suspected infection of any IPP component, revision surgeries without complete device replacement have resulted in higher rates of infection than those in which the entire IPP is removed, washed out, and replaced. This is likely due to suspected bacterial biofilm formation [18].

Surgeons must be diligent in staying current on updates to antibiotic infection prevention guidelines published by the American Urological Association and European Urologic Association, as well as latest IPP infection prophylaxis literature. Techniques to decrease the incidence of postoperative infection include using antibiotic-coated reservoirs, avoiding prolonged wound exposure, and minimizing surgeon and assistant contact with prosthesis components [29]. Recent studies identify antibiotic-resistant microorganisms in infected implant cultures, emphasizing how important it is for surgeons to minimize risk of infection [23, 30]. Revision surgery, including an antibiotic solution washout, is recommended in cases of infection of the reservoir.

Organ and Tissue Damage

Reservoir erosion into adjacent tissues is a rare but serious adverse event associated with IPP implant surgery. In a review of all reservoir-related tissue damage publications through 2013, the majority of cases were bladder/neobladder or bowel injury.

The study identified that 15/37 (41%) of cases were related to bladder erosion, while erosion into an ileal conduit, neobladder, or small bowel obstruction accounted for 8/37 (22%) of cases [31].

Two primary issues may cause postoperative bladder erosion: consistent friction from a reservoir on bladder tissue caused by taut tubing pulled in the direction of the bladder or pressure placed on the bladder from too small of a reservoir implantation cavity. In the case of any bladder injury that has been repaired, care should be taken to prevent further damage by leaving a Foley catheter or suprapubic cystostomy in place to supplement tissue healing. When revision surgery is performed, the reservoir can be replaced on the opposite side of the pelvis in the SOR or in an ectopic location.

Postoperative bowel injuries are rare, with only a few documented cases in the literature [32]. In most of these cases, patients were at increased risk due to a history of pelvic surgery or radiation. If a reservoir migrates intraperitoneally and there is enough tubing for it to reach the mid-abdomen, there is potential for the bowel to loop around it and cause a bowel obstruction. Misplaced intraperitoneal reservoirs may erode into nearby bowel segments, causing another surgical injury.

In the event of any bladder or bowel injury, the damaged tissue or organ needs to be repaired as soon as the patient can undergo surgical revision. Prompt intervention is associated with favorable outcomes [33]. Although many urologic surgeons have experience working with bowel in urologic surgeries, i.e., ileal conduit, consulting a general surgeon is always advised [17, 34]. Reservoir revision surgery options depend on surgeon experience and time since implantation of the reservoir, as the formation of a fibrous capsule around a reservoir can be a limiting factor in easily replacing or accessing the device. If the prosthesis is >3 years old, most surgeons elect to replace the entire IPP device.

Herniation

Reservoir migration from its originally implanted position is a postoperative complication estimated to occur in 0.9–1.2% of SOR placements and 1.4% of ectopic placements [35]. Results from one retrospective survey indicated 97% of reservoir herniations were associated with a penoscrotal surgical approach [36].

Postoperatively, forceful and repetitive Valsalva maneuvers, including coughing and straining, may increase intra-abdominal pressure and cause reservoir migration. Reservoir migration due to insufficient tubing length between IPP reservoir and pump, such that a patient may accidentally pull a reservoir caudally through the inguinal canal, is also reported in the literature [15]. As such, and to aid in the general healing process after IPP placement, patients should avoid any strenuous activity during the postoperative recovery period (4–6 weeks). Other potential causes and risk factors for reservoir migration cited in the literature include inguinal ring weakness, respiratory disorders, obesity, smoking, and penoscrotal placement approach [36].

Reservoir herniation typically presents in the immediate postoperative period. Surgical techniques/approaches published to minimize the possibility of reservoir herniation for at-risk patients include HSM location and placement of radial inguinal ring purse-string sutures [9, 37]. A Foley catheter can be used to dilate the retropubic space during SOR reservoir placement and decrease the potential risk for herniation. It has been suggested that surgeons place reservoirs ≥4 inches cephalad to the inguinal ring and ensure that the reservoir is filled to capacity to secure placement [17]. In cases of acute and chronic reservoir herniation, it is recommended to replace the reservoir through the original incision.

Mechanical Failure

Reported IPP mechanical survival ranges from 78.5 to 94.7% and 78.2 to 85% at 5- and 10-year post-surgical timelines, respectively [24, 38–41]. There are limited studies comparing incidences of mechanical dysfunction between IPP device components. One study of 82 patients reported that mechanical failure is associated with cylinder leakage as five times as prevalent as mechanical failure of the reservoir [42].

Leakage

Reservoir leakage is a rare complication in both traditional and ectopic reservoir placements. A 2018 study of 612 ectopic reservoirs reported that the most common complication was reservoir leakage ($n = 5$; 0.8%). Interestingly, the implanted reservoirs in these patients in this series were observed to be folded with a pinpoint hole noted at the apex of the fold. A significant correlation was found with respect to reservoir leakage and underfilling, as leaks were found to be correlated with underfilled reservoirs at the time of implantation (67.5 mL vs. 89 mL; $P = 0.00018$). The authors of the study recommended that the 100 mL Conceal™ Reservoir (Boston Scientific; Marlborough, MA) be filled with at least 80 mL to prevent folding and the occurrence of leakage [43].

Auto-Inflation

Estimated auto-inflation rates in the literature are approximately 2–3% for the AMS 700 CX™ (Boston Scientific; Marlborough, MA) and 1.3% for Coloplast prostheses [7, 44]. Auto-inflation is uncomfortable and embarrassing for patients, and the increased/consistent pressure on penile tissue could theoretically result in erosion

[45]. Auto-inflation may occur if the reservoir is placed in a location that is too small, causing a pressure overload. It typically occurs early in the postoperative period [7, 46]. The presence of scar tissue or formation of a scar tissue capsule around the reservoir can also cause auto-inflation, though post RP patients have been observed to have similar rates of auto-inflation as non-RP patients. This has been attributed to improved lockout valve technology [47]. In a recent study of HSM reservoir placement, the authors noted that tissue capsule formation around a reservoir may actually protect the reservoir from compression in close proximity to abdominal musculature [48].

If auto-inflation is believed to be caused by a constrictive capsule, the patient may require revision surgery by open or laparoscopic capsulotomy. In a capsulotomy, electrocautery is used to separate fat from the reservoir capsule. Before cutting the capsule around the reservoir, it is recommended to minimize reservoir volume by fully inflating the corporal cylinders. Electrocautery should be used on the "cut" setting to free the reservoir from the capsule. Once the reservoir has been fully freed of surrounding capsule, the IPP is cycled to check device integrity and function. Surgeons should advise their patients to not use the device for 4–6 weeks following the procedure. Other revision options in the setting of device auto-inflation include reservoir relocation an reservoir volume reduction [44].

Penile prosthesis manufacturers have made design changes to IPP models in order to reduce the occurrence of auto-inflation. Both Coloplast and AMS have released lock-out valves which do not respond to positive pressures from abdominal compression. The development of kink-free tubing prevents tubing torsion, further reducing the risk of auto-inflation [42]. A case report highlights the rare occurrence, whereby a Conceal reservoir became folded in half, locking fluid on one side of the crease – researchers noted that filling below reservoir capacity and/or incomplete emptying between cycling may have been predisposing factors for this incident [49].

Tubing Torsion

Non-kink tubing has nearly eliminated tubing torsion risk in penile implants, though, in the rare occurrence of this mechanical malfunction, it is recommended to replace the device if it has been in place for longer than 1 year [17]. A recent study described cases of tubing torsion between the IPP reservoir and pump, collectively termed "telephone cord syndrome," in which patients were unable to inflate their IPP. Of 974 implanted IPPs (612 ectopic; 362 traditional SOR), 3 cases (0.5%) occurred in patients with ectopic reservoir placement, and 1 case (0.3%) occurred in a patient with a traditional reservoir placement. The study authors hypothesized that a synergistic combination of caudal migration of tubing and increased abdominal wall pressures may have caused this complication [43].

Palpability

Reservoir palpability is of particular concern with ectopic placement. A 2013 survey noted that 65% of patients or physicians noticed a bulge on the exterior of a patient's body following ectopic reservoir placement [35]. To reduce palpability/visibility, both Coloplast (Cloverleaf reservoir) and AMS (Conceal reservoir) have updated their IPP models to maintain a flat orientation when filled (or partially filled). With the increasing use of ectopic reservoir placements, patients may be able to palpate the reservoir in the abdominal musculature; however, palpability is rarely bothersome so as to require surgical revision. Surgical revision rates to fix reservoir palpability range from 0% to 0.45%, as reported in larger study samples [8, 9, 37]. In a recent study of 142 patients with HSM or SOR reservoir placement, reservoir palpability was found to be correlated with a patient's BMI in both primary ($n = 125$) and replacement ($n = 17$) implantations [12]. Of patients with HSM reservoir placement, 63% ($n = 45$; BMI: 18.5–28.8) indicated that they could palpate the reservoir. After assumed capsule formation around the reservoir 3 months postoperatively, palpability diminished in patients with BMI > 26.5. Palpability did not appear to affect patient satisfaction in either HSM or SOR cohorts.

Explantation of IPP

When an IPP is explanted, the surgeon must decide whether to remove the reservoir with the rest of the device. As previously stated, removing a reservoir can be a challenging process, placing the patient at potential risk of vascular or organ damage. For this reason, many surgeons opt for a "drain and retain" strategy in which the fluid is removed from the reservoir and it is left in place [50]. Cefalu et al. performed a study in 2013 comparing outcomes of IPP/artificial urinary sphincter (AUS) surgery in 55 patients with "retained reservoirs" vs 352 patients without. They reported that the patients with the retained reservoirs were *not* at increased risk of complication during re-operative IPP/ AUS surgery [50].

While rare, there are case reports throughout the literature of complications caused by retained reservoirs. There is a report of a 79-year-old man who developed an infection of his retained reservoir after his IPP was replaced due to mechanical failure [20]. Munoz et al. and Brusky et al. each present a male with genitourinary issues secondary to erosion of a retained reservoir into the bladder [51, 52]. There is a report of a patient presenting with right upper quadrant pain secondary to a herniated retained reservoir next to the liver [53]. Lastly, there have been several reported cases of cyst or mass formation around a retained reservoir interfering with nearby bowel or bladder function [54, 55].

Of course, it is not possible to completely eradicate the risk of retained reservoir complications, but there are a variety of techniques that can be utilized to minimize risk. Reddy et al. reviewed several strategies meant to optimize patient outcomes:

tubing should be placed on traction and cut as close to the reservoir as possible to minimize the amount left within the body cavity; the reservoir should be completely drained to reduce the risk of mass effect on nearby structures; strict infection minimization protocols should be followed; and the patient needs to be educated about the location of their retained hardware, as well as any alarm symptoms for which they should see a doctor [56]. Patient education is of particular importance, as many patients receive their IPP at a hospital outside of their normal network. A properly educated patient can inform future surgeons of the retained reservoir, allowing for preoperative imaging. This imaging provides the surgeon with a more thorough understanding of the patient's pelvic anatomy and location of the retained reservoir, decreasing the likelihood of intraoperative complications.

Conclusion

Reservoir placement is the most variable part of inflatable penile prosthesis surgery. There are several locations a surgeon can choose to place the reservoir, each with its advantages and disadvantages. A well-taken patient history is paramount in helping the surgeon decide which location will work best for his patient. Once a location is decided, the surgeon can decide what approach to take and review potential intraoperative complications. After surgery, consistent follow-up with patients ensures that any postoperative complications are identified and treated promptly. When a patient is undergoing prosthesis explantation for a reason other than infection, the surgeon can remove the reservoir or leave it within the patient utilizing the "drain and retain" strategy. If the reservoir is retained, proper patient education about the retained device can reduce the risk of future complications.

Acknowledgements We give special thanks to Jessica Daigle for her assistance in the preparation and submission of this chapter.

References

1. Deho F, Henry GD, Marone EM, et al. Severe vascular complication after implantation of a three-piece inflatable penile prosthesis. J Sex Med. 2008;5(12):2956–9.
2. Sadeghi-Nejad H, Munarriz R, Shah N. Intra-abdominal reservoir placement during penile prosthesis surgery in post-robotically assisted laparoscopic radical prostatectomy patients: a case report and practical considerations. J Sex Med. 2011;8(5):1547–50.
3. Henry G, Hsaio W, Karpman E, et al. A guide for inflatable penile prosthesis reservoir placement: pertinent anatomical measurements of the retropubic space. J Sex Med. 2014;11(1):273–8.
4. Eldefrawy A, Kava BR. An unusual complication during inflatable penile prosthesis implantation. Urology. 2010;76(4):847.
5. Kramer AC, Chason J, Kusakabe A. CASE REPORTS: report of two cases of bladder perforation caused by reservoir of inflatable penile prosthesis. J Sex Med. 2009;6(7):2064–7.

6. Perito P, Wilson S. The history of nontraditional or ectopic placement of reservoirs in prosthetic urology. Sex Med Rev. 2016;4(2):190–3.
7. Wilson SK, Henry GD, Delk JR, Cleves MA. The mentor Alpha 1 penile prosthesis with reservoir lock-out valve: effective prevention of auto-inflation with improved capability for ectopic reservoir placement. J Urol. 2002;168(4, Part 1):1475–8.
8. Stember DS, Garber BB, Perito PE. Outcomes of abdominal wall reservoir placement in inflatable penile prosthesis implantation: a safe and efficacious alternative to the space of Retzius. J Sex Med. 2014;11(2):605–12.
9. Morey AF, Cefalu CA, Hudak SJ. High submuscular placement of urologic prosthetic balloons and reservoirs via transscrotal approach. J Sex Med. 2013;10(2):603–10.
10. Ziegelmann MJ, Viers BR, Lomas DJ, Westerman ME, Trost LW. Ectopic penile prosthesis reservoir placement: an anatomic cadaver model of the high submuscular technique. J Sex Med. 2016;13(9):1425–31.
11. Clavell-Hernández J, Aly SG, Wang R, Sadeghi-Nejad H. Penile prosthesis reservoir removal: surgical description and patient outcomes. J Sex Med. 2019;16(1):146–52.
12. Osmonov D, Chomicz A, Tropmann-Frick M, Arndt KM, Jünemann KP. High-submuscular vs. space of Retzius reservoir placement during implantation of inflatable penile implants. Int J Impot Res. 2020;32(1):18–23.
13. Garber BB, Bickell M. Subcutaneous placement of inflatable penile prosthesis reservoirs. Urology. 2016;88:93–6.
14. Henry GD, Mahle P, Caso J, Eisenhart E, Carrion R, Kramer A. Surgical techniques in penoscrotal implantation of an inflatable penile prosthesis: a Guide to increasing patient satisfaction and surgeon ease. Sex Med Rev. 2015;3(1):36–47.
15. Levine LA, Hoeh MP. Review of penile prosthetic reservoir: complications and presentation of a modified reservoir placement technique. J Sex Med. 2012;9(11):2759–69.
16. Henry G, Jones L, Carrion R, et al. Pertinent anatomical measurements of the retropubic space: a guide for inflatable penile prosthesis reservoir placement shows that the external iliac vein is much closer than thought: 027. J Sex Med. 2012;9.
17. Mulcahy JJ. The prevention and management of noninfectious complications of penile implants. Sex Med Rev. 2015;3(3):203–13.
18. Wintner A, Lentz AC. Inflatable penile prosthesis: considerations in revision surgery. Curr Urol Rep. 2019;20(4):18.
19. Hartman RP, Kawashima A, Takahashi N, LeRoy AJ, King BF. Inflatable penile prosthesis (IPP): diagnosis of complications. Abdom Radiol (NY). 2016;41(6):1187–96.
20. Hsi RS, Hotaling JM, Spencer ES, Bollyky PL, Walsh TJ. Isolated infection of a decommissioned penile prosthesis reservoir with Actinomyces neuii. J Sex Med. 2011;8(3):923–6.
21. Wilson SK, Delk JR 2nd. Inflatable penile implant infection: predisposing factors and treatment suggestions. J Urol. 1995;153(3 Pt 1):659–61.
22. Silverstein AD, Henry GD, Evans B, Pasmore M, Simmons CJ, Donatucci CF. Biofilm formation on clinically noninfected penile prostheses. J Urol. 2006;176(3):1008–11.
23. Gross MS, Phillips EA, Carrasquillo RJ, et al. Multicenter investigation of the micro-organisms involved in penile prosthesis infection: an analysis of the efficacy of the AUA and EAU guidelines for penile prosthesis prophylaxis. J Sex Med. 2017;14(3):455–63.
24. Carson CC, Mulcahy JJ, Govier FE. Efficacy, safety and patient satisfaction outcomes of the AMS 700CX inflatable penile prosthesis: results of a long-term multicenter study. AMS 700CX Study Group. J Urol. 2000;164(2):376–80.
25. Lokeshwar SD, Bitran J, Madhusoodanan V, Kava B, Ramasamy R. A surgeon's guide to the various antibiotic dips available during penile prosthesis implantation. Curr Urol Rep. 2019;20(2):11.
26. Mandava SH, Serefoglu EC, Freier MT, Wilson SK, Hellstrom WJ. Infection retardant coated inflatable penile prostheses decrease the incidence of infection: a systematic review and meta-analysis. J Urol. 2012;188(5):1855–60.

27. Eid JF, Wilson SK, Cleves M, Salem EA. Coated implants and "no touch" surgical technique decreases risk of infection in inflatable penile prosthesis implantation to 0.46%. Urology. 2012;79(6):1310–5.
28. Gross MS, Stember DS, Garber BB, Perito PE. A retrospective analysis of risk factors for IPP reservoir entry into the peritoneum after abdominal wall placement. Int J Impot Res. 2017;29(5):215–8.
29. Pineda M, Burnett AL. Penile prosthesis infections-a review of risk factors, prevention, and treatment. Sex Med Rev. 2016;4(4):389–98.
30. Gross MS, Phillips EA, Balen A, et al. The malleable implant salvage technique: infection outcomes after Mulcahy salvage procedure and replacement of infected inflatable penile prosthesis with malleable prosthesis. J Urol. 2016;195(3):694–7.
31. Simon R, Hakky TS, Henry G, et al. Tips and tricks of inflatable penile prosthesis reservoir placement: a case presentation and discussion. J Sex Med. 2014;11(5):1325–33.
32. Clavell-Hernández J, Shah A, Wang R. Non-infectious reservoir-related complications during and after penile prosthesis placement. Sex Med Rev. 2019;7(3):521–9.
33. Park JK, Jang SW, Lee SW, Cui Y. Rare complication of multiple revision surgeries of penile prosthesis. J Sex Med. 2005;2(5):735–6.
34. Luks FI, Huntley HN, Tula JC, Pizzi WF. Small-bowel obstruction by an inflatable penile prosthesis reservoir. Surgery. 1989;106(1):101–4.
35. Karpman E, Sadeghi-Nejad H, Henry G, Khera M, Morey AF. Current opinions on alternative reservoir placement for inflatable penile prosthesis among members of the Sexual Medicine Society of North America. J Sex Med. 2013;10(8):2115–20.
36. Sadeghi-Nejad H, Sharma A, Irwin RJ, Wilson SK, Delk JR. Reservoir herniation as a complication of three-piece penile prosthesis insertion. Urology. 2001;57(1):142–5.
37. Karpman E, Brant WO, Kansas B, et al. Reservoir alternate surgical implantation technique: preliminary outcomes of initial PROPPER study of low profile or spherical reservoir implantation in submuscular location or traditional prevesical space. J Urol. 2015;193(1):239–44.
38. Kim DS, Yang KM, Chung HJ, Choi HM, Choi YD, Choi HK. AMS 700CX/CXM inflatable penile prosthesis has high mechanical reliability at long-term follow-up. J Sex Med. 2010;7(7):2602–7.
39. Chung E, Van CT, Wilson I, Cartmill RA. Penile prosthesis implantation for the treatment for male erectile dysfunction: clinical outcomes and lessons learnt after 955 procedures. World J Urol. 2013;31(3):591–5.
40. Wilson SK, Delk JR, Salem EA, Cleves MA. Long-term survival of inflatable penile prostheses: single surgical group experience with 2,384 first-time implants spanning two decades. J Sex Med. 2007;4(4 Pt 1):1074–9.
41. Dick B, Tsambarlis P, Reddy A, Hellstrom WJ. An update on: long-term outcomes of penile prostheses for the treatment of erectile dysfunction. Expert Rev Med Devices. 2019;16(4):281–6.
42. O'Rourke TK Jr, Erbella A, Zhang Y, Wosnitzer MS. Prevention, identification, and management of post-operative penile implant complications of infection, hematoma, and device malfunction. Transl Androl Urol. 2017;6(Suppl 5):S832–s848.
43. Hernández JC, Trost L, Köhler T, et al. Emerging complications following alternative reservoir placement during inflatable penile prosthesis placement: a 5-year multi-institutional experience. J Urol. 2019;201(3):581–6.
44. Abbosh PH, Thom MR, Bullock A. Laparascopic capsulotomy to treat autoinflation of inflatable penile prostheses. J Sex Med. 2012;9(4):1212–5.
45. Kobayashi K, Hisasue S, Shimizu T, Itoh N, Tsuksamoto T. Erosion of an inflatable penile prosthesis due to autoinflation. Hinyokika Kiyo. 2004;50(7):515–7.
46. Wilson SK, Salem EA, Costerton W. Anti-infection dip suggestions for the Coloplast Titan Inflatable Penile Prosthesis in the era of the infection retardant coated implant. J Sex Med. 2011;8(9):2647–54.

47. Hollenbeck BK, Miller DC, Ohl DA. The utility of lockout valve reservoirs in preventing autoinflation in penile prostheses. Int Urol Nephrol. 2002;34(3):379–83.
48. Chung PH, Morey AF, Tausch TJ, Simhan J, Scott JF. High submuscular placement of urologic prosthetic balloons and reservoirs: 2-year experience and patient-reported outcomes. Urology. 2014;84(6):1535–40.
49. Navarrete RA, Cui T, Carson C, Terlecki R. Failure of the inflatable penile prosthesis due to abnormal folding of a low-profile reservoir – a selected case from an overall series and systematic review. Urol Case Rep. 2017;14:56–8.
50. Cefalu CA, Deng X, Zhao LC, Scott JF, Mehta S, Morey AF. Safety of the "drain and retain" option for defunctionalized urologic prosthetic balloons and reservoirs during artificial urinary sphincter and inflatable penile prosthesis revision surgery: 5-year experience. Urology. 2013;82(6):1436–9.
51. Munoz JJ, Ellsworth PI. The retained penile prosthesis reservoir: a risk. Urology. 2000;55(6):949.
52. Brusky J, Dikranin A, Aboseif S. Retrieval of inflatable penile prosthesis reservoir from the bladder. Int J Impot Res. 2005;17(3):302–3.
53. Cui T, Terlecki R, Mirzazadeh M. Infrequent reservoir-related complications of urologic prosthetics: a case series and literature review. Sex Med. 2015;3(4):334–8.
54. Abboudi H, Bolgeri M, Nair R, Chetwood A, Symes A, Thomas P. 'A reservoir within a reservoir' – an unusual complication associated with a defunctioned inflatable penile prosthesis reservoir. Int J Surg Case Rep. 2014;5(10):758–60.
55. Jiann BP, Ou CW, Lin JT, Huang JK. Compression of ureter caused by a retained reservoir of penile prosthesis. Int J Impot Res. 2006;18(3):316–7.
56. Reddy AG, Tsambarlis PN, Akula KP, Dick BP, Hong J, Hellstrom WJG. Retained reservoirs of inflatable penile prosthesis: a systematic review of the literature and a guide to perioperative management. Sex Med Rev. 2020;8(2):355–63.

Chapter 7
The Hostile Penis: Managing the Patient with Corporal Fibrosis

Benjamin M. Dropkin, Nathan A. Chertack, Samantha W. Nealon, Gregory A. Joice, and Allen F. Morey

Introduction

Fibrosis of the corpora cavernosa occurs when pathologic tissue insult triggers a cellular response that ultimately leads to the replacement of healthy sinusoidal tissue with inelastic connective tissue [1]. Inciting events include penile implant infection [2, 3], prolonged tissue ischemia as may be seen in ischemic priapism [4, 5], Peyronie's disease [6], and tissue trauma such as penile fracture [7] or repeated intracavernosal injections [8]. The extent of corporal fibrosis can range in severity and domain from weak scarring in sub-centimeter corporal segments (e.g., after intracavernosal therapy) to dense fibrosis involving the entirety of both corporal bodies (e.g., after prolonged ischemic priapism). The incidence and prevalence of corporal fibrosis are not well defined.

Management options for patients with erectile dysfunction and corporal fibrosis are determined by the degree of erectile dysfunction, medical comorbidities, and patient preference. Vacuum erection devices (VED), oral phosphodiesterase-5 inhibitors (PD5-i), intraurethral alprostadil, intracavernosal injections of vasoactive agents, and penile prosthesis (PP) insertion may be considered. The majority of patients with clinically significant corporal fibrosis suffer from venous leak [9] and will not be able to achieve erections sufficient for intercourse without PP insertion.

B. M. Dropkin (✉) · N. A. Chertack · G. A. Joice · A. F. Morey
Department of Urology, UT Southwestern Medical Center, Dallas, TX, USA

S. W. Nealon
Department of Urology, University of South Florida, Tampa, FL, USA

E. P. Miranda, J. P. Mulhall (eds.), *Penile Implant Surgery*, https://doi.org/10.1007/978-3-030-82363-4_7

Here we review the preoperative, operative, and postoperative management of men with corporal fibrosis seeking PP insertion with a focus on intraoperative strategies and complication prevention and management.

Prevention

Several preventative measures have the potential to spare men from the onset and detrimental effects of corporal fibrosis. In the setting of penile prosthesis infection, two different strategies have gained popularity: salvage PP insertion and antibiotic cast insertion. Mulcahy first described the single-stage salvage procedure, in which device removal is followed by thorough irrigation using combination antibiotic and antiseptic solutions, exchange of gowns and gloves, and immediate IPP replacement without drain placement [10]. In contemporary practice, salvage insertion of a malleable penile prosthesis (MPP) has gained popularity [11, 12]. An alternative approach is to pack the corporal bodies with an antibiotic (vancomycin/tobramycin) infused calcium sulfate paste that hardens into a "cast" within the corpora and is meant to maintain the corporal space until a PP can be inserted at a later date. The cast slowly dissolves over 5–6 weeks while locally releasing antibiotics and reducing scar formation [11, 13]. Corporal body installation with mitomycin C immediately following cylinder explant and washout was also recently reported with good success in a small series of five patients [14].

In the context of ischemic priapism, expedient resolution using sympathomimetics, corporal aspiration and irrigation, and/or shunting procedures may prevent fibrosis and potentially preserve erectile function [15]. If these efforts fail, immediate PP insertion may also be considered depending on patient preference, surgeon comfort, and product availability [16]. We favor penoscrotal decompression (PSD) over distal shunts for ischemic priapism refractory to sympathomimetics and corporal aspiration because PSD keeps the distal tunica albuginea intact, which becomes advantageous if the patient ultimately elects PP insertion [17, 18]. While a detailed review of these preventative approaches is beyond the scope of this chapter, these options do warrant careful consideration by the implanting urologist.

Preoperative Management

History

A thorough history is needed to maximize the chance of achieving a successful outcome. Prior attempts at treating erectile dysfunction should be determined. Operative reports from all prior genitourinary surgeries should be obtained and reviewed. In cases where the patient had a prior PP explant for infection, operative reports will help determine [1] the timing of explant, [2] prior surgical approach(es) (i.e., infrapubic or penoscrotal), [3] type and length of prior devices (including information on rear tip extenders), [4] prior reservoir location (e.g., space of Retzius or high submuscular) and management at the time of device explant (i.e., removed or "drain and retain"), and [5] the presence or absence of cylinder extrusion or urethral erosion at time of PP explant. For patients with a history of priapism, it is important to determine if and in which locations prior shunts were created.

For any patient electing PP insertion, it is also important to understand the patient's prior non-penile surgical history with a focus on inguinal surgery, procedures that may have violated the space of Retzius, and other lower abdominal and pelvic surgeries. We use this information to help guide the location of reservoir placement. The medical history should focus on cardiovascular health sufficient for sexual activity, the presence and control of diabetes mellitus, the use of anticoagulation, and the ability to tolerate general anesthesia [19]. We find it useful to rule out gross hematuria and significant voiding dysfunction prior to PP insertion, as indicated transurethral procedures should be performed prior to PP insertion whenever possible. The patient should also be asked about perceived loss of penile length, and this information should be documented in the medical record for medicolegal purposes.

Physical Exam

The examination begins with the patient in the supine position. The surgeon should palpate the entire length of each corporal body to evaluate for firm areas suggestive of corporal fibrosis. It is important to examine for abdominal, suprapubic, and penoscrotal scars as patients may forget about prior operations until prompted when asked about specific surgical scars. We measure the stretched penile length (SPL) by measuring from the pubic symphysis to the urethral meatus with the penis on full stretch. We demonstrate SPL to the patient and document it in the medical record. The inguinal rings should be evaluated for evidence of hernia bilaterally. The patient's manual dexterity and grip strength should be assessed if penile prosthesis insertion is being considered.

Imaging

Non-contrast computed tomography should be considered preoperatively in patients who have undergone a prior IPP explant in order to definitely determine if and which device component(s) were left behind at the time of explantation [20].

Patient Counseling

It has been said that "success equals results minus expectations," and this truism certainly applies to IPP insertion in the context of corporal fibrosis. This is a significantly more difficult operation than virgin IPP insertion and the outcomes are unequivocally inferior. The patient should be informed that the length of the cylinders implanted is determined strictly by patient anatomy – "this is not a penile lengthening operation." They should be informed that their new implant may be shorter than a prior implant due to scar tissue [2]. Penile girth may be reduced if the patient previously had a larger caliber device (e.g., AMS 700 CX or Coloplast Titan) and goes on to receive a narrow-base device (e.g., AMS 700 CXR and Titan Narrow-base). The patient should know that their penoscrotal incision will likely be longer than the incision used for a virgin IPP insertion and that a distal counter incision may be required for adequate distal corporal dilation and safe cylinder placement.

A thorough discussion of surgical risks should be held (Table 7.1). Patients need to understand that implant infection becomes more likely in the presence of corporal fibrosis [21] and with each successive implant procedure [22]. They must know that an infected implant needs to be explanted and that changes in penile sensation are possible postoperatively [23]. Additionally, proximal and distal perforation are understandably more likely in the setting of penile fibrosis [24].

Patients frequently inquire about preoperative strategies to maximize the length of the IPP that can be implanted. Several retrospective studies have demonstrated an improvement in IPP cylinder length with preoperative daily use of the vacuum erection device [25, 26]. Tsambarlis et al. found that 3 months of vacuum therapy (10–15 min sessions twice daily) prior to IPP insertion led to an increase in SPL of 0.92 ± 0.76 cm compared to baseline SPL in 13 men with a history of corporal fibrosis [26]. Levine et al. reported similar results among ten men with a history of penile shortening who used an external penile traction device (FastSize® Penile Extender; Aliso Viejo, CA, USA) for at least 2 h daily in the 2–4 months prior to IPP insertion. Post-IPP erect length increased by 0.9 cm compared to pre-traction SPL. In light of these results, we encourage motivated patients with corporal fibrosis to use vacuum therapy for 15 min twice daily for 3 months leading up to IPP insertion.

Operative Management

Surgical Instruments and Equipment

Optimizing exposure of the corporal bodies is critical in virgin IPP insertion and becomes essential in the context of corporal fibrosis.

Table 7.1 Summary of series reporting on IPP insertion in setting of corporal fibrosis

Publication (year)	Source(s) of fibrosis	Prosthesis type(s)	No. patients	Mean f/u (mo.)	Infection (%)	Mech. failure (%)	Other reported complications (e.g., perforation)	Surgical technique
Hebert (2019) [27]	Infection (79%)	Not reported	72	12	4	0	Erosion (15%)	Tunneling with backward-cutting scissors
	Priapism (21%)						Revision (6%)	
Tsambarlis (2017) [26]	Infection (85%)	Not reported	13		8	0	Erosion (8%)	Preoperative vacuum therapy
	Priapism (15%)							
Garber (2016) [28]	Infection (80%)	Titan narrow (11/13)	13	25	15	0	N/R	Limited corporal excavation
	Priapism (20%)	Titan regular (2/13)						
Sansalone (2012) [29]	Infection (100%)	AMS 700CX (78%)	18	26	0	0	Elective revision (22%)	Excavation with grafting
		AMS 650 11 mm (22%)						
Lopes (2009) [30]	Priapism (60%)	Malleable (100%)	5	32	0	0	N/R	Bovine pericardial graft corporoplasty
	Infection (40%)							
Brusky (2008) [31]	Infection (100%)	Malleable (100%)	3	91	0	0	N/R	Combined perineal and penoscrotal approach
Shaeer (2008) [32]	Infection (42%)	Malleable 13 mm (66%)	12	1–12	0	0	N/R	Ultrasound-guided endoscopic excavation over a guidewire
	Priapism (33%)	Inflatable (33%)						
	ICI (17%)							
	Unknown (8%)							

(continued)

Table 7.1 (continued)

Publication (year)	Source(s) of fibrosis	Prosthesis type(s)	No. patients	Mean f/u (mo.)	Infection (%)	Mech. failure (%)	Other reported complications (e.g., perforation)	Surgical technique
Montague (2006) [33]	Infection (44%)	AMS 700CXM (78%)	9	44	0	11	N/R	Extended ventral corporotomies
	Priapism (44%)	AMS 700CX (22%)						
	DM + Tx (11%)							
Pathak (2005) [23]	PD (47%)	AMS 700 (53%)	15	18	0	0	Penile hypoesthesia (14%)	Rectus fascia grafting
	Erosion (27%)	Alpha-1 (47%)						
	Infection (20%)							
	Explantation (7%)							
Park (2002) [34]	Priapism (100%)	Mentor-NB (100%)	1	12	0	0	N/R	Electrovaporization
Palese (2001) [35]	Erosion (100%)	Not reported	4	10	0	0	N/R	Pericardium allograft
Ghanem (2000) [36]	Infection (71%)	Malleable 9.5 mm (47%)	17	3	0	0	Crural perforation (6%)	Corporal counterincisions
	Priapism (29%)	Duraphase 10 mm (41%)						
		Malleable 11 mm (12%)						
Rajpurkar (1999) [37]	Infection (82%)	Alpha-1 (44%)	34	24	0	3	Revision (12%)	Scar excision, corporal dilation
	Priapism (12%)	AMS 600 (21%)					Crural perforation (3%)	
	ICI (6%)	AMS 700 (21%)						
		Semirigid (12%)						
		Mark-2 (3%)						

Mooreville (1999) [38]	Infection (81%)	Alpha-NB (75%)	16		0	0	Crural perforation (38%)	Dilation with cavernotomes
	Priapism (19%)	Alpha-1 (13%)					Distal perforation (25%)	
		AMS 700CXM (13%)					Crossover (19%)	
George (1996) [39]	Infection (83%)	Semirigid (58%)	12	22	0	8	Revision (25%)	PTFE grafting
	Priapism (17%)	Inflatable (42%)						
Knoll (1995) [21]	Infection (90%)	AMS 700CXM (100%)	20	20	5	0	Revision (5%)	Downsizing
	Priapism (10%)							
Herschorn (1995) [40]	Infection (36%)	AMS 700CX (82%)	11	46	0	0	Revision (27%)	Synthetic grafting
	Explant (27%)	Jonas 9.5 mm (18%)						
	Priapism (18%)							

Abbreviations: *AMS* American Medical Systems, *DM* diabetes mellitus, *ICI* intracavernosal injection, *PD* Peyronie's disease, *PTFE* polytetrafluoroethylene, *TX* renal transplantation

Retraction

A self-retaining retractor such as the Lone Star system (Cooper Surgical, Trumbull, CT) is of significant value in these cases. Multi-prong "rake" retractors are helpful in retracting the scrotal contents inferiorly away from the proximal corpora. We typically place a glans stitch using 2–0 silk in a longitudinal fashion to help provide superior retraction of the penis.

Scissors

Reverse-cutting Facelift scissors employ a sharp outer edge that incises the surrounding tissue when the scissors are spread and withdrawn. These scissors can be of major help in developing the corporal dissection just deep to the tunica albuginea at the proximal and distal apices of the corporotomy.

Cavernotomes

Cavernotomes are bladed dilators that are specifically designed to facilitate dilation of a fibrotic corporal body. Two types of cavernotomes are currently manufactured (Fig. 7.1; Table 7.2). The Carrion-Rossello cavernotome (Coloplast Corporation, Minneapolis, MN, USA) [41] employs sharp circumferential barbs and the Uramix-Mooreville cavernotome (Uramix, Inc. Lansdowne, PA, USA) utilizes (a) longitudinal 1 mm cutting blade(s) [38]. Cavernotome selection is determined by surgeon preference. No head to head trials have compared the effectiveness of these instruments.

Narrow-Base Inflatable Penile Prosthesis

Narrow-base IPPs allow for proximal device insertion with a lower degree of proximal dilation than is required for insertion of a standard IPP. They have gained popularity for use in the setting of corporal fibrosis. Two models are currently available

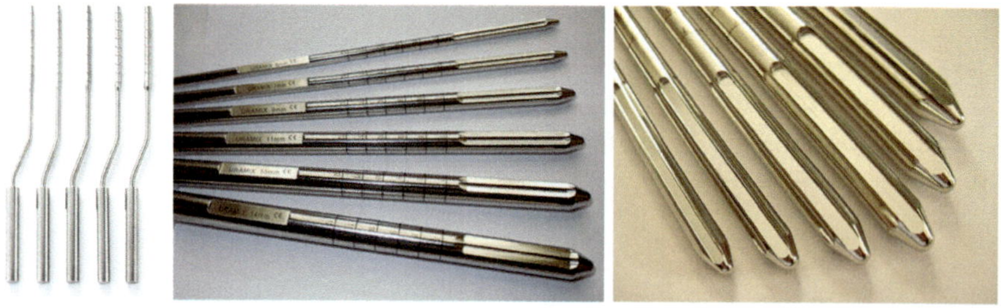

Fig. 7.1 Commercially available cavernotomes: Carrion-Rosselo (Coloplast Corporation, Minneapolis, MN) (left), Uramix-Mooreville (Uramix Incorporated, Lansdowne, PA) bladed cavernotome (center) and double-bladed advanced cavernotome (right)

Table 7.2 Comparison of commercially available cavernotomes

Cavernotome	Carrion-Rosselo	Uramix-Mooreville
Current manufacturer	Coloplast Corporation, Minneapolis, MN	Uramix Incorporated, Lansdowne, PA
Year introduced	1995	1999 (bladed cavernotome)
		2014 (double-bladed advanced cavernotome)
Mechanism	Rotational advancement forms tunnel, forceful removal disrupts fibrotic bands	Laterally oriented cutting blade(s) incise(s) fibrosis; if needed, rotational motion causes shaving of fibrosis
Shape	Bayonet	Straight
Diameter (mm)	8, 9, 10, 11, 12 (stainless steel)	6, 7, 9, 11, 13 (original model)
		6, 7, 8, 9, 10, 11 (double-bladed advanced model)
Length (cm)	9 (barbed dilator), 31.2 (total length)	23 (classic model)
		23.5 (double-bladed advanced model)

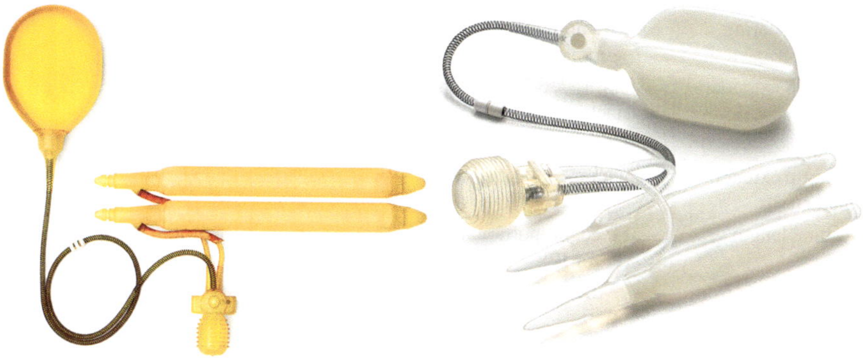

Fig. 7.2 Narrow-base IPPs: AMS 700 CXR (Boston Scientific, Marlborough, MA) (left) and Titan Narrow-base (Coloplast Corporation, Minneapolis, MN) (right)

(Fig. 7.2, Table 7.3): the AMS 700 Controlled Expansion Restricted (CXR) IPP (Boston Scientific, Marlborough, MA) and the Coloplast Titan Narrow-base (Coloplast Corporation, Minneapolis, MN). Both narrow-base implants utilize a narrow, 3 cm non-inflatable proximal cylinder. The proximal dilation required for device insertion is less for the CXR (9 mm) and Coloplast Titan Narrow-base (10 mm) than for their standard model counterparts, which are known as the AMS 700 CX (13 mm) and Coloplast Titan (13 mm) [42]. The tubing length for both devices is proportional to cylinder length and planned surgical approach (i.e., infrapubic or penoscrotal) [43]. When a patient's corporal measurements call for the use of multiple rear tip extenders (RTE), it should be noted that the 1.5 cm RTE is the only RTE in the AMS CXR product line that can be "stacked upon." In our experience, the CXR has provided axial rigidity sufficient for intercourse and high satisfaction among patients with corporal fibrosis.

Table 7.3 Comparison of commercially available narrow-base IPPs

IPP	AMS 700 CXR	Titan Narrow-base
Manufacturer	Boston Scientific, Marlborough, MA	Coloplast Corporation, Minneapolis, MN
Year introduced	2003	2000
Narrow base	3 cm non-inflatable proximal cylinder	5 cm non-inflatable proximal cylinder
Base diameter	9 mm	10 mm
Inflatable cylinder diameter	9.5 mm deflated (all cylinder lengths)	11–13 mm deflated (proportional to length)
	14.5 mm inflated (all cylinder lengths)	12–15 mm inflated (proportional to length)
Cylinder length, volume	10 cm, 8.7 ml	11 cm, 10.3 ml
	12 cm, 12 ml	14 cm, 11.3 ml
	14 cm, 16.4 ml	16 cm, 14.8 ml
	16 cm, 18.8 ml	18 cm, 25.5 ml
	18 cm, 22.3 ml	
Reservoir volume	65 ml or 100 ml	75 ml or 125 ml
Device coating	Rifampin/minocycline	Hydrophilic (surgeon selects antibiotic(s))
Rear tip extender length	0.5, 1, 2, 3, 4, 5, 6 cm (cannot stack upon)	1, 1.5, 2, 3 cm (can stack upon)
	1.5 cm (can stack upon)	
Rear tip extender diameter	9 mm	9 mm
Tubing length	Fixed, proportional to approach (PS or IP)	Fixed, proportional to approach (PS or IP)
Tubing angle from cylinder	22 degrees	0 degrees
Lock-out valve location	Pump	Reservoir

PS penoscrotal, *IP* infrapubic

Operative Technique

Patient Positioning and Preparation

Following the induction of general anesthesia, the patient is positioned in the supine position with arms out and all pressure points padded. Sequential compression devices are applied to the lower extremities bilaterally; we do not routinely utilize pharmacologic deep vein thrombosis prophylaxis in these cases. Broad-spectrum parenteral antibiosis is achieved with weight-based cefazolin and gentamicin per recommendations from the American Urological Association Best Practice Statement on Urologic Procedures and Antibiotic Prophylaxis [44]. The genitalia are shaved in an atraumatic fashion using surgical clippers. A 14Fr silicone catheter is placed to maximize the ease of urethral identification during the penoscrotal dissection. A surgical headlight is used to assist with visualization during dissection of the proximal corpora. We place a glans stitch using 2-0 silk if we anticipate that it will enhance penile stability during the procedure. When possible, based on the degree of corporal fibrosis, we perform an artificial erection with 30 cc of 0.25% plain bupivacaine mixed with 30 cc of normal saline. The artificial erection can help to identify any substantial penile curvature that may warrant correction in conjunction with IPP insertion.

Incision

We prefer a 3 cm, longitudinal, penoscrotal incision because it provides access to the majority of the ventral corporal bodies and can easily be extended if additional distal exposure is required to facilitate cylinder placement. Other high-volume implanters have reported good success with a transverse penoscrotal incision [45]. To our knowledge, there have not been any published reports describing the use of the infrapubic approach for IPP insertion in cases of corporal fibrosis.

Penoscrotal Dissection and Corporotomy Creation

Next we dissect sharply down through the tunica dartos and onto the corporal body. We place a medial stay suture using absorbable 2-0 polydioxanone (Johnson and Johnson, New Brunswick, NJ) 0.5 cm lateral to the urethra and a lateral stay suture 1 cm further lateral. We use a minimum of three sets of stay sutures per corpora in cases complicated by corporal fibrosis and often place up to six or seven sets of stay sutures, as needed, depending on the degree of fibrosis (Fig. 7.3). We then perform a corporotomy between the stay sutures using a fresh 15 blade and extend the corporotomy proximally and distally using curved Mayo scissors.

Corporal Dilation +/− Excavation

Since the early 1990s, multiple advancements have been made toward the goal of safe and effective dilation of the fibrotic corporal body. Extensive wide excision of corporal fibrosis from the surrounding tunica albuginea using Metzenbaum scissors was the first technique described to facilitate IPP insertion in the context of corporal fibrosis [33, 46, 47]. Subsequently, the conception and development of cavernotomes allowed the surgeon to drill into the corpora to facilitate dilation without the need for excision of fibrosis [38, 41]. Penoscopic resection of fibrosed cavernosal tissue using a resectoscope was also described; this technique has not been widely adopted [32, 34, 48]. Finally, a novel extracorporeal implantation technique was described in 2018 for use in cases where cavernosal dilation was deemed impossible after attempts using the previously described techniques. A single malleable rod is placed in a “U” configuration on the ventral aspect of the penis superficial to the ventral corporal bodies with the base of the “U” placed through both corporal

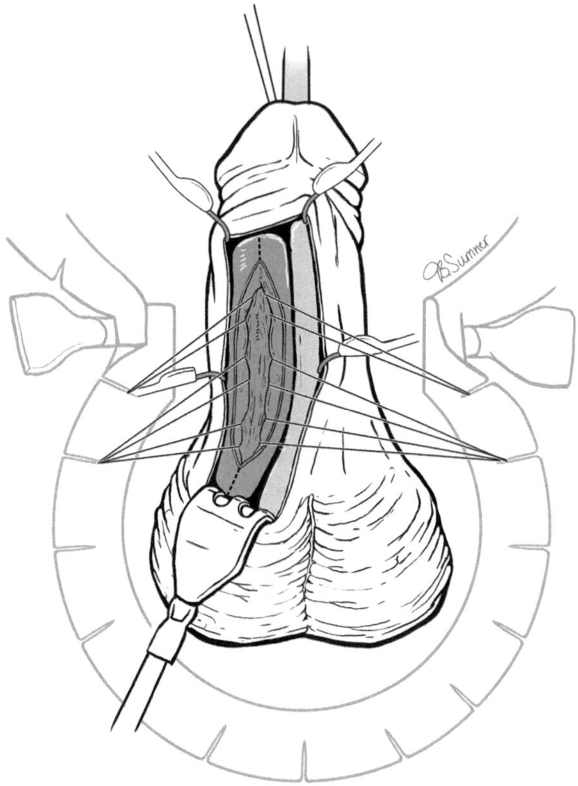

Fig. 7.3 An extended corporotomy is usually necessary to facilitate corporal dilation and cylinder insertion in cases of corporal fibrosis. Three pairs of 2-0 PDS stay sutures are placed initially. The corporotomy is extended, as needed, to facilitate dilation (dashed lines)

bodies and a septal window at the penoscrotal junction [49]. The distal limbs are anchored to the proximal glans.

We start the corporal dilation by inserting the closed reverse-cutting Facelift scissors into the scarred cavernosal tissue just deep to the tunica albuginea at the apex of the corporotomy. This is done with a twisting motion to help advance the tips into the scar. The surgeon should keep his/her elbow close to the torso to maximize control over the scissor tips. Once the scissor tips have been advanced 1 cm or so into the corporal fibrosis, the scissors are aggressively opened and withdrawn. This process is repeated several times until the dilation tract can accommodate the smallest diameter cavernotome. The total length of the corporotomy will be longer than for virgin cases. A perineal counter incision to enhance access to the proximal corpora may also be considered in cases where dense fibrosis prevents the surgeon from confidently dilating in this region [31].

We prefer the Carrion-Rosselo cavernotomes (Coloplast Corporation, Minneapolis, MN) (Fig. 7.1) to further dilate the corporal body proximally and distally. We typically start with the 8 Fr cavernotome and dilate up to 10 or 11 Fr. If the cavernotome cannot be inserted into the corporal body due to dense fibrosis, then the corporotomy should be extended proximally and/or distally. Additional sets of stay sutures should be placed as the corporotomy is extended.

Once the corporal dilation is complete, we use the Furlow introducer to measure the total length of the corporal bodies. We then test for evidence of urethral injury by filling the corpora with antibiotic irrigant through each corporotomy and ensuring that no fluid leaks out of the meatus around the urethral catheter. We then insert the Furlow introducer into the mid glans via the corporotomy and pass the Keith needle through the distal tunica and out through the glans. We insert the proximal aspect of the implant cylinder into the corporal body prior to the distal. We place small pieces of oxidized regenerated cellulose (Surgicel Fibrillar, Johnson and Johnson, New Brunswick, NJ) onto the implanted cylinder that is visible through the corporotomy in order to minimize bleeding from the cut edges of the corporotomy after closure. The distal corporotomy is closed by tying each set of stay sutures together. The proximal corporotomy is closed after placement of additional oxidized regenerated cellulose (Surgicel Fibrillar, Johnson and Johnson, New Brunswick, NJ), and the device is inflated to ensure satisfactory positioning.

A distal counter incision should be considered if a distal area of dense fibrosis precludes controlled dilation into the mid glands (Fig. 7.4). This technique was initially described with high success in 30 patients by Rajpukar et al. in 1999 [37]. A lateral hemi-circumscribing incision is made over the area where the dilator meets resistance. We then dissect down through the tunica dartos and directly onto the tunica albuginea, ensuring that the dissection remains lateral to the urethra. 2-0 polydioxanone stay sutures are placed transversely into the tunica albuginea. At this point a 2 cm transverse corporotomy is made to allow for further dilation into the mid glans with the use of reverse cutting scissors and cavernotomes. This step becomes easier with the additional leverage provided by being closer to the area of fibrosis. The Furlow introducer is then used to pass the Keith needle through the

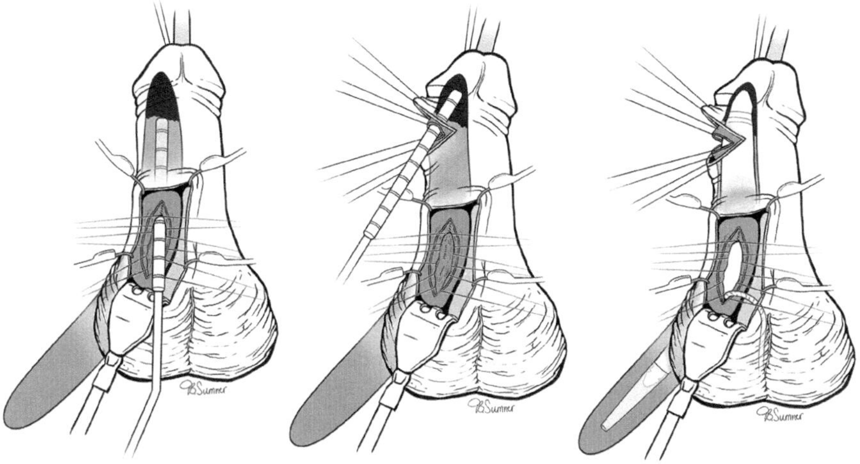

Fig. 7.4 Dense scarring of the distal corpora may prevent dilation into the mid-glands (left). A distal counter incision can facilitate controlled dilation of the distal scar tissue into the mid glans (center) and ultimately allow for adequate seating of the cylinder (right)

glans. If difficulty is encountered when passing the distal implant cylinder into the glans, it may be helpful to bring the cylinder tip out of the distal corporotomy. It can then be inserted into the glans, while the surgeon has the opportunity to apply pressure to the proximal aspect of the cylinder tip.

Selection of Cylinder Length

We measure corporal length using the Furlow introducer. We pick a stay suture and use this as the basis for our proximal and distal measurements. We choose not to aggressively size the device in cases of corporal fibrosis in order to minimize the risk of distal cylinder extrusion. Knoll previously reported a decreased risk of device infection (30 vs 5%) by selecting an undersized implant in cases where corporal grafting would have otherwise been required to facilitate corporotomy closure [21]. Wilson et al. later showed that undersized devices can often be removed and replaced with wider and longer cylinders at a later date, suggesting that the undersized device may function as a tissue expander over time [50].

Cylinder Insertion

We palpate the tip of the Furlow introducer in the mid glans and use a hemostat or Kelly clamp to optimize the exit site for the Keith needle so as to avoid injury to fossa navicularis and maximize glans support. We then insert the proximal aspect of the cylinder into the proximal corpora with the aid of the blue enhancing tool prior to inserting the distal cylinder.

Corporotomy Closure

Reapproximation of the tunica albuginea after device insertion can be difficult in the presence of substantial corporal fibrosis. Inadequate tunical closure puts the device at risk of cylinder herniation out of the corporotomy. We combat this challenge by (1) incising into the fibrosed cavernosal tissue with a 15 blade, (2) creating an adequate corporal dilation with the use of reverse cutting scissors and cavernotomes, (3) utilizing a narrow-base IPP, and (4) utilizing ample sets of stay sutures. By utilizing these techniques, we have not found tunical reapproximation to be a significant problem.

While not used in our practice, multiple implanters have described the utilization of grafts to facilitate corporotomy closure. Options for graft closure include bovine pericardium [30, 51], cadaveric pericardium (*Tutoplast*, Coloplast Corporation, Minneapolis, MN, USA) [35], rectus fascia [23, 31], and polytetrafluoroethylene (PTFE) [39].

Reservoir Insertion and Fill

Reservoir insertion does not typically differ substantially from virgin cases. We place the reservoir in the high submuscular space (HSM) using the five-step technique via the external inguinal ring or further superiorly in the HSM via a lower abdominal counter incision if both inguinal rings have previously been violated [52]. We utilize the 100 cc rifampin/minocycline-coated Conceal reservoir (Boston Scientific, Marlborough, MA) and typically fill the reservoir with around 70 cc of normal saline for use with the AMS 700 CXR.

Tubing Passage and Connection

When a counter incision is required for reservoir placement, we utilize the curved AMS Tubing Passer (Boston Scientific, Marlborough, MA) to pass the reservoir tubing down into the penoscrotal incision. Reservoir and pump tubings are then cut to size to minimize redundancy and connected via the Quick Connect system (Boston Scientific, Marlborough, MA).

Pump Insertion

Pump insertion may be more challenging in patients with a history of prior device infection. We sharply develop a pocket deep to the anterior scrotal skin in the midline. Following pump placement, we close the overlying dartos tissue in two layers prior to skin closure.

Drain Insertion

In cases involving corporal fibrosis, we routinely utilize a closed suction 10 Fr round silicone drain, which we pass through the suprapubic skin several centimeters superolateral to the base of the penis on the side opposite the reservoir.

Postoperative Care

While we favor same-day surgery for the vast majority of virgin IPP insertions, we routinely admit corporal fibrosis patients overnight to facilitate drain and catheter removal on the morning of the first postoperative day.

While limited retrospective evidence has not identified a benefit of postoperative antibiotics [53–55], patients with corporal fibrosis are at increased risk for infection.

We feel this justifies the use of postoperative antibiotics in this setting. Our standard regimen is a 3-day course of oral ciprofloxacin and simultaneous 3-day course of oral cephalexin.

We see patients back 6 weeks postoperatively for a device activation visit and 3 months after that to ensure successful use of the implant. Thereafter patients are seen on an as-needed basis.

Management of Selected Complications

We suspect that the following complications are more likely to occur in the setting of corporal fibrosis based on the limited published literature and our own experience.

Injury to the Ventral Corpus Spongiosum +/– Urethra

Corpus spongiosal and/or urethral injury during the penoscrotal dissection are rare in the context of IPP insertion [56]. They are more likely to occur in reoperative cases where normal anatomical planes between the corporal bodies and urethra are distorted by fibrosis [57]. The keys to preventing injury of the urethra are early identification of its location and cautious dissection through scarred tissue planes. We place a 14Fr silicone urethral catheter in every patient undergoing IPP insertion to assist in urethral identification. It is critical that any urethral injury is recognized and immediately repaired to prevent postoperative urinary extravasation, which would place the patient at high risk of subsequent implant infection. We prefer sharp dissection over electrocautery during the penoscrotal dissection to avoid the potential for delayed presentation of urethral cauterization injuries.

Injuries to the urethra in this location should be managed with a two-layer repair using fine absorbable sutures. Management options after repair include aborting the case or proceeding with implantation. This decision is dependent on the extent of the injury, surgeon experience, and comfort level. A recently conducted survey of implanting urologists regarding management of urethral injuries at time of penile prosthesis placement showed that 43% of respondents would continue the procedure with primary repair with either unilateral or bilateral cylinder placement, while 57% would abort the procedure [58]. After urethral repair, confirmation of watertight repair can be confirmed if desired prior to implant placement by flushing saline through the urethral meatus [59]. In this scenario, we recommend leaving a Foley catheter in place for at least 1 week as well as consideration of suprapubic urinary diversion for 4 weeks depending on the degree of injury [57].

Proximal (Crural) Perforation

Proximal crural perforation is a well-known complication during corporal dilation but injury rates are infrequently reported in the literature. In the setting of corporal fibrosis due to prior infection or ischemic priapism, crural perforation rates of 3%, 6%, and 38% have been reported [36–38]. We attempt to minimize the risk of proximal perforation by (1) dilating immediately deep to the tunica albuginea, (2) dilating in a lateral direction onto the ischiopubic ramus, (3) maximizing control of all instruments by keeping the surgeon's elbow in toward the torso, (4) avoiding the use of excessive force, and (5) electing to place a shorter device if dense fibrosis is encountered in the final 1–3 cm of the proximal corporal body. In our experience, a shorter device placed for proximal fibrosis will not affect the aesthetics of the implant distally or its ultimate functionality.

Proximal perforation can be identified in several ways. Typically there will be a sudden decrease in resistance that allows the dilator to pass into the gluteal fat without resistance. If a tunical defect is already present from prior prosthesis placement, the dilator will pass without resistance from the outset, and there will be a discrepancy in corporal measurements [60]. In our experience, the Furlow introducer will provide a proximal measurement of >14 cm if perforation has occurred. There will not be a feeling of stability when the dilator is "bounced" up and down in this location. In the setting of a proximal perforation, a Brooks dilator inserted into the perforated corpora will travel posterior to the ischiopubic ramus and a "Field Goal" shape will not be formed when both dilators are placed simultaneously (a failed "Field Goal" test) [61].

It is important to identify and address a crural perforation at the time of injury in order to prevent subsequent proximal cylinder migration. Historically, a formal proximal corporal repair was performed via perineal exploration [24]. Contemporary approaches to managing a proximal perforation include: (1) an attempt to re-dilate into the correct space under direct vision or (2) "U-stitch" suture sling surrounding cylinder tubing at the exit site from the corporotomy. Measurement of the non-perforated corporal body is used to select the correctly sized implant. Postoperatively a fibrous capsule forms around the implant and helps to stabilize it in place despite the corporal defect. A rear tip extender sling, in which a Prolene stitch is thrown through each side of the corporotomy and the tip of the rear tip extender, is another popular approach to proximal perforation management [62]. Other described management techniques include the use of a synthetic "windsock" that is wrapped around the proximal cylinder and fixed to the corporal body and the use of a polyglycolic acid "Plug and Patch" [24, 63].

Distal Urethral Perforation

Urethral perforation at the level of the distal corpora is more likely to occur in the setting of corporal fibrosis. These injuries typically occur during overaggressive dilation or during penile remodeling for curvature. Surgeons should have a high index of suspicion for distal perforation, especially if any blood is seen per urethra. Corporal integrity can be easily tested with saline flush into the corporotomy while looking for a rush of fluid from the urethra. This complication is an indication to abort ipsilateral placement of a prosthetic cylinder. If the injury to the urethra is distal enough to be seen via the urethral meatus, a two-layer closure can be attempted. If the contralateral corpora has already been dilated, a single inflatable or malleable cylinder can be placed as a placeholder to prevent further fibrosis. However, if the perforation occurs and is recognized during the initial dilation, there is little advantage to attempting contralateral cylinder placement and will only increase the risk of bilateral perforation or subsequent device infection [24]. We recommend urethral catheterization for a duration of 1 week and consideration of repeat attempt at implant insertion no sooner than 6 months after the injury [64].

Various approaches have been proposed in the literature for management of urethral injuries based on anatomical location along the urethra [56]. For injuries along the distal urethra (fossa navicularis to meatus), the injury can be repaired primarily with at least 2 layers of closure with absorbable suture. An extended meatotomy can be performed to the level of the injury for better visualization of the repair. Perito et al. described a staged repair in which a hypospadias defect is purposely created, the urethra repaired, and the implant cylinders placed bilaterally with planned return to the OR for delayed repair of the hypospadias [65]. Shah et al. described a series of 9 urethral injuries out of a group of 871 patients from a high-volume center. All were managed with primary urethral repair with either bilateral or unilateral cylinder placement. They reported a 100% infection-free rate at a mean follow-up of 253 days [66]. While this technique has been successfully employed, it is important to note that it should only be employed in experienced hands. Standard of care after distal perforation is to abort cylinder placement with or without urethral repair and delayed reattempt at prosthesis placement.

Distal Crossover

Distal crossover refers to a cylinder tip that inadvertently crossed through the intracorporal septum into the contralateral corporal body during corporal dilation or cylinder passage. This complication can be subtle but can usually be identified after cylinder placement during implant cycling by carefully palpating over the length of the cylinders on the dorsal and ventral aspects of the penis. It can usually be seen clearly from the side as one cylinder will appear to tilt in front of the other. For a proximal crossover, the ipsilateral cylinder will have a diagonal trajectory from the base of the shaft toward the contralateral cylinder. A distal crossover can be identified by palpating the cylinder tips in the glans which will feel crowded together to one side. Management involves removal of the malpositioned cylinder and repeat dilation of the tract in a more lateral trajectory. A Hegar dilator can be placed in the unaffected corpora during re-dilation to facilitate correction of the deviated cylinder.

Infection

For virgin implant placement, infection rates range from 1% to 4% [67]. In the presence of corporal fibrosis, incidence of infection is much higher, ranging from 0% to 30% in the literature [21, 23, 36, 37, 39–41]. Infections are largely due to bacterial seeding of the device either before or during implantation [68]. Bacteria then create a biofilm that is impenetrable by antibiotics, making conservative treatment of infections unlikely to succeed [69]. Known risk factors for prosthesis infection include poorly controlled diabetes, immunosuppression, spinal cord injury, decreased penile sensation, and concomitant AUS insertion [70]. Jarow et al. reviewed infection rates in patients undergoing virgin implant surgery vs revision for mechanical reasons vs revision with reconstruction (neophallus, Peyronie's plaque reconstructions, or extensive corporal reconstruction due to corporal fibrosis), finding infection rates of 1.8%, 13.3%, and 21.7%, respectively [71]. The higher infection rates in revision surgery were thought to be due to release of bacteria from the biofilm, decreased penetration of preoperative antibiotics to the surgical area due to fibrosis, and longer operative times and implant/corporal exposure to the environment.

Infection prevention includes the use of preoperative IV antibiotic administration per AUA guidelines, hair removal with clippers, chlorhexidine-based skin prep, and meticulous attention to sterile technique [72]. Penile prostheses should be coated with broad-spectrum antibiotics. AMS devices are pre-coated with rifampin and minocycline (InhibiZone ®), while Coloplast devices can be custom coated with antibiotics based on surgeon preference or local antibiograms [73]. Generous utilization of antibiotic irrigation (e.g., 80 mg gentamicin in 1 L normal saline) should be utilized during implantation to wash out all surgical spaces.

Device infections are present similarly in the hostile penis and virgin settings. Typical symptoms include pain, swelling, purulent drainage, and pump adherence to the skin. If an isolated superficial skin infection is suspected, the patient can be treated with oral or IV antibiotics in an attempt to preserve the prosthesis. However, if a device infection is identified, then the entire system will need to be explanted. It is important to note that many of these patients are on their second or third implants and the recurrence of device infection can be a particularly distressing event. It is critical to counsel patients preoperatively of all expected outcomes and what salvage plans are in place should the device need to be explanted.

As discussed above, several adjunctive measures can be considered at the time of explanation including immediate insertion of a new IPP [10], MPP [11, 12], or antibiotic-infused cast [11, 13]. Corporal installation of mitomycin C was also recently reported with success observed in all five patients treated [14]. Serious consideration should be given to these techniques as a corporal placeholder since complete device explantation will only worsen the degree of corporal fibrosis. It should be discussed with patients that, although rare, some patients may progress to an "end-stage" penis with severe fibrosis after multiple infections that would preclude future attempts at safe prosthesis insertion. Emotional, sexual, or psychiatric support may be necessary as many patients will experience a significant sense of loss at the inability to have further erections.

Supersonic Transformer (SST) Deformity and Intrinsic Glanular Hypermobility (IGH)

The term "supersonic transport" deformity is based on the downward tilted nose of the Concorde civilian supersonic transport aircraft, which is replicated by an inadequately supported glans penis. It is also referred to as "floppy glans syndrome" [74]. This physical exam finding can also occur in the setting of adequate cylinder sizing in which case it is referred to as intrinsic glanular hypermobility (IGH). This complication can be particularly troublesome with corporal fibrosis as it is more difficult to fully dilate the distal corpora due to scarring. It can be very frustrating for patients and their partners due to issues with penetration and/or appearance. If an SST is detected intraoperatively during cycling, a longer cylinder can be placed or further distal dissection using a counter incision can be performed.

If this complication occurs postoperatively, it may be due to proximal migration of a cylinder or due to incorrect sizing at time of surgery. SST deformity may be corrected by reoperation with cylinder upsizing or by glanulopexy [75]. Ziegelmann et al. described their modified glanulopexy technique to repair SST and IGH in which small incisions are made along the distal penile shaft, either ventrally or dorsally, depending on the direction of glans tilt. Dissection is carried down to Buck's fascia. Proximal and distal dissection along the shaft creates a space through which permanent sutures are secured proximally on either corporal body taking care to avoid puncturing the implant. A third stitch is passed from one incision to the other, distally through the mid glans, and then the suture ends are tied together, securing the glans in the desired straight position. This technique is minimally invasive with high success rates [75].

Distal or Lateral Extrusion

Cylinder extrusion occurs when a cylinder tip erodes through the tunica albuginea. It is more likely in the context of corporal fibrosis, overly aggressive dilation or device sizing, passage of the dilator in an exaggerated lateral path, and when a small caliber dilation device is used (e.g., Metzenbaum scissors or narrow Brooks dilator) [24, 76]. Additionally, distal extrusion can occur in patients with a history of prolonged ischemic priapism who have undergone a distal shunting procedure that has violated the tunica albuginea. Extrusion occurs more commonly on the distal, ventral corpora which may be explained by the fact that the tunica albuginea of the distal corpora is thinner than along the penile shaft [77]. Once an extrusion has occurred, the goal becomes preventing erosion through the skin, which necessitates explant. Patients may report pain at the site of extrusion, or their partners may report painful intercourse due to the protrusion of the device causing a bump or edge on the phallus.

Various management strategies for cylinder extrusion warrant consideration in the setting of fibrosis. Smith et al. were the first to describe the successful use of a distal windsock using PTFE graft [78]. Subsequent series reported infection rates ranging from 5% to 42% [24]. Due to infection risk, the use of graft material is generally avoided in contemporary practice [79]. A two-stage rectus fascia, tunica vaginalis flap procedure, was also described to create an additional layer between the distal cylinder and tunica albuginea [80]. In patients with corporal fibrosis and multiple prior devices, we prefer to avoid multiple surgeries and graft material insertion in favor of minimally invasive approaches. Mulcahy described a lateral hemi-circumscribing incision that is followed by a lateral corporotomy and cylinder tip evacuation. A new dilation tract is then developed medial to the pseudo capsule. Finally, the Furlow introducer and Keith needle are utilized to insert the cylinder tip into the medialized position within the glans. This technique obviates the need for infection-prone graft material and reduces operative time when compared to graft-based procedures [81]. Lue further simplified this technique using a transglanular approach to anchor the prosthesis to the fibrotic capsule opposite the side of erosion [82] (Table 7.4).

Conclusions

Corporal fibrosis represents a major challenge for patients and surgeons. Most patients with extensive corporal fibrosis will be dependent on a penile prosthesis for adequate erectile function. While difficult, controlled development of an accommodating channel within the scarred corporal body is possible with the use of modern surgical instruments. Narrow-base penile implants have decreased the degree of proximal corporal dilation required for implant insertion. Complications are more likely with IPP insertion in the setting of corporal fibrosis. Fortunately, the vast majority of patients achieve a satisfactory result and are able to regain sexual function.

Table 7.4 Management of intraoperative and postoperative complications

Complication	Complication rates in the setting of corporal fibrosis	Prevention strategies	Diagnosis	Management options
Injury to corpus spongiosum and/or urethra during initial – penoscrotal dissection	N/R	Place urethral catheter at start of case	Bleeding	Multilayer closure, proceed with implant, prolonged catheterization
			Visualization of urethral mucosa and/or catheter	Abort case and delay IPP insertion
Proximal (crural) perforation	3–38% [36–38]	Dilate immediately deep to the tunica albuginea	Dilator and/or Furlow measuring device passes without resistance into the gluteal fat	Attempt to re-dilate into the correct space directly
		Dilate laterally down onto the ischiopubic ramus	Lack of resistance at proximal most aspect of dilation tract	U-stitch "suture sling" surrounding cylinder tubing at the exit site from the corporotomy +/− incorporation of the RTE
		Maximize control of all instruments by keeping the surgeon's elbow in toward the torso	Abnormal "field goal" test	Synthetic windsock
		Avoid excessive force		
		Select a shorter cylinder length if dense fibrosis is encountered in the final 1–3 cm of the corporal body		
Urethral perforation during distal dilation	N/R	Perform distal dilation with the tip of the dilator angled laterally, away from the urethra	Intraoperative fluid challenge via both corporotomies – fluid should fill corpora without leaking out of meatus around catheter	Abort case, prolonged catheterization, consider reattempt at later date
				Primary repair or injury, proceed with IPP insertion

Distal crossover	19% [38]	Perform distal dilation with the tip of the dilator angled laterally, away from the urethra	Palpate cylinders and cylinder tips after insertion. A small space between the cylinder tips should be present	Re-dilate more laterally on the side that produced the crossover. Consider placing metal dilator in corpora on the side that received the crossover
Device infection	0–30% [21, 23, 36, 37, 39–41]	Sterile technique	Patient history	Device removal, extensive washout +/− insertion of a malleable prosthesis or IPP
		Perioperative antibiotics	Physical exam	
		Antibiotic-coated implant	Laboratory values	
		Alcohol-based skin prep	Cross-sectional imaging	
Supersonic transformer deformity	N/R	Dilate into mid glans, ensure adequate glans support intraoperatively	Patient history	Glanulopexy
			Physical exam	Revision surgery to upsize cylinders
Distal or lateral extrusion	N/R	Avoid overaggressive distal dilation	Physical exam reveals a palpable cylinder, typically ventral or lateral to distal corpora	Device removal if device eroded through skin
		Ensure adequate corporal dilation		Corporoplasty +/− autologous flap

N/R not reported

References

1. Rockey DC, Bell PD, Hill JA. Fibrosis--a common pathway to organ injury and failure. N Engl J Med. 2015;372:1138–49.
2. Wilson SK. Reimplantation of inflatable penile prosthesis into scarred corporeal bodies. Int J Impot Res. 2003;15(Suppl 5):S125–8.
3. Gasser TC, Larsen EH, Bruskewitz RG. Penile prosthesis reimplantation. J Urol. 1987;137:46–7.
4. Stember DS, Mulhall JP. Ischemic priapism and implant surgery with sharp corporal fibrosis excision (CME). J Sex Med. 2010;7:1987–90.
5. Bertram RA, Carson CC 3rd, Webster GD. Implantation of penile prostheses in patients impotent after priapism. Urology. 1985;26:325–7.
6. Levine LA, Benson J, Hoover C. Inflatable penile prosthesis placement in men with Peyronie's disease and drug-resistant erectile dysfunction: a single-center study. J Sex Med. 2010;7:3775–83.
7. Orvis BR, McAninch JW. Penile rupture. Urol Clin North Am. 1989;16:369–75.
8. Larsen EH, Gasser TC, Bruskewitz RC. Fibrosis of corpus cavernosum after intracavernous injection of phentolamine/papaverine. J Urol. 1987;137:292–3.
9. Jordan GH, Angermeier KW. Preoperative evaluation of erectile function with dynamic infusion cavernosometry/cavernosography in patients undergoing surgery for Peyronie's disease: correlation with postoperative results. J Urol. 1993;150:1138–42.
10. Mulcahy JJ. Long-term experience with salvage of infected penile implants. J Urol. 2000;163:481–2.
11. Gross MS, Phillips EA, Balen A, et al. The malleable implant salvage technique: infection outcomes after Mulcahy salvage procedure and replacement of infected inflatable penile prosthesis with malleable prosthesis. J Urol. 2016;195:694–7.
12. Chandrapal J, Harper S, Davis LG, Lentz AC. Penile implant infection: experience with expanded salvage criteria and a shortened course of postoperative antibiotics. Sex Med Today. 2020;8:383–7.
13. Swords K, Martinez DR, Lockhart JL, Carrion R. A preliminary report on the usage of an intracorporal antibiotic cast with synthetic high purity CaSO4 for the treatment of infected penile implant. J Sex Med. 2013;10:1162–9.
14. Shaeer O, Abdel Rahman IFS, Shaeer K. Shaeer's anti-scarring technique: a preventive measure against corporal fibrosis upon explantation of infected penile implants. Sex Med Today. 2019;7:357–60.
15. Muneer A, Alnajjar HM, Ralph D. Recent advances in the management of priapism. F1000Res. 2018;7:37.
16. Ralph DJ, Garaffa G, Muneer A, Freeman A, Rees R, Christopher AN, Minhas S. The immediate insertion of a penile prosthesis for acute ischaemic priapism. Eur Urol. 2009;56:1033–8.
17. Fuchs JS, Shakir N, McKibben MJ, Mathur S, Teeple S, Scott JM, Morey AF. Penoscrotal decompression-promising new treatment paradigm for refractory ischemic priapism. J Sex Med. 2018;15:797–802.
18. Baumgarten AS, VanDyke ME, Yi YA, et al. Favorable multi-institutional experience with penoscrotal decompression for prolonged ischemic priapism. BJU Int. 2020; https://doi.org/10.1111/bju.15127.
19. Nehra A, Jackson G, Miner M, et al. The Princeton III Consensus recommendations for the management of erectile dysfunction and cardiovascular disease. Mayo Clin Proc. 2012;87:766–78.
20. Kava BR, Burdick-Will J. Complications associated with retained foreign bodies from infected penile implants: proposal for the use of an implant-specific checklist at the time of device removal. J Sex Med. 2013;10:1659–66.
21. Knoll LD, Furlow WL, Benson RC Jr, Bilhartz DL. Management of nondilatable cavernous fibrosis with the use of a downsized inflatable penile prosthesis. J Urol. 1995;153:366–7.

22. Montgomery BD, Lomas DJ, Ziegelmann MJ, Trost LW. Infection risk of undergoing multiple penile prostheses: an analysis of referred patient surgical histories. Int J Impot Res. 2018;30:147–52.
23. Pathak AS, Chang JH, Parekh AR, Aboseif SR. Use of rectus fascia graft for corporeal reconstruction during placement of penile implant. Urology. 2005;65:1198–201.
24. Stember DS, Kohler TS, Morey AF. Management of perforation injuries during and following penile prosthesis surgery. J Sex Med. 2015;
25. Sellers T, Dineen M, Salem EA, Wilson SK. Vacuum preparation, optimization of cylinder length and postoperative daily inflation reduces complaints of shortened penile length following implantation of inflatable penile prosthesis. Adv Sex Med. 2013;3(1):14–8.
26. Tsambarlis PN, Chaus F, Levine LA. Successful placement of penile prostheses in men with severe corporal fibrosis following vacuum therapy protocol. J Sex Med. 2017;14:44–6.
27. Hebert KL, Yafi FA, Wilson S. Inflatable penile prosthesis implantation into scarred corporal bodies: timing may decrease postoperative problems. BJU Int. 2020;125:168–72.
28. Garber BB, Lim C. Inflatable penile prosthesis insertion in men with severe intracorporal fibrosis. Curr Urol Rep. 2017;10:92–6.
29. Sansalone S, Garaffa G, Djinovic R, Antonini G, Vespasiani G, Ieria FP, Cimino S, Loreto C, Ralph DJ. Simultaneous total corporal reconstruction and implantation of a penile prosthesis in patients with erectile dysfunction and severe fibrosis of the corpora cavernosa. J Sex Med. 2012;9:1937–44.
30. Lopes EJA, Kuwano AY, Guimaraes AN, Flores JP, Jacobino MAO. Corporoplasty using bovine pericardium grafts in complex penile prosthesis implantation surgery. Int Braz J Urol. 2009;35:49–53; discussion 53–5
31. Brusky JP, Tran VQ, Rieder JM, Aboseif SR. A preliminary report on combined penoscrotal and perineal approach for placement of penile prosthesis with corporal fibrosis. Adv Urol. 2008:524392.
32. Shaeer O. Implantation of penile prosthesis in cases of corporeal fibrosis: modified Shaeer's excavation technique. J Sex Med. 2008;5:2470–6.
33. Montague DK, Angermeier KW. Corporeal excavation: new technique for penile prosthesis implantation in men with severe corporeal fibrosis. Urology. 2006;67:1072–5.
34. Park JK, Kim HJ, Kang MH, Jeong YB. Implantation of penile prosthesis in a patient with severe corporeal fibrosis induced by cavernosal injection therapy. Int J Impot Res. 2002;14:545–6.
35. Palese MA, Burnett AL. Corporoplasty using pericardium allograft (Tutoplast) with complex penile prosthesis surgery. Urology. 2001;58:1049–52.
36. Ghanem H, Ghazy S, El-Meliegy A. Corporeal counter incisions: a simplified approach to penile prosthesis implantation in fibrotic cases. Int J Impot Res. 2000;12:153–6.
37. Rajpurkar A, Li H, Dhabuwala CB. Penile implant success in patients with corporal fibrosis using multiple incisions and minimal scar tissue excision. Urology. 1999;54:145–7.
38. Mooreville M, Adrian S, Delk JR. Implantation of inflatable penile prosthesis in patients with severe corporeal fibrosis: introduction of a new penile cavernotome. J Urol. 1999;162(6):2054–7.
39. George VK, Shah GS, Mills R, Dhabuwala CB. The management of extensive penile fibrosis: a new technique of "minimal scar-tissue excision.". Br J Urol. 1996;77:282–4.
40. Herschorn S, Ordorica RC. Penile prosthesis insertion with corporeal reconstruction with synthetic vascular graft material. J Urol. 1995;154:80–4.
41. Barbara MR, Carrion H. Cavernotomy. Arch Esp Urol. 1991;44:185–6.
42. Martínez-Salamanca JI, Mueller A, Moncada I, Carballido J, Mulhall JP. Penile prosthesis surgery in patients with corporal fibrosis: a state of the art review. J Sex Med. 2011;8:1880–9.
43. Garber BB. Inflatable penile prostheses for the treatment of erectile dysfunction: an update. Expert Rev Med Devices. 2008;5:133–44.
44. Lightner DJ, Wymer K, Sanchez J, Kavoussi L. Best practice statement on urologic procedures and antimicrobial prophylaxis. J Urol. 2020;203:351–6.

45. Helo S, Clavell-Hernandez J, Wilson SK. Penile prosthesis implantation in complex and previously failed settings. In: Textbook of male genitourethral reconstruction. Cham: Springer; 2020.
46. Wilson SK, Terry T, Delk JR. Improved implant survival in patients with severe corporal fibrosis: a new technique without necessity of grafting. J Urol. 1995;153:359.
47. Fishman IJ. Corporeal reconstruction procedures for complicated penile implants. Urol Clin North Am. 1989;16:73–90.
48. Shaeer O, Shaeer A. SURGERY: Corporoscopic excavation of the fibrosed corpora cavernosa for penile prosthesis implantation: optical corporotomy and trans-corporeal resection, Shaeer's technique. J Sex Med. 2007;4:218–25.
49. Shaeer O, Shaeer K. Extracorporeal transseptal penile prosthesis implantation for extreme cases of corporeal fibrosis: Shaeer implantation technique. J Sex Med. 2018;15:1350–6.
50. Wilson SK, Delk JR, Mulcahy JJ, Cleves M, Salem EA. Upsizing of inflatable penile implant cylinders in patients with corporal fibrosis. J Sex Med. 2006;3:736–42.
51. Lopes EJ, Santos TC, Jacobino M. Bovine pericardium in penile prosthesis reimplantation. Int Braz J Urol. 2007;33:74–6.
52. Morey AF, Cefalu CA, Hudak SJ. High submuscular placement of urologic prosthetic balloons and reservoirs via transscrotal approach. J Sex Med. 2013;10:603–10.
53. Dropkin BM, Kaufman MR. Antibiotics and inflatable penile prosthesis insertion: a literature review. Sex Med Rev. 2020; https://doi.org/10.1016/j.sxmr.2020.04.005
54. Dropkin BM, Chisholm LP, Dallmer JD, Johnsen NV, Dmochowski RR, Milam DF, Kaufman MR. Penile prosthesis insertion in the era of antibiotic stewardship-are postoperative antibiotics necessary? J Urol. 2020;203:611–4.
55. Adamsky MA, Boysen WR, Cohen AJ, Ham S, Dmochowski RR, Faris SF, Bales GT, Cohn JA. Evaluating the role of postoperative oral antibiotic administration in artificial urinary sphincter and inflatable penile prosthesis explantation: a nationwide analysis. Urology. 2018;111:92–8.
56. Carlos EC, Sexton SJ, Lentz AC. Urethral injury and the penile prosthesis. Sex Med Rev. 2019;7:360–8.
57. Yi YA, Fuchs JS, Davenport MT, McKibben MJ, Bergeson RL, Morey AF. Synchronous urethral repair during prosthetic surgery: safety of planned and damage control approaches using suprapubic tube urinary diversion. J Sex Med. 2019;16:1106–10.
58. Sexton SJ, Granieri MA, Lentz AC. Survey on the contemporary management of intraoperative urethral injuries during penile prosthesis implantation. J Sex Med. 2018;15:576–81.
59. Bettocchi C, Ditonno P, Palumbo F, Lucarelli G, Garaffa G, Giammusso B, Battaglia M. Penile prosthesis: what should we do about complications? Adv Urol. 2008;573560
60. Pearlman AM, Terlecki RP. Proximal corporal perforation during penile prosthesis surgery: prevention, recognition, and review of historical and novel management strategies. J Sex Med. 2018;15:1055–60.
61. Gupta NK, Ring J, Trost L, Wilson SK, Köhler TS. The penoscrotal surgical approach for inflatable penile prosthesis placement. Transl Androl Urol. 2017;6:628–38.
62. Wilson SK. Rear tip extender sling: a quick and easy repair for crural perforation. J Sex Med. 2010;7:1052–5.
63. Szostak MJ, DelPizzo JJ, Sklar GN. The plug and patch: a new technique for repair of corporal perforation during placement of penile prostheses. J Urol. 2000;163:1203–5.
64. Sharma D, Smith RP. Troubleshooting intraoperative complications of penile prosthesis placement. Transl Androl Urol. 2017;6:S892–7.
65. Perito P. Urethral injury during inflatable penile prosthesis: a new repair. Video J Prosthet Urol. 2014;1:034.
66. Shah B, Loeb A, Beilan J, Baumgarten A, Slongo J, Parker J, Carrion R. 334 Intraoperative management algorithm for urethral injury at the time of PP placement. J Sex Med. 2018;15:S260.
67. Narang GL, Figler BD, Coward RM. Preoperative counseling and expectation management for inflatable penile prosthesis implantation. Transl Androl Urol. 2017;6:S869–80.

68. Wilson SK, Costerton JW. Biofilm and penile prosthesis infections in the era of coated implants: a review. J Sex Med. 2012;9:44–53.
69. Lotan Y, Roehrborn CG, McConnell JD, Hendin BN. Factors influencing the outcomes of penile prosthesis surgery at a teaching institution. Urology. 2003;62:918–21.
70. Pineda M, Burnett AL. Penile prosthesis infections-a review of risk factors, prevention, and treatment. Sex Med Rev. 2016;4:389–98.
71. Jarow JP. Risk factors for penile prosthetic infection. J Urol. 1996;156:402–4.
72. Hebert KJ, Kohler TS. Penile prosthesis infection: myths and realities. World J Mens Health. 2019; https://doi.org/10.5534/wjmh.180123
73. Lokeshwar SD, Bitran J, Madhusoodanan V, Kava B, Ramasamy R. A surgeon's guide to the various antibiotic dips available during penile prosthesis implantation. Curr Urol Rep. 2019;20:11.
74. Bickell M, Manimala N, Parker J, Steixner B, Wiegand L, Carrion R. Floppy glans syndrome: pathogenesis and treatment. Sex Med Rev. 2016;4:149–56.
75. Ziegelmann MJ, Alom M, Bole R, Kohler T, Trost L. Modified glanulopexy technique for supersonic transporter deformity and glanular hypermobility in men with penile prostheses. J Sex Med. 2018;15:914–9.
76. Fuentes JL, Yi YA, Davenport MT, Bergeson RL, Ward EE, Morey AF. Long-term sequelae of inflatable penile prosthesis: clinical characteristics of patients who develop distal cylinder tip extrusion. Transl Androl Urol. 2020;9:38–42.
77. Hsu GL, Brock G, Martínez-Piñeiro L, von Heyden B, Lue TF, Tanagho EA. Anatomy and strength of the tunica albuginea: its relevance to penile prosthesis extrusion. J Urol. 1994;151:1205–8.
78. Smith CP, Kraus SR, Boone TB. Management of impending penile prosthesis erosion with a polytetrafluoroethylene distal wind sock graft. J Urol. 1998;160:2037–40.
79. Jordan GH, Alter GJ, Gilbert DA, Horton CE, Devine CJ Jr. Penile prosthesis implantation in total phalloplasty. J Urol. 1994;152:410–4.
80. Alter GJ, Greisman J, Werthman PE, Seid AS, Joseph BJ. Use of a prefabricated tunica vaginalis fascia flap to reconstruct the tunica albuginea after recurrent penile prosthesis extrusion. J Urol. 1998;159:128–32.
81. Mulcahy JJ. Distal corporoplasty for lateral extrusion of penile prosthesis cylinders. J Urol. 1999;161:193–5.
82. Shindel AW, Brant WO, Mwamukonda K, Bella AJ, Lue TF. Transglanular repair of impending penile prosthetic cylinder extrusion. J Sex Med. 2010;7:2884–90.

Chapter 8
Considerations in the Management of Visceral and Vascular Injury During Penile Implant Surgery

Kristina Buscaino, Raul E. Fernandez-Crespo, and Rafael Carrion

Introduction

Since its invention in the 1970s, the inflatable penile prosthesis (IPP) has been successful in treating erectile dysfunction (ED) [1]. Although the semirigid penile prosthesis (SRPP) is an option for the treatment of ED with less complications and mechanical failure rates, there is a higher satisfaction rate, among patients and their partners, with the IPP when compared to the SRPP [2]. Among these two models, in the United States, the IPP is the most used and implanted device [3]. The overall mechanical survival rate of an IPP is >95% and 80% at 5 and 10 years, respectively [4]. Although the IPP has adequate durability, 1–3% of penile prosthetics become infected requiring removal of all components [5]. Complications may occur with any of the IPP components during its placement and/or removal. However, reservoir placement and/or removal is one of the most critical parts of this surgery, as it has the highest risk of injuries and/or complications including potential bladder, bowel, and vascular injury. The best approach against any complication is prevention, as well as being prepared with the proper armamentarium in case they are encountered [6].

K. Buscaino · R. E. Fernandez-Crespo · R. Carrion (✉)
Morsani College of Medicine, University of South Florida, Tampa, FL, USA
e-mail: carriore@usf.edu

E. P. Miranda, J. P. Mulhall (eds.), *Penile Implant Surgery*,
https://doi.org/10.1007/978-3-030-82363-4_8

Anatomy

Normal Anatomy

In patients without altered pelvic anatomy, either secondary to previous surgeries, trauma, or radiation therapy, the traditional reservoir placement has been within the retropubic space of Retzius (SOR) (Fig. 8.1). It is critical for the implanting surgeon to be aware of the anatomical relationships of the inguinal ring and all the surrounding structures when placing the reservoir in this space, not only for adequate placement, but for prevention of complications as well. Despite the importance for detailed measurements in this anatomical area, no data regarding this was available to aid the prosthetic surgeon. This all changed after a group of prosthetic surgeons performed multiple cadaveric dissections and measurements between key landmarks were obtained and published [8].

Henry et al. [8] used the inguinal ring as their landmark and published that the distance to a decompressed bladder is 5–8 cm (average of 6.4 cm) at 15–25 degrees (average 23 degrees) medially, while the distance to a distended bladder with 200 cc instilled is 1.5–4 cm (average 2.4 cm) medially, and the distance from the ring to the external iliac vein is 2.5–4.5 cm (average 3.4 cm) at 20–57.5 degrees (average 35.3 degrees) laterally. Placing a patient in approximately 20 degrees of Trendelenburg may beneficially alter a patient's normal anatomy. This position may increase a

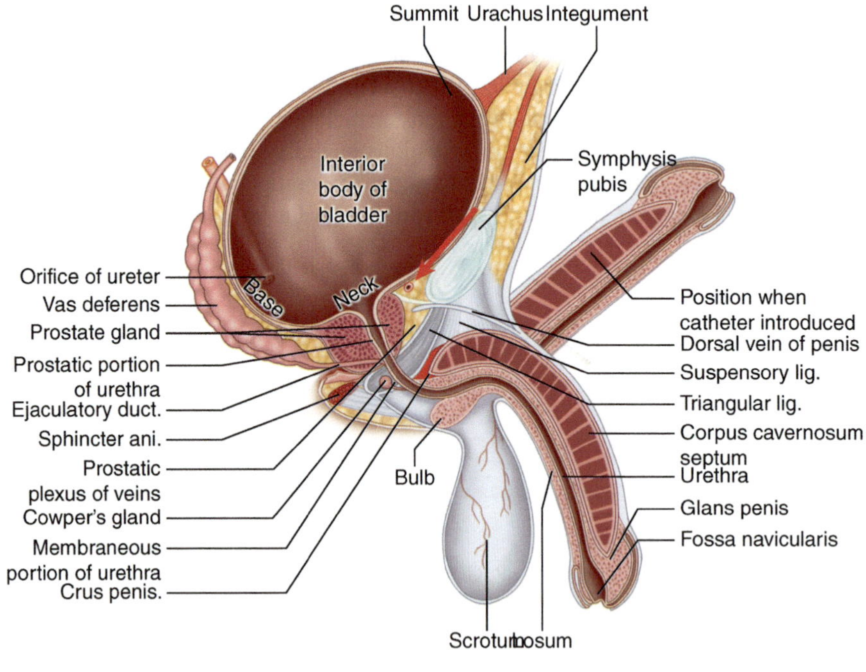

Fig. 8.1 Illustration of SOR (red arrow) [7]

distended bladder distance from the inguinal ring to 2.6 cm (versus 2.0 cm in non-Trendelenburg position) and decompress the external iliac vein.

Altered Anatomy

Anatomic changes can be appreciated after pelvic surgery, trauma and radiation therapy. Therefore, the implanting surgeon must perform a thorough medical history, as well as a physical exam in order to identify any previous surgeries or conditions that can alter the pelvic/abdominal wall anatomy. This information will directly impact and dictate the approach that will be used for a safe reservoir placement.

Post-prostatectomy

Before the introduction of robotic surgery, open radical prostatectomies historically remained in the extraperitoneal space [9]. Extraperitoneal prostatectomies avoid the intraperitoneal cavity, isolate vesicourethral anastomotic leaks, and allow an easier approach if the patient had a history of prior abdominal surgeries [9]. Although an extraperitoneal approach may still be achieved robotically, it has limitations due to decreased working space, higher CO2 absorption, and increased tension on the vesicourethral anastomosis due to the bladder remaining attached to the urachus [9]. Therefore, transperitoneal robotic-assisted radical prostatectomy (RALP) has been increasingly utilized, as approximately 70% of all prostatectomies are now performed robotically [10]. This requires the transection of the medial and median umbilical ligaments, the parietal peritoneum, ultimately dividing the urachus and obliterating the SOR [9]. The peritoneal veil is not re-established, and because of the division of the urachus, the bladder sits more dependently [9, 11] and the SOR is exposed to the peritoneal cavity [12]. The previous allows the reservoir to sit on top of the bladder versus laterally, increasing the risk of inadvertent perforation or erosion over time [9]. Bowel may migrate into the SOR or into the internal inguinal ring and become fixated due to adhesions [13, 14].

Post-cystectomy

Similarly to RALP, the SOR is obliterated after a radical cystectomy (RC). Therefore, placement of the reservoir into the SOR is extremely challenging due to adhesions, translocation of bowel, fibrosis, and urinary diversion in this space [15]. When a cystectomy is performed through a midline incision, the space between the rectus abdominis and transversalis fascia may also be disrupted due to the division of the urachus and mobilization of the of the bladder from anterior structures, potentially allowing peritoneal structures and urinary diversion to sit immediately posterior to the rectus abdominis [16]. This may be avoided by performing the procedure robotically [16]. If a neobladder is present, the inferior portion of the peritoneum is not closed, therefore intraperitoneal structures may enter the pelvic cavity [17].

Radiation

Radiation has immediate and long-term impacts on soft tissue [18]. Free radical generation and ionization will impair cellular processes, causing a pro-inflammatory cascade that will inevitably cause small vessel obliteration and injury, activation of coagulation cascades, and tissue fibrosis, ultimately effecting vascular regeneration and wound healing [15, 19]. These tissue changes may increase adjacent organ injury during reservoir placement, surgical site, and IPP infection as well as erosion of any of the IPP components [15, 19]. There have been no reports regarding optimal timing for IPP placement after radiation therapy [20].

Renal Transplant

Placement of a renal transplant is dependent on many patient factors such as previous surgeries, other abdominal transplants, laterality, and anomalies of the donor kidney. Traditionally, the renal transplant is placed in the right iliac fossa due to the more anterior external iliac vein [21]. However, the left iliac fossa is preferred if there is a simultaneous kidney-pancreas transplant, and the abdominal fossa is preferred if a pediatric patient is receiving from an adult donor [21]. Typically, in order to allow the anastomosis of the external iliac artery and vein, the retroperitoneal space is entered [21].

Inguinal Hernia Repair

Inguinal hernia repairs make it nearly impossible to place the reservoir through the external inguinal ring. Often, a mesh is used for inguinal hernia repairs, closing the external inguinal ring. If a mesh it not used, and the hernia is repaired primarily, there will be scar tissue present [22]. In both repairs, bowel may be directly posterior to the hernia repair [22].

Reservoir Placement

The ideal insertion of the IPP reservoir is a location that is safe for the patient and within a space that does not have excessive pressure on the reservoir [11]. Depending on a patient's history and surgeon preference, the IPP reservoir can be placed in the traditional SOR or an alternate location. The different techniques are discussed below. Being familiar with each can assist with surgical planning contingent on the patient's history, ultimately decreasing the risk of intraoperative injuries.

Traditional Reservoir Placement

Traditionally, the IPP reservoir is placed in the SOR as introduced by Dr. Scott in 1973 [23]. With time and adjustments made to the surgical techniques, multiple modifications have emerged to safely develop this space. If a "hostile" pelvis is not present, the SOR is easy to access and provides a low-pressure space. When placed in this location, it is not palpable to the patient due to its retropubic location [12]. When IPPs were initially performed, the reservoirs were placed through a midline counter incision and through the inferior portion of the linea alba [13]. The reservoir can be placed blindly in the SOR via the external inguinal ring after piercing the transversalis fascia through the same surgical incision [11, 24, 25]. However, a counter incision may need to be made in some instances to ensure the reservoir is placed properly and securely.

At our institution, the external inguinal ring is palpated on either side. An S retractor is placed inside the external inguinal ring and is pulled anteriorly allowing tension on the tissue below. The external inguinal ring and the overlying tissue is bluntly swept away with the index finger, while repositioning the S retractor until transversalis fascia is palpated (Fig. 8.2). The transversalis fascia is then punctured with the index finger, and the SOR is entered. Confirmation of correct position is performed by feeling the pubic bone posteriorly as well as the pre-/perivesical fat. At this time, the S retractor is repositioned into the SOR and left here until the reservoir is placed. If the transversalis fascia is tough, the finger can be used as a drill

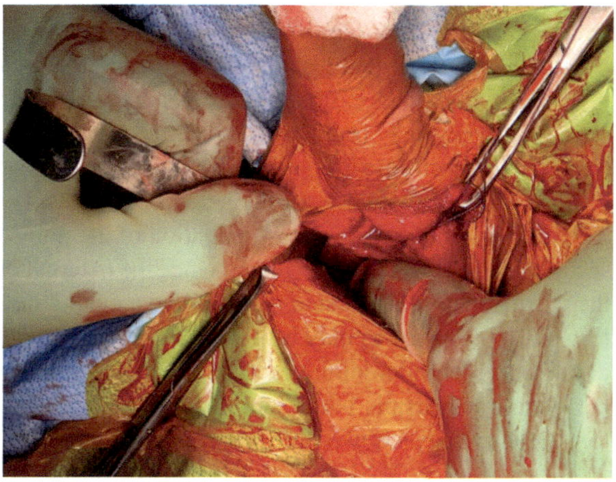

Fig. 8.2 Entering the SOR with anterior traction of the S retractor in the external inguinal ring with the contralateral index finger dissecting through transversalis fascia

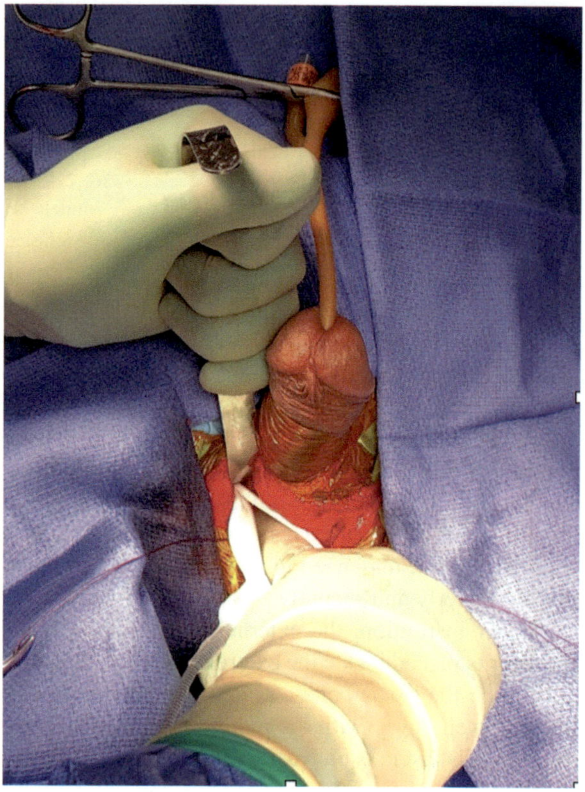

Fig. 8.3 Insertion of reservoir into the SOR with anterior traction of the S retractor in the external inguinal ring

motion to find an area where the fibers give way [26]. The reservoir is then placed with an index finger in the retropubic space with anterior retraction of the S retractor (Fig. 8.3). After the reservoir is confirmed to be in the correct space, the S retractor is then removed while the finger still in the SOR. This ensures the reservoir remains in place, and is not moved or pulled out, while the S retractor is being removed. Other surgeons use a nasal speculum, Jorgenson scissors (Fig. 8.4) with the tips pointing medially, or a tonsil clamp to puncture the transversalis fascia [1, 25–28].

If the transversalis fascia is not amendable for entry via the external ring, the retropubic space may be entered above the pubic tubercle. In these cases, a fasciotomy may be performed to assist with the reservoir placement [29]; this can safely be done with adequate exposure. As described by Mykoniatis et al. [29], Deaver and S retractors are utilized to allow palpation of the pubic tubercle, and layers are dissected bluntly with the index finger. Once the external oblique muscle fascia is seen, the spermatic cord is isolated laterally and a medial incision over the fascia is made (Fig. 8.5). Stay sutures may be placed at this time, to allow closure after placement of the reservoir and minimize needle injury to the reservoir. A finger may be used to perforate transversalis fascia, but if this is difficult, a nasal speculum, scissors, or tonsil clamp may be used [28]. At our institution, this space is typically further

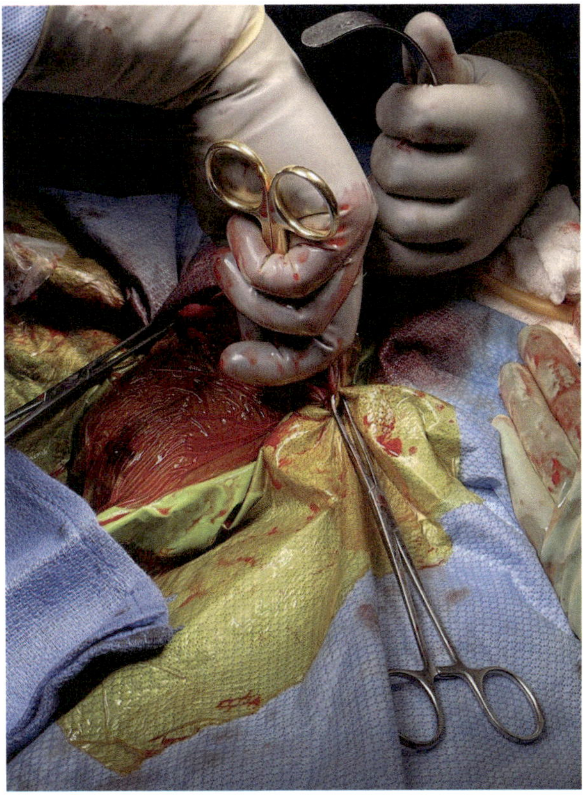

Fig. 8.4 Jorgenson scissors tips placed superior to pubic tubercle using index finger; the scissors are then used to perforate the transversalis fascia, using the pubic tubercle as a fulcrum

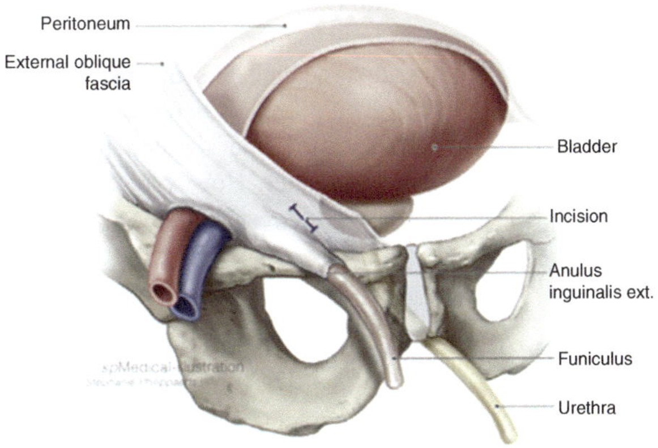

Fig. 8.5 External oblique fasciotomy medial to the spermatic cord [29]

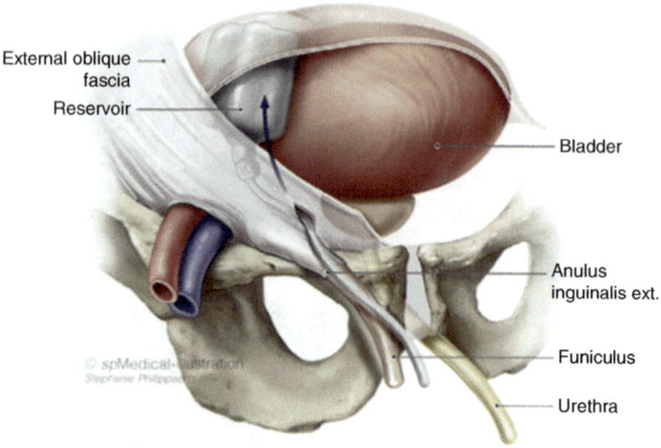

Fig. 8.6 Reservoir inserted through the external oblique fasciotomy after puncturing the transversalis fascia [29]

developed with index finger dissection. The reservoir is then inserted (Fig. 8.6). The medial incision allows direct visualization and protects the inguinal ring as it is not entered, decreasing the risk of inguinal hernias or damaging inguinal canal structures. This same incision can potentially increase risk of injury to the bladder because of the medial fasciotomy [29]; however, the bladder should always be drained prior to reservoir placement to prevent this.

A midline counter incision may also be made to develop the SOR (Fig. 8.7), similar to the incision used for the open retropubic radical prostatectomies. The tissue is dissected down until the anterior rectus fascia above the pubic symphysis is located. A small incision is made through the fascia and stay sutures are placed on each side. The rectus abdominis muscle is the spread gently with curved Mayo scissors or a right-angled clamp. Once transversalis fascia is palpated and seen, it is bluntly dissected and entered downward and laterally utilizing an index finger, clamp, or nasal speculum [28].

One idea to prevent injury adjacent structures during SOR reservoir placement is to preoperatively over distend and subsequently drain the bladder if retropubic scarring is suspected [22]. The intention is to detach the bladder wall from local scarring, forming a space to allow the surgeon to develop the SOR, decreasing the potential of injuring the bladder. However, the space is limited as the bladder is drained prior to developing the reservoir space [22].

Alternate Reservoir Placement

Many surgeons believe that if there has been any violation of the SOR, reservoir placement within the SOR should not be attempted due obliteration of this space and intra-peritonialization of the retropubic space [29, 30]. Due to the increasing amounts of radical pelvic surgery, alternate reservoir placement is becoming more in favor [25]. Over 90% of prosthetic surgeons believe an alternative reservoir placement is the safest option [30] as it limits visceral or vascular injury due to its limitation of violating fascial planes [12]. 80% of high-volume implanters believed

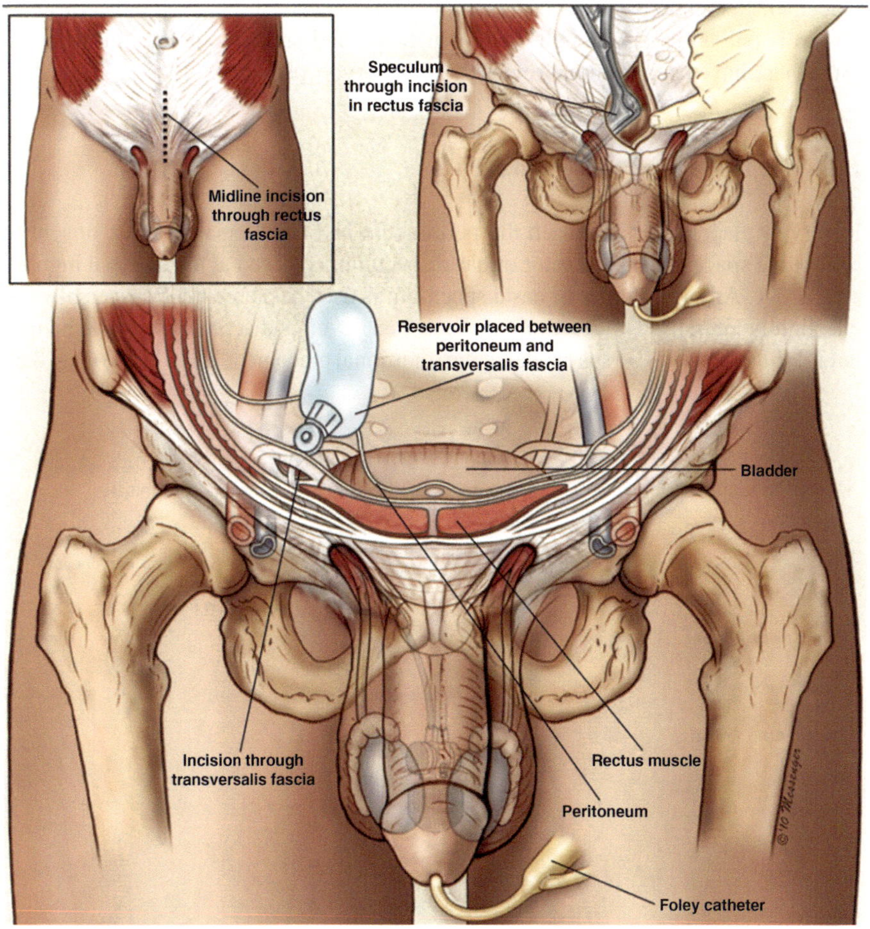

Fig. 8.7 Midline incision for reservoir placement in the SOR. Incise rectus fascia midline and split the rectus muscle. Once the pubic tubercle is felt midline, pass an index finger slightly lateral to feel transversalis fascia, piercing with either an index finger, clamp, or nasal speculum [28]

that reservoir placement into the SOR after RALP was more difficult, indicating that an alternative reservoir placement is beneficial to this patient population [30]. Originally, alternative reservoir placement was limited due to auto-inflation from high pressure being exerted on the reservoir [37]. However, this all changed in 2000, when Mentor introduced a lockout valve in their reservoir [31]. Then in 2002, Wilson et al. [32] published their 1-year follow-up after alternative reservoir placement using this type of reservoir.

The modern reservoirs currently available are the American Medical Systems' (AMS) spherical and Conceal™ Low-Profile reservoir and Coloplast's Cloverleaf reservoir. Both systems have a lockout valve to mitigate auto-inflation concerns. The lockout valve for AMS is located within their pump (AMS Momentary Squeeze™ pump). Whereas the lockout valve for Coloplast exists at the reservoir tubing junction, and also within the Coloplast Touch® pump [13]. As some alternative reservoir placement techniques place the reservoir more anteriorly, there is concern about reservoir palpability. Although 79% of patients and surgeons notice the reservoir [30], there have been minimal revisions for reservoir palpability [2, 33, 34].

Posterior to Transversalis Fascia (PTF)

Reservoir placement is between the peritoneum and transversalis fascia, not in the retropubic space [28]. A retractor or nasal speculum is placed at the external inguinal ring above. An index finger or nasal speculum is used to pierce the transversalis fascia slightly laterally. The reservoir space is then developed cephalad toward the ipsilateral shoulder [28] (versus caudal in the traditional placement in the SOR) (Fig. 8.8).

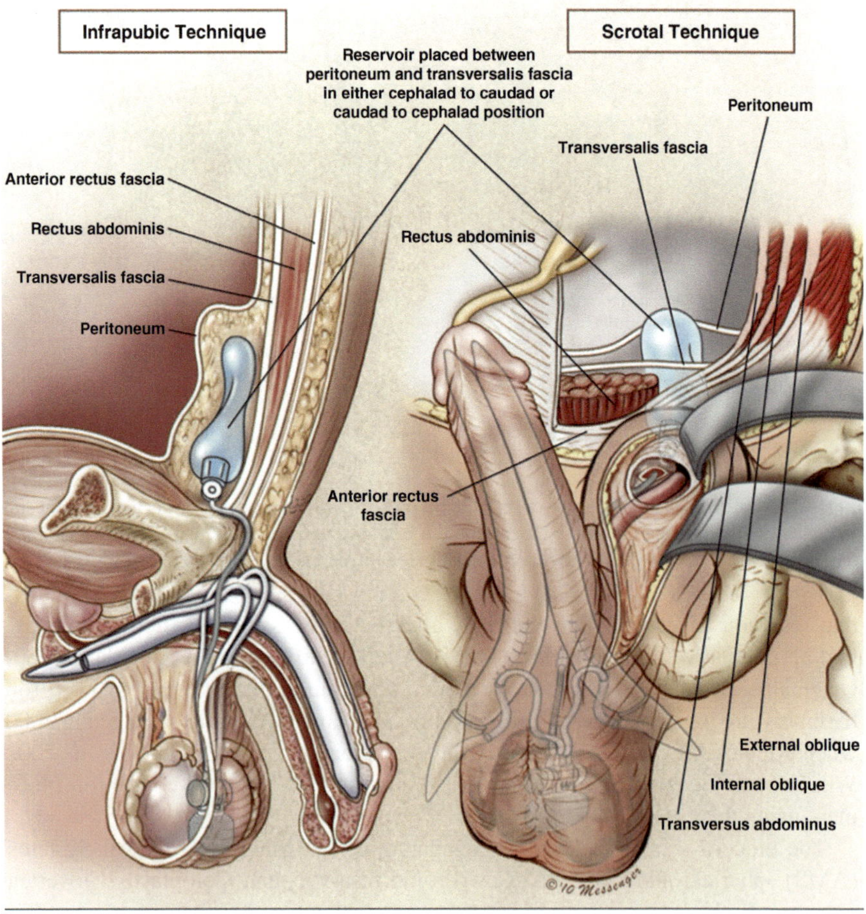

Fig. 8.8 PTF [28]

Anterior to the Transversalis Fascia (ATF)

For this approach, as described by Perito [35], placement of the reservoir is between the transversalis fascia posteriorly and rectus abdominis anteriorly. A retractor or nasal speculum is placed at the external inguinal ring above [35, 36]. Either an index finger or nasal speculum is placed above the transversalis fascia and driven upward and toward the ipsilateral shoulder to develop the reservoir space. If using the latter, the nasal speculum blades should be turned in an anterior-posterior orientation and spread to develop the reservoir space [25, 35] (Fig. 8.9). The reservoir must be pushed in a cephalad direction; if pushed posteriorly, there is risk of piercing the transversalis fascia; and if pushed laterally, the reservoir may be too superficial as the fascia becomes thinner laterally [35].

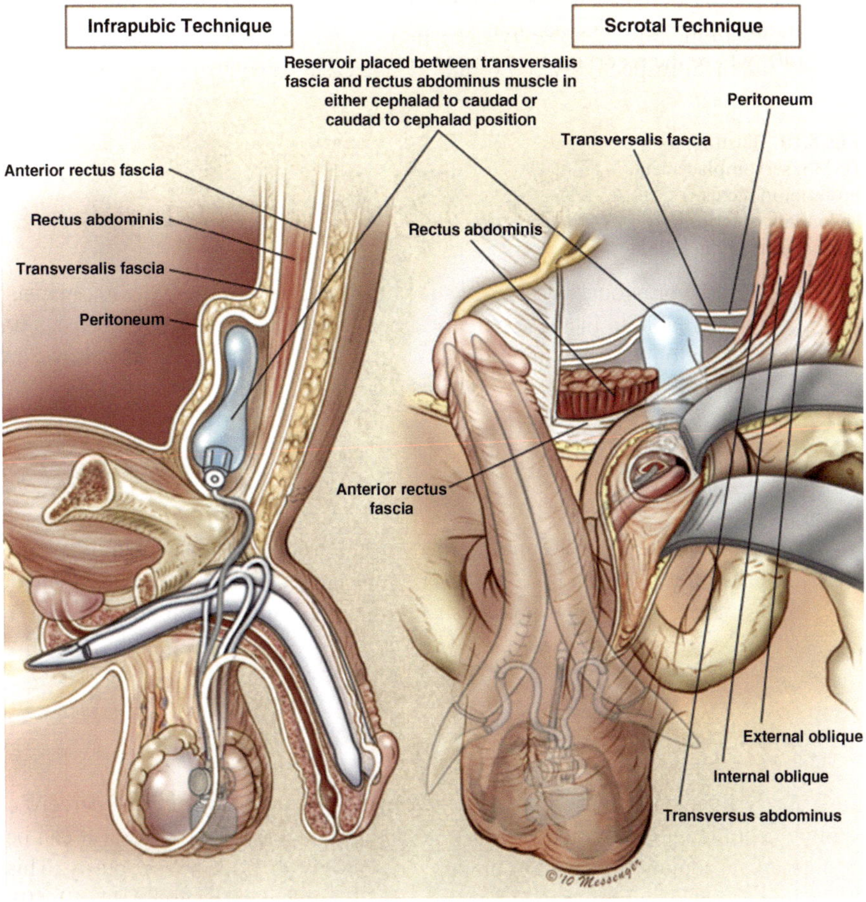

Fig. 8.9 ATF placement of reservoir [35]

High Submuscular (HSM)

Initially described by Morey et al. [34] in 2012, reservoir placement is more cephalolateral compared to the ATF (Fig. 8.10). The external ring is identified and using a small Deaver retractor, the ring is elevated anteriorly. Using an index finger, the submuscular space between transversus abdominis and transversalis fascia is developed. Once completed, the Deaver retractor is readjusted into this space, which allows retraction of the entire abdominal wall. The space is further developed using a 14 Brooks dilator toward the ipsilateral nipple with gentle, smooth, and constant pressure to avoid perforation through transversalis fascia or the peritoneum. If there is resistance, one should redirect dilation more anteriorly. The Foerster clamp is used to grasp the reservoir and advance it through the developed space. Once in position, the reservoir is filled to its maximum volume. This allows the reservoir to rid of folds that may form when advancing the reservoir. The reservoir volume is then adjusted to the desired volume. It may be readjusted if it is too inferior or lateral. Due to the transversalis being more delicate superiorly, unintentional placement in another/potential space may occur. This was demonstrated by Ziegelmann et al. [40] where the reservoir was placed between the internal and external oblique

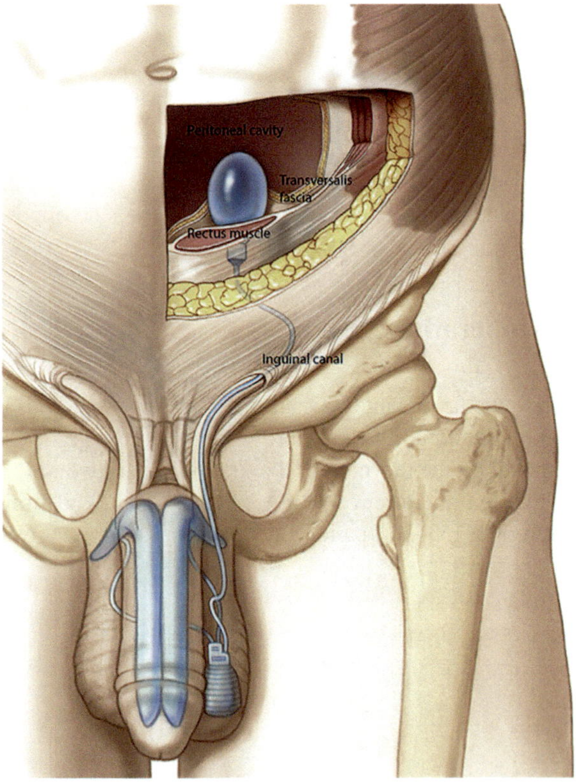

Fig. 8.10 Illustration of HSM reservoir placement, posterior to rectus abdominis, anterior to transversalis fascia [40]

(45%), in the retroperitoneum (10%), above the peritoneum (5%), and in the intraperitoneal space (5%). Prior to modifying the HSM technique, there were complications, including six reservoir herniations and one bowel obstruction due to intraperitoneal reservoir placement [34, 38]. Reservoir herniation may be prevented by placing a purse-string suture around the inguinal ring as published by Karpman et al. [33]. Baumgarten et al. further refined the technique for high submuscular reservoir placement with their five-step technique (FST) in 2014, noting an improvement in reservoir-related complications without visceral or vascular complications [38].

The FST utilizes the following steps: First, proper position and inguinal ring access is necessary. The second and third step develop the lower and high submuscular pocket, respectively. The fourth step allows the reservoir delivery ("fill and fine tune"). The fifth step is to confirm and connect the reservoir. Steps 1 and 5 remain the same as described above. The development of the high submuscular muscle differs slightly. The development of the lower two-thirds of the high submuscular pocket is performed by using digital dissection, initially with the index finger, followed by the middle finger. Development of the upper two-thirds of the high submuscular pocket is performed with a curved sponge stick, toward the ipsilateral nipple, spreading the clamp to separate the two muscle layers. By the end of these two steps, the reservoir pocket is at least 10 cm long. Rather than using a Foerster clamp, step 4 utilizes an angled sponge stick for reservoir delivery. The angled sponge stick has a smaller spread radius, allowing more controlled space dissection [38].

Trans-Fascial Placement of HSM

Kava et al. [41] first introduced this procedure for patients who have undergone RC. The anterior rectus sheath is exposed, and a Kelly clamp is used to pierce the fascia approximately 1 cm laterally from midline. A Kelly clamp is then used to spread laterally to further expose the rectus muscle. At this time, a retractor is placed superiorly under the anterior rectus fascia, and the rectus muscle is further divided until transversalis fascia is identified. The submuscular space is then developed above the transversalis fascia. The reservoir is placed under direct vision (versus ATF, HSM/FST). There were no intraoperative complications and no episodes of auto-inflation. However, post-implantation imaging was performed in ten patients. In seven patients, the reservoir was in correct position, one patient had reservoir herniation into the scrotum, and two patients had part of their reservoir in the lateral rectus muscle and posterior to the external oblique fascia. It was noted that in one of the latter scenarios, the reservoir was intentionally placed in this area due to extensive rectus muscle scarring from previous surgeries.

Intraperitoneal

Intraperitoneal placement of the reservoir remains controversial [42]. This was initially practiced in Germany without significant complications, with the main purpose of preventing auto-inflation, as no capsule forms around the intraperitoneal reservoir [9, 39, 43]. Mulcahy [14] points that if the reservoir is placed in the peritoneal cavity, it must be brought anteriorly against the pelvic wall without any excess tubing in order to prevent negative sequelae. Since redundant tubing can cause reservoir migration elsewhere within the abdominal cavity, the bowel may become entangled around it, could form adhesions, or could cause intussusception, consequently leading to bowel obstruction [14, 34, 45]. If adhesions form around the reservoir, pressure-induced ischemia on surrounding structures when the cylinders are fully deflated may occur [46–49]. Also, intraperitoneal reservoirs have the potential to cause erosion into adjacent bowel segments [14].

Epigastric

To avoid the pelvic area entirely, an epigastric location for reservoir placement was first introduced by Riemenschneider in 1981 [50]. This is achieved by making a left subcostal incision. The aponeurosis of the external oblique muscle is incised, with subsequent separation of the internal oblique and transversus abdominis, allowing the reservoir to be placed above omentum [50].

Lateral Retroperitoneal

This technique has been regularly utilized in patients with history of radical cystectomy with urinary diversion, radical prostatectomies, prior open pelvic surgery, and significant fibrosis from radiation therapy [13, 16, 19, 22]. Loh-Doyle et al. [16] published their reasoning and recommendations upon choosing the laterality, as this will be dictated by the patient's past surgical history and the type of urinary diversion they have. They recommend in patients with an ileal conduit, the opposite side of the stoma should be used (usually the left); however, if a neobladder is present, the right or left side may be utilized. A counter incision is made to minimize injury to the intestine or urinary diversion. This separate counter incision is 2 cm medial and 2 cm inferior to the anterior superior iliac spine (ASIS) and is extended 3 cm inferior and parallel to the inguinal crease [16]. After identifying the external oblique fascia, a 2 cm incision is made following the direction of the fibers. After stay sutures are placed, local anesthetic is injected, and muscle fibers are spread with either a tonsil or curved Mayo scissors until the transversalis fascia is identified. Finally, the retroperitoneal space is entered after the transversalis fascia is bluntly dissected [16].

There is concern that a second incision may increase operative time and post-op discomfort; however, it may save time due to surgical difficulty and potential surgical complications if attempting to develop reservoir space in the SOR [22].

Loh-Doyle et al. [16, 19] reports a single colonic injury in a patient with history of colon surgery, RC, and a catheterizable conduit diversion constructed by the right colon but reports no other injuries, including the subset of patients with history of radiation. Hartman et al. [22] had no intraoperative or postoperative complications with this technique.

Preperitoneal

Placement of the reservoir in the preperitoneal area was initially described in a patient with history of cystoprostatectomy with orthotopic Studer neobladder by Kim et al. [17]. In their publication, they report that placement in this space may be performed to minimize reservoir palpability and risk of injury to the neobladder. First, a vertical counter incision is made 2 fingerbreadths lateral to the umbilicus, and layers are dissected down until the anterior fascia is encountered. Afterward, an incision over the anterior rectus fascia is made, and the rectus muscle is mobilized within its sheath to access the posterior rectus sheath, incising the posterior rectus sheath as well. The transversalis fascia is entered, allowing entry into the preperitoneal space, visualizing yellow preperitoneal fat. The preperitoneal space is developed utilizing the index finger by sweeping circumferentially laterally and medially. A flat reservoir is preferred and is filled to amount needed for the cylinders. Both rectus fascias must be closed to prevent herniation.

Scrotal

Fein [51] described placement of the reservoir in the scrotum in 1986. Since its introduction, no other reports of scrotal insertion has been documented. In his publication, the patient had a history of RC with urinary diversion, abdominal vascular surgery, and multiple intestinal surgeries, making SOR or abdominal wall reservoir placement difficult. At the time of reservoir placement, a left orchiectomy had to be performed. The left spermatic cord was covered with lining of the scrotum and the reservoir tubing was brought to the right hemiscrotum, reuniting with the right scrotal pump tubing. An angulated Quick-Connect was used to connect the reservoir and pump tubing. The angle connector was then covered to assure it would not rub against the reservoir or pump.

Subcutaneous

Specifically preserved for obese or severely obese patients, subcutaneous reservoir placement (SRP) is a promising option as adipose tissue decreases palpability of the reservoir [52, 53]. Obesity continues to increase in prevalence; from 1999–2000 through 2017–2018, age-adjusted obesity (BMI $\geq$30) and severe obesity (BMI $\geq$40) had increased from 30.5% to 42.4% and 4.7–9.2%, respectively [54]. In this population, it may be difficult to develop a reservoir space in the previously discussed techniques due to their abdominal size, increasing in difficulty if the patient has had previous abdominal or pelvic surgeries [53]. Necessary criteria for SRP are a thick abdominal wall adipose layer that can conceal the reservoir and difficulty developing reservoir space in the SOR or other abdominal wall layers [53]. If the patient is planning future weight loss, or experiences weight loss after SRP, the reservoir will become palpable and may require surgical intervention if bothersome [53].

In 2016, Garber et al. [53] published their surgical approach for subcutaneous placement of IPP reservoirs as well as their results. When the SRP is placed through a penoscrotal approach, it should be directed medially, and the neck of the tunnel is approximated with absorbable suture. If the SRP is placed infrapubically, Scarpa's and Camper's fascia are approximately in multilayered fashion anterior to the reservoir with absorbable suture. If not performed, reservoir herniation may occur [9]. In their published series, none of the eight patients who underwent SRP complained of palpability, and on physical exam, they showed no evidence of a palpable, visible, or herniated reservoir. SRP utilized in this study was a 125 cc Coloplast Cloverleaf and filled to the minimal amount of saline required for cylinder inflation, allowing the reservoir to remain flat in the subcutaneous space [53].

Reservoir Removal

If the initial operative is not available, our institution recommends obtaining cross-sectional imaging (CT or MRI) for further evaluation of all the components, and surgical planning. This was further emphasized by Reddy et al. [7] when evaluating patients with multiple surgeries and suspected retained reservoirs. This assists with assessing the location of the reservoir and its proximity to vital organs or vessels. Although the Coloplast and the AMS reservoirs are made or covered in inert materials, Bioflex [55] and an outer silicone and an inner Parylene [56], respectively, an inflammatory response can still occur, making removal difficult [57, 58]. If necessary, a second incision may be utilized.

Traditional Reservoir Removal

Due to risk of bladder, vascular, or bowel injury with removal of the reservoir, the "drain and retain" approach is becoming more accepted for traditional reservoirs, whenever an infection is not present or suspected. If the reservoir removal is due to malfunction, and it is not easily accessible or firmly adherent to surrounding structures, the "drain and retain" approach may be utilized. This eliminates operative time and the risk of trauma or injury to the pelvic structures from adhesiolysis [59]. There is some limited literature that has shown that retained reservoirs do not increase subsequent infections and have limited risk of erosion [59, 60]. Cefalu et al. [59] compared infections rates in retained reservoirs versus virgin IPP and AUS placements with no difference in infection rate. A 2012 comprehensive review by Levine et al. [1] demonstrated that retained reservoirs may become infected, herniate, obstruct bowel, or erode into the bladder or bowel. In 2020, a literature review performed by Reddy et al. [7] concluded that despite there being a low risk for complications after leaving behind a reservoir, serious complications can arise. In their publication, they emphasized about making sure that the patient is aware when a reservoir is not removed.

If the reservoir is not removed, it is important to cut the tubing as proximal as possible on traction, allowing proximal migration of the tubing when it is released [61]. Prior to release, all the reservoir fluid within it must be drained. It is recommended to cap or tie off the tubing to occlude the tubing to prevent fluid from entering the reservoir. The distal tie will also allow for easier intraoperative location of the reservoir if removal is necessitated later. To prevent reservoir relocation, a 2-0 Ethibond may be used to suture the tissue over the pubic bone and through an additional tubing connector and then connected to the remaining reservoir tubing as described by Yang et al. [44] (Fig. 8.11). Our institution has removed defunctionalized purulent filled uncapped reservoirs, indicating the importance of capping or occluding the tubing if the reservoir will not be removed (Fig. 8.12). Many

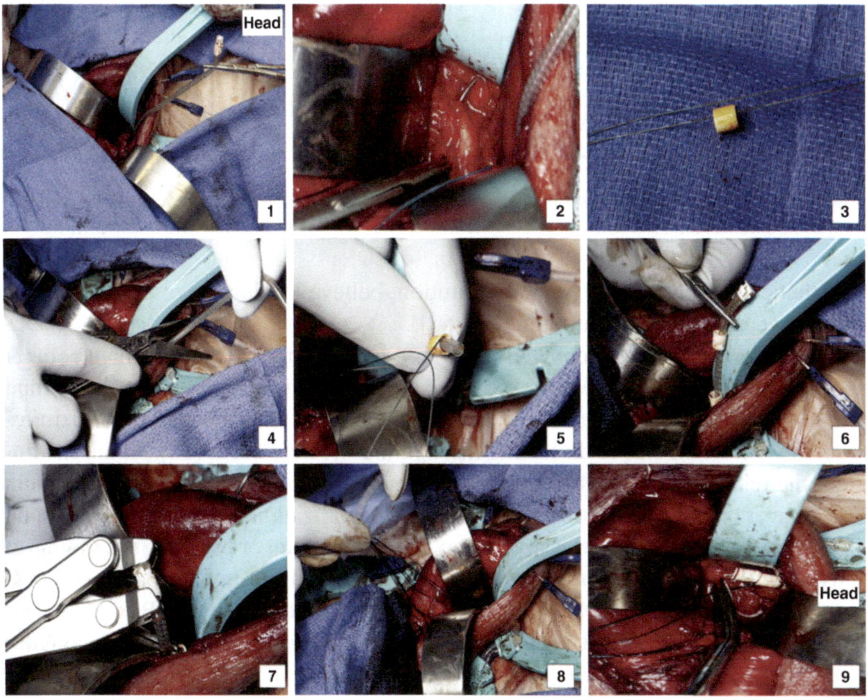

Fig. 8.11 THALIA technique for retained reservoir. (1) exposure of tubing and the left pubic tubercle with retraction of spermatic cord medially, (2) hitch bite of overlying pubic tubercle tissue with 2-0 ethibond, (3) Lasso through extra tubing connector with ethibond stitch, (4) complete drainage of old reservoir and tubing cut without letting it retract away, (5) put collar through remaining tubing, (6) place second collar and cap, (7) crimp two plugs together, (8) tie ethibond suture down, (9) complete technique to prevent retained reservoir migration [44]

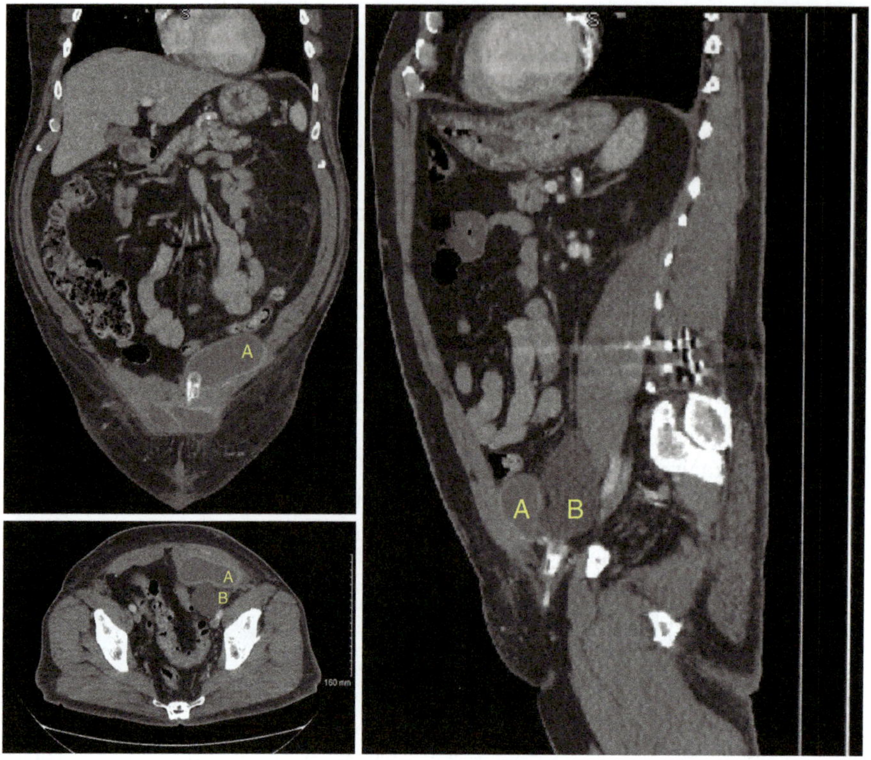

Fig. 8.12 Cross-sectional imaging of (*A*) defunctionalized infected retained reservoir and (*B*) functioning reservoir

prosthetic surgeons, including our institution, believe leaving the reservoir in place can only cause issues in the future [62, 63].

The reservoir may be removed through a penoscrotal, infrapubic, or a counter incision made over the reservoir. If there is dense fibrotic scar tissue, it is important not to be too aggressive, as tissue may be adhered to the surrounding structures. Excessive bleeding due to dissecting through muscle may occur [13]. At our institution, the reservoir tubing is followed superiorly, and a combination of S retractors and Deaver retractors are utilized to maximize visualization. The tubing is pulled on firm tension, however, not too strongly to avoid damaging or breaking the tubing. If tension is too excessive, the tubing may tear, ultimately losing the pathway to the reservoir. As described by Clavell et al. [57], while on tension, long Bovie tip electrocautery is used to dissect the tissue anterior to the tubing, following it proximally (Fig. 8.13). This is performed until the thick portion of the tubing, distal to the lockout valve, is palpated and visualized (Fig. 8.14). An index finger is then placed through the inguinal ring to identify the reservoir, feeling for any adhesions or dense

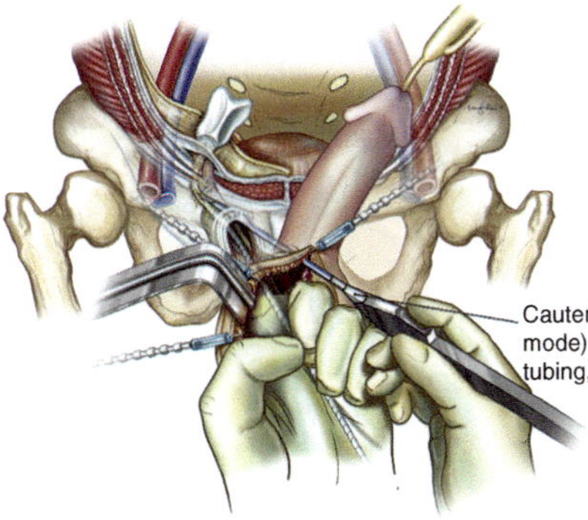

Fig. 8.13 Utilizing long tip bovie electrocautery to follow reservoir tubing proximally [57]

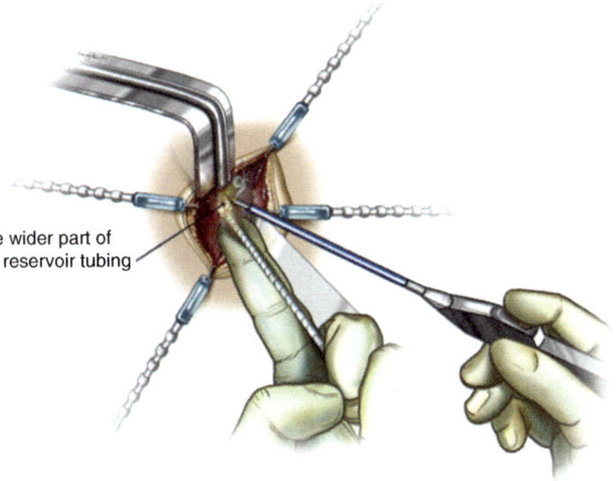

Fig. 8.14 Utilizing long tip bovie electrocautery to follow reservoir tubing until the wider part of the tubing is encountered [57]

scar tissue. If present, the adhesions are gently freed with an index finger. The reservoir tubing is then cut proximal to the connector. Drainage of the reservoir is achieved with a disposable Yankauer and angiocatheter attached to a 60 cc syringe. The reservoir is then removed and placed off the field. A Kelly clamp may also be used to grab the thick portion of the reservoir tubing for removal (Fig. 8.15) [57], while also utilizing Bovie electrocautery to free the reservoir capsule (Fig. 8.16).

If a counter incision is necessary due to noted adherence, the index finger is used to follow the tubing superiorly, while applying anterior pressure toward the abdominal wall. An incision is made over the pubic bone while feeling the index finger from below. The tubing is then regrasped from the new incision and may be followed into the retropubic space [57]. It is our belief that an experienced surgeon knows when to employ a counter incision without unnecessary delay to help minimize the risk or prevent any surgical complication.

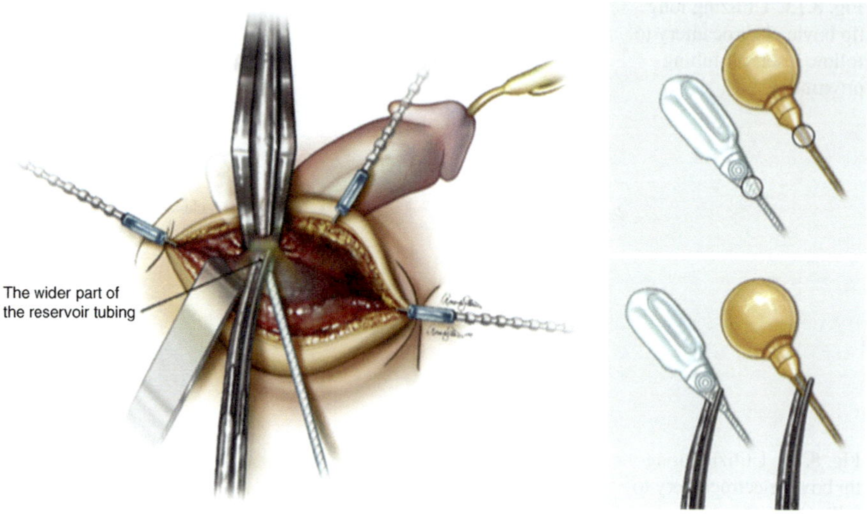

Fig. 8.15 Kelly clamp grasping the wide part of the reservoir tubing for removal [57]

Fig. 8.16 Kelly clamp grasping the wide part of the reservoir tubing for removal, with utilization of bovie electrocautery to free the reservoir capsule

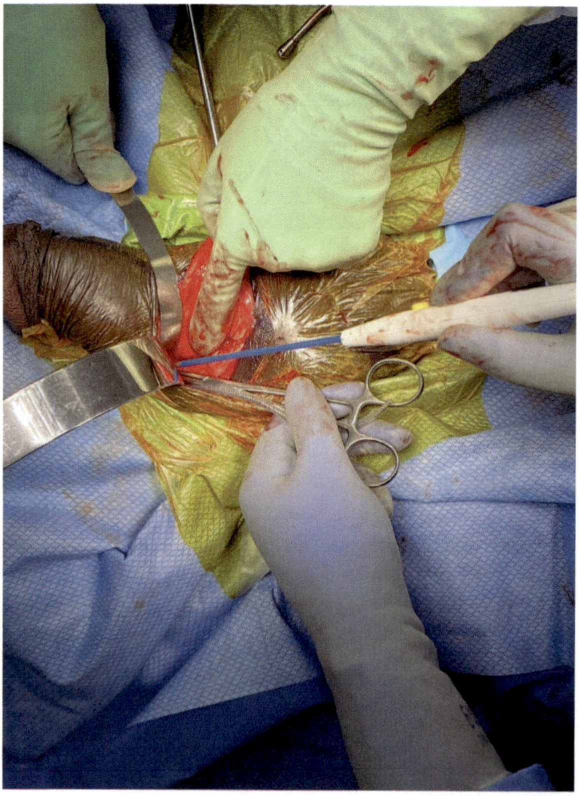

Alternative Reservoir Removal

It is hypothesized that if the reservoir is placed above the transversalis fascia, the continuous plane allows for easy delivery [61]. If the reservoir is placed HSM, delivery of the reservoir requires a longer distance [61]. Firm traction on the tubing will often deliver the reservoir. However, as inadvertent placement of the any ectopic/alternative placed reservoir is possible, and the reservoir may not be easily removed. If this occurs, a counter incision may be performed over the reservoir with palpation or intraoperative ultrasound [12, 61, 64]. Use of laparoscopic instruments may also prove useful [65]. If the reservoir is intraperitoneal, an exploratory laparotomy is indicated.

Intraoperative Injuries

Although rare, bladder, vascular, and/or bowel injuries can be devastating complications. The following will discuss how to minimize injury to these injuries, recognize, and manage them properly. Placing the patient in Trendelenburg can decrease injuries to these structures, since it increases the distance from the bladder, pelvic vessels, bowel, and to the SOR (if present), and decompresses the iliac vein [8, 11].

Bladder Injuries

To decrease bladder injury intraoperatively, it is highly recommended to always drain the bladder prior to developing the reservoir space, especially when the reservoir will be placed in the SOR. At our institution, a Foley catheter is placed prior to our incision and is drained with a disposable plastic Yankauer, which is then discarded from the field. When transversalis fascia is pierced and there is concern for bladder injury, the Foley catheter is drained and/or irrigated to assess for gross hematuria. Hematuria is concerning for bladder injury [6, 11, 24]. To further evaluate, pack the SOR and fill the bladder with methylene blue and saline [66]. If there is dye visible on the packing, bladder injury is confirmed [66]. Identifying the location of the injury will require cystoscopy or surgical exploration via separate suprapubic incision [24, 57, 66, 67] (Fig. 8.17).

If the same reservoir or reservoir space is utilizing during revision surgery, it is important to note that the previous capsule is likely contracted [11]. The capsule is contracted and thickened due to fluid leak [68]. To minimize formation of a contracted capsule, it is imperative to perform revision surgery as soon as fluid leakage is noted [67]. Inflation with new saline in the old or new reservoir may cause the capsule to rupture, resulting in laceration of the bladder [11]. If there is noted resistance with reservoir filling, the old or previous reservoir space should not be utilized

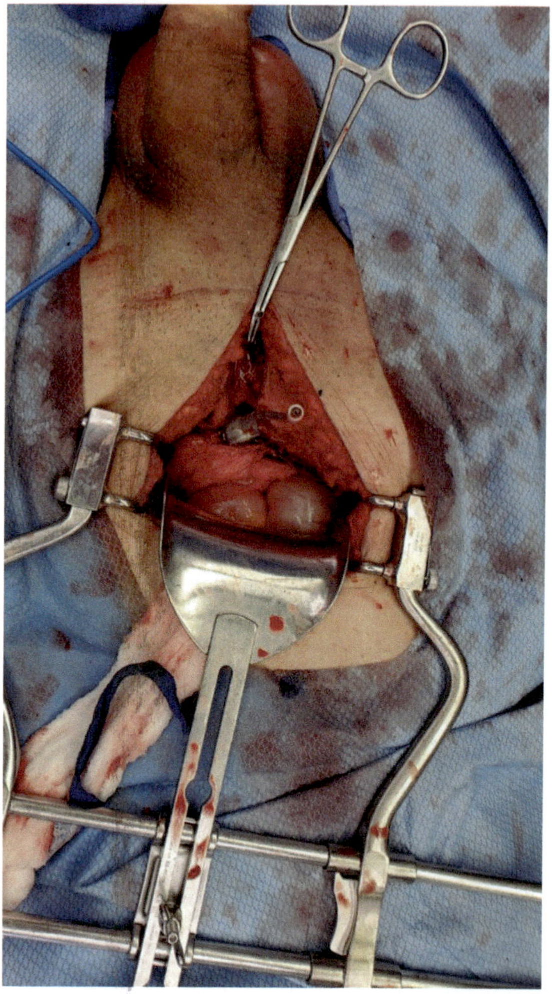

Fig. 8.17 Suprapubic incision to explore an unnoticed bladder injury with reservoir placement, which eventually eroded/migrated intravesically

[68]. If a popping noise is heard during inflation, there should be immediate concern for capsule rupture [67, 68]. Reports have shown that the capsule may burst or break into the lumen of the adjacent bladder [68]. Gross hematuria may be noted immediately or postoperatively [11, 24, 26, 68, 69].

The reservoir may be noted intravesically by inadvertent placement or erosion into the bladder [11, 46, 62, 67, 70, 71]. Unintentional placement may occur if the reservoir was placed in the traditional manner, with a patient history of prior pelvic surgery, radiation or if the bladder is not drained prior to development of the SOR [62, 70] (Fig. 8.17). Erosion may occur immediately or remotely [52]. Symptoms may present as lower urinary tract symptoms, dysuria, pyuria, hematuria, or recurrent urinary tract infection [1, 24, 70, 63]. In some cases, a retained reservoir may erode into the bladder and completely heal off [63, 71], and if present in the bladder

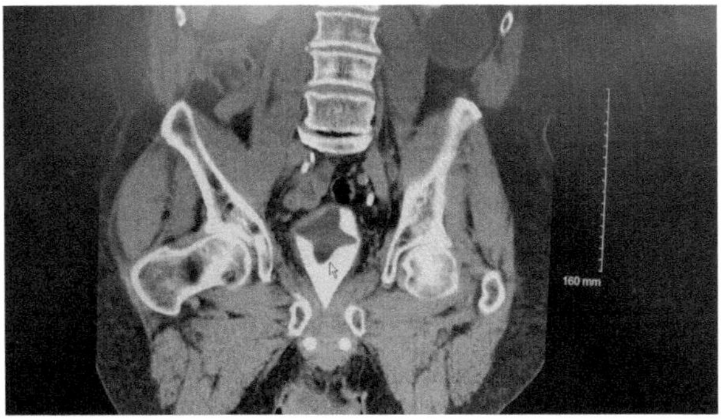

Fig. 8.18 CT confirming intravesical Coloplast cloverleaf reservoir

for a prolonged period of time, may present as a bladder calculus [72]. Intravesical reservoirs are confirmed with cystoscopy, cystogram, and/or cross-sectional imaging (Fig. 8.18). The defect size may help differentiate timing of the injury, since wide or small can likely represent an acute or chronic injury, respectively [68].

In all bladder injury or intravesical reservoir scenarios, the bladder is repaired in two layers with absorbable suture. The surgeon may choose to abort or proceed with reservoir placement on the contralateral side of bladder injury; regardless of the approach, the bladder should be repaired [70]. The Foley catheter may be placed while the cystotomy heals; however, there may be increased risk for IPP infection or cylinder erosion. Therefore, suprapubic tube catheter placement at the time of repair may be beneficial [63, 67].

Vascular Injury

Injury to the pelvic vessels have been documented, including avulsion of branches of the external iliac vein and venous compression syndrome [1, 6, 11, 73]. When developing the SOR, it is important not to perform digital or sharp dissection laterally [1]. It is imperative to stay medial when entering the external inguinal ring, as well as when placing an S retractor in the space. If any resistance is noted during creating the reservoir space, a new position should be considered.

A vascular tear may occur with placement or removal of a virgin or revision implant reservoir, respectively [1], as the iliac vessels may be as close as 1 inch lateral to the SOR reservoir [8, 13]. The most common lacerated vessel is an external iliac vein branch (inferior epigastric vein, external superficial vein, pudendal vein or cremasteric vein) [1]. If the injury is a small venous branch, it may be ligated [1] or a combination of fibrinogenic products and direct pressure may stop the bleeding [3, 11]. However, if there is noticeable blood filling the surgical field, there is obvious concern for injury of a major vessel, adequate visualization must be achieved quickly. If the primary incision does not provide adequate exposure and visualization, a secondary incision must be made, whether a midline or Gibson incision [1, 11], while maintaining pressure on the vessels to prevent further bleeding [1]. If pressure is not sufficient to stop the hemorrhage, it is crucial to have proximal and distal control of the major vessel with Satinsky clamps [74]. Vascular surgery must be consulted, and if not available, the major vessel may be closed primary with running 4-0 or 5-0 Prolene [29, 74]. Immediate type and cross should be drawn if not performed pre-operatively [11], and the anesthesia team needs to be aware of blood loss to plan transfusion of blood products if necessary.

External iliac vessel compression may occur if placement of the reservoir is too lateral and/or if the reservoir is overfilled [1, 11, 73, 76, 77]. Presentation occurs with subsequent ipsilateral lower extremity edema [1, 73]. This can be avoided by creating an adequate reservoir space anterolaterally to the bladder, thus avoiding the lateral pelvic vessels [1]. Compression of the iliac vein can be life-threatening, as it may cause a prethrombotic state, forming venous clots and may subsequently lead to pulmonary embolism [1, 73]. If the former occurs, an inferior vena cava filter may be placed to prevent this sequela [14, 73]. Compression of the iliac artery can cause limb ischemia [73]. The IPP should be fully activated to decrease vascular compression if surgery is delayed [73], but ultimately, the reservoir must be repositioned whether more medially, on the contralateral side, or in an alternative position [75].

Bowel Injuries

Direct bowel injury is extremely rare. Bowel injury may occur if a reservoir or its tubing erodes into the bowel and ultimately cause a bowel obstruction [46, 47]. The bowel segment near a newly placed reservoir is usually small intestine, where contents are sterile [14]. Colon in the pelvis is normally behind the bladder and too posterior to be near the location of the reservoir [14]. However, as previously stated, anatomy is altered after any pelvic surgery. Postoperative ileus or mechanical obstruction may demonstrate a bowel perforation or erosion [14, 24, 45]. If suspected, cross-sectional imaging is necessary [24]. If only obstruction is noted due to compression, the reservoir may be removed without bowel resection [45]. If there is noted injury, whether ischemia or erosion, the bowel incorporated must be resected, either anastomosing the two bowel segments or creating an ostomy [14, 47], depending on the general surgeon.

Reservoirs eroding into neobladders and ileal conduits require a different approach. Chronic compression in adjunction with pelvic and reservoir adhesions are a major contributing factor for this occurrence [48]. Both scenarios require removal of the eroded reservoir and repair of appropriate urinary diversion [48, 49, 75]. Tran et al. [48] reported one case where it was noted that the reservoir's pseudocapsule and neobladder were nearly fused around a 1–2 cm defect. To repair this, the pseudocapsule surrounding the defect was excised and a plane was developed to separate the pseudocapsule from the neobladder, allowing closure with absorbable sutures. In another case report by Godiwalla et al. [49], a patient presented with left flank pain due to an eroded reservoir into an ileal conduit, compressing the left ureteroileal anastomosis. A suprapubic incision was made and was dissected down until reservoir tubing was encountered. The tubing was cut and endoscopically, the reservoir was removed through the ileal conduit. Even after removal, the patient had persistent left flank pain and loopogram confirmed persistent obstruction, and a new ileal conduit had to be created. Kelly et al. [77] reported on a patient that presented with asymptomatic stone disease, and upon CT imaging, was found to have a calcified reservoir within their ileocecal continent urinary reservoir. Pouchoscopy confirmed the urinary reservoir. The patient subsequently underwent exploratory laparotomy for removal of the reservoir.

Conclusion

The reservoir placement of an IPP can be the most stressful portion of the procedure, especially if placed in the SOR as it may come in proximity of the bladder, bowel, and iliac vessels. Numerous techniques have been created and modified to prevent injuries to these structures, including alternative reservoir placement. It is of utmost importance for the implanting surgeon to be aware of all the different techniques used for reservoir placement, since the patient's history, anatomy, and previous surgery can dictate the approach to be used in order to decrease the risks for visceral complications. Advanced anatomic knowledge of all the pelvic and abdominal structures and its spatial relationship are required to safely place the reservoir in every patient and provide the best outcomes. A wise surgeon once said, "the surgeon that says that he/she has no complications, is a liar or not operating enough". This is because despite everything, complications can occur. Being able to prevent and recognize these complications intraoperatively and postoperatively will help yield the best patient outcomes.

References

1. Levine LA, Hoeh, MP. Review of penile prosthetic reservoir: complications and presentation of a modified reservoir placement technique. J Sex Med. 2012;9:2759–2769; Gupta NK, Ring J, Trost L, et al. The penoscrotal surgical approach for inflatable penile prosthesis placement. Transl Androl Urol. 2017;6(4):628–38. https://doi.org/10.21037/tau.2017.07.32
2. Stember DS, Garber BB, Perito PE. Outcomes of abdominal wall reservoir placement in inflatable penile prosthesis implantation: a safe and efficacious alternative to the space of Retzius. J Sex Med. 2014;11:605.
3. Scherzer B, Dick B, Gabrielson A, et al. Penile prosthesis complications: planning, prevention, and decision making. Sex med Rev. 2019;7:349–59.
4. Ziegelmann M, Kohler TS, Bailey GC, et al. Surgical selection and counseling. Transl Androl Urol. 2017;6:509.
5. Mulcahy JJ. Current approach to the treatment of penile implant infections. Ther Adv Urol. 2010;2:69–75.

6. Sharma D, Smith R. Troubleshooting intraoperative complications of penile prosthesis placement. Transl Androl Urol. 2017;6(Suppl 5):S892–7. https://doi.org/10.21037/tau.2017.07.13.
7. Reddy AG, Tsambarlis PN, Akula KP, et al. Retained reservoirs of inflatable penile prosthesis: a systematic review of literature. Sex Med Rev. 2020;8:355–63.
8. Henry G, Hsaio W, Karpman E, et al. A guide for inflatable penile prosthesis reservoir placement: pertinent anatomical measurements of the retropubic space. J Sex Med. 2014;11:273–8.
9. Sadeghi-Nejard H, Munarriz R, Shah N. Intra-abdominal reservoir placement during penile prosthesis surgery in post-robotically assisted laparoscopic radical prostatectomy patients: a case report and practical considerations. J Sex Med. 2011;8:1547–50. https://doi.org/10.1111/j.1743-6109.2011.02229.x.
10. Lowrance WT, Eastham JA, Savage C, et al. Contemporary open and robotic radical prostatectomy practice patterns among urologists in the United States. J Urol. 2012;187:2087.
11. Yang DY, Kohler TS. Damage control considerations during IPP surgery. Curr Urol Rep. 2019;20:10. https://doi.org/10.1007/s11934-019-0872-x.
12. Hudak S. Reservoir placement considerations during inflatable penile prosthesis surgery. Curr Urol Rep. 2019;20:8.
13. Mellon M, Mulcahy J. Surgery for erectile dysfunction. In: Partin A, Peters C, Dmonchowski R, et al., editors. Campbell Walsh Wein urology. 12th ed. Philadelphia: Elsevier Inc.; 2020. p. 1582–99.
14. Mulcahy JJ. The prevention and management of noninfectious complications of penile implants. Sex Med Rev. 2015;3:203–13.
15. Loh-Doyle J. Penile implant considerations in the bladder cancer survivor. Curr Urol Rep. 2019;20:7.
16. Loh-Doyle J, Patil MB, Sawkar H, et al. 3 pieces inflatable penile prosthesis placement following radical cystoprostatectomy and urinary diversion: technique and outcomes. J Sex Med. 2018;15:907–13.
17. Kim JK, Cho MC, Ku JH, et al. Preperitoneal placement of an inflatable penile prosthesis reservoir for postoperative erectile dysfunction after radical cystoprostatectomy with orthotopic neobladder. Investig Clin Urol. 2016;57:364–6.
18. Stone HB, Coleman CN, Anscher MS, et al. Effects of radiation on normal tissue: consequences and mechanisms. Lancet Oncol. 2003;4:529–36.
19. Loh-Doyle J, Patil MB, Nakhoda Z, et al. Three pieces inflatable penile prosthesis placement following pelvic radiation: technical considerations and contemporary outcomes. J Sex Med. 2013;15:1049–54.
20. Golan R, Patel NA, Sun T, et al. Impact of pelvic radiation therapy on inflatable penile prosthesis reoperation rates. J Sex Med. 2018;15:1653–8.
21. Kakaei F, Nikeghbalian S, Malekhosseini SA. Kidney transplantation techniques. In: Current issues and future direction in kidney transplantation. IntechOpen; 2013.
22. Hartman RJ, Helfand BT, McVary KT. Outcomes of lateral retroperitoneal reservoir placement of three-piece penile prosthesis in patients following radical prostatectomy. Int J Impot Res. 2010;22:279–83.
23. Scott FB, Bradley WE, Timm GW. Management of erectile impotence. Use of implantable inflatable prosthesis. Urology. 1973;2:80–2.
24. Langston JP, Muneer A, Garaffa G, et al. Complications of penile prosthesis surgery. In: Prosthetic surgery in urology. Cham: Springer; 2016. p. 223–34. https://doi.org/10.1007/978-3-319-13859-6_19.
25. Langston JP, Muneer A, Ralph D. Penile prosthesis surgery. In: Prosthetic surgery in urology. Cham: Springer. p. 203–21. https://doi.org/10.1007/978-3-319-13859-6_18.
26. Gupta JK, Ring J, Trost L, et al. The penoscrotal surgical approach for inflatable penile prosthesis placement. Transl Androl Urol. 2017;6(4):628–38.
27. Capoccia EM, Phelps JN, Levine LA. Modified inflatable penile prosthesis reservoir placement into space of retzius: comparing outcomes in men with or without prior pelvic surgery. J Sex Med. 2017;14:968–73.

28. Perito PE, WIlson SK. Traditional (retroperitoneal) and abdominal wall (ectopic) reservoir placement. J Sex Med. 2011;8:656–9.
29. Mykoniatis I, Osmonov D, van Renterghem K. A modified surgical technique for reservoir placement during inflatable penile prosthesis implantation. Sex Med. 2020;8:378–82. https://doi.org/10.1016.j.esxm.2020.04.004
30. Karpman E, Sadeghi-Nejad H, Henry G, et al. Current opinions on alternative reservoir placement for inflatable penile prosthesis among members of the sexual medicine society of North America. J Sex Med. 2013;10:2115–20.
31. Levine LA, Becher E, Bella A, et al. Penile prosthesis surgery: current recommendations from the international consultation on sexual medicine. J Sex Med. 2016;13:489–518.
32. Wilson SK, Henry GD, Delk JR Jr, et al. The Mentor alpha I penile prosthesis with reservoir lock-out valve: effective prevention of auto-inflation with improved capability for ectopic reservoir placement. J Urol. 2002;168:1475–8.
33. Karpman E, Brant WO, Kansas B. Reservoir alternate surgical implantation technique: preliminary outcomes of initial PROPPER study of low profile or spherical reservoir implantation in submuscular location or traditional prevesical space. J Urol. 2015;193:239–44.
34. Morey AF, Cefalu CA, Hudak SJ. High submuscular placement of urologic prosthetic balloons and reservoirs via transscrotal approach. J Sex Med. 2013;10:603–10.
35. Perito P. Ectopic reservoir placement – no longer in the space of retzius. J Sex Med. 2011;8:2395–8.
36. Vollstedt A, Gross M, Antonini G, et al. The infrapubic surgical approach for inflatable penile prosthesis placement. Transl Androl Urol. 2017;6(4):620–7. https://doi.org/10.21037/tau.2017.07.14.
37. Gross MS, Stember DS, Garber BB, et al. A retrospective analysis of risk factors for IPP reservoir entry into the peritoneum after abdominal wall placement. Int J Impot Res. 2017;00:1–4.
38. Baumgarten AS, Kavoussi M, VanDyke ME, et al. Avoiding deep pelvic complications using a "five-step" technique for high submuscular placement of inflatable penile prosthesis reservoirs. BJU Int. 2020;126(4):457–63.
39. Pagliara TJ, Viers BR, Scott J, et al. Extended experience with high submuscular placement of urological prosthetic balloons and reservoirs: refined technique for optimal outcomes. Urol Pract. 2018;5:293–8.
40. Ziegelmann MJ, Viers BR, Lomas DJ. Ectopic penile prosthesis reservoir placement: an anatomic cadaver model of the high submuscular technique. J Sex Med. 2016;13(9):1425–31.
41. Kava BR, Lopategui DM, Levine A, et al. Trans-fascial placement of a high, submuscular reservoir in patients following radical cystectomy: safety, efficacy, and predictability of final reservoir location verified with abdominal imaging. J Sex Med. 2019;16:338–45.
42. Clavell-Hernandez J, Trost L, Kohler T, et al. Emerging complications following alternative reservoir placement during inflatable penile prosthesis placement: a 5-year multi-institutional experience. J Urol. 2019;201:581–6.
43. Perito P, Wilson S. The history of nontraditional or ectopic placement of reservoirs in prosthetic urology. Sex Med Rev. 2016;4:190–3.
44. Yang D, Heslop DH, Houlihan M. The tubing, hitch and lasso, intussusception anchor (THALIA) technique: a novel approach to fixate the penile implant reservoir. J Sex Med. 2021;18:224–9.
45. Johnson M, Johnson F. Small bowel obstruction from a displaced penile prosthesis reservoir: case report and review of the literature. Br J Med Med Res. 2014;4(22):4025–9.
46. Leach GE, Shapiro CE, Hadley R, et al. Erosion of inflatable penile prosthesis reservoir into bladder and bowel. J Urol. 1984;131:1177–8.
47. Singh I, Godec CJ. Asynchronous erosion of inflatable penile prosthesis into small and large bowel. J Urol. 1992;147:709–10.
48. Tran CN, Boncher N, Montague DK, et al. Erosion of inflatable penile prosthesis reservoir into neobladder. J Sex Med. 2013;10:2343–6.
49. Godiwalla SY, Beres J, Jacobs S. Erosion of an inflatable penile prosthesis reservoir into an ileal conduit. J Urol. 1987;137:297–8.

50. Riemenschneider HR. Epigastric placement of reservoir for inflatable penile prosthesis. Urology. 1981;27:79–81.
51. Fein RL. Scrotal placement of reservoir of inflatable penile prosthesis. Urology. 1986;28(5):430–1.
52. Smaldone M, Cannon G, Benoit M. Subcutaneous reservoir placement during penile prosthesis implantation. Can J Urol. 2006;13:3351–2.
53. Garber BB, Bickell M. Subcutaneous placement of inflatable penile prosthesis reservoirs. Urology. 2016;88:93–6.
54. Hales CM, Carroll MD, Fryar CD, Ogden CL. Prevalence of obesity and severe obesity among adults: United States, 2017–2018. NCHS Data Brief, no 360. Hyattsville: National Center for Health Statistics; 2020.
55. Coloplast titan bioflex infographic. 2017. Available at: https://www.coloplastmd.com/wp-content/uploads/2017/06/PM00479-Titan-Bioflex-Infographic.pdf.
56. AMS Conceal low profile reservoir. 2017. Available at: https://www.amsmenshealth.com/content/dam/bostonscientific/uro-wh/general/ams/Resources/MH-402906-AA_Conceal%20Physician%20Sell%20Sheet-final.pdf.
57. Clavell-Hernandez J, Aly SG, Wang R, et al. Penile prosthesis reservoir removal: surgical description and patient outcomes. J Sex Med. 2019;16:146–52.
58. Thirumavalavan N, Gross M, Munarriz R. Techniques of ectopic reservoir placement and their pitfalls. J Sex Med. 2017;14:1451–4.
59. Cefalu CA, Deng Xiangrong D, Zhao LC, et al. Safety of the "drain and retain" option for defunctionalized urologic prosthetic balloons and reservoirs during artificial urinary sphincter and inflatable penile prosthesis revision surgery: 5-year experience. Urology. 2013;82:1436–9.
60. Rajpurkar A, Bianco FF, Al-Omar O, et al. Fate of the retained reservoir after replacement of 3-piece penile prosthesis. J Urol. 2004;172:664–6.
61. Kavoussi M, Bhanvadia RR, VanDyke ME, et al. Explanation of high submuscular reservoirs: safety and practical considerations. J Sex Med. 2020;17:2488–94.
62. Garber BB, Morris A. Intravesical penile implant reservoir: case report, literature review, and strategies for prevention. Int J Impot Res. 2012;25:41–4. https://doi.org/10.1038/ijir.2012.31.
63. Munoz JJ, Ellsworth PI. The retained penile prosthesis reservoir: a risk. Urology. 2000;55:949viii–49ix.
64. Baten E, Vandewalle T, van Renterghem K. Stretch due to penile prosthesis reservoir migration. Urol Case Rep. 2016;5:20–1.
65. Staller AL, Chang CM, Wagenheim GN, et al. A novel approach for removal of an inflatable penile prosthesis reservoir using laparoscopic instruments. Asian J Androl. 2017;19:132–4.
66. Pathak RA, Broderick GA. Inflatable penile prosthesis implantation. In: Smith JA, Howards SS, Preminger GM, et al., editors. Hinman's atlas of urologic surgery. 4th ed. Philadelphia: Elsevier, Inc.; 2018. p. 890–9.
67. Fitch WP, Roddy T. Erosion of inflatable penile prosthesis reservoir into bladder. J Urol. 1986;136:1080.
68. Kramer AC, Chason J, Kusakabe A. Report of two cases of bladder perforation caused by reservoir of inflatable penile prosthesis. J Sex Med. 2009;6:2064–7.
69. Eldefrawy A, Kava BR. An unusual complication during inflatable penile prosthesis implantation. Urology. 2010;76:847.
70. Reznicek DG, Bryson R, Kramer AC. Review: alternative placement of penile prosthesis reservoir and AUS pressure regulating balloon. Sex Med Rev. 2015;3:48–55.
71. Brusky J, Dikranin A, Aboseif S. Retrieval of inflatable penile prosthesis reservoir from the bladder. Int J Impot Res. 2005;17:302–3.
72. Dupont MC, Hochman HI. Erosion of an inflatable penile prosthesis reservoir into the bladder, presenting as bladder calculi. J Urol. 1988;139:367–8. (not printed, cited in #62)
73. Deho F, Henry GD, Marone EM, et al. Severe vascular complication after implantation of a three-pieces inflatable penile prosthesis. J Sex Med. 2008;5:2956–9.

74. Kobayashi LM, Costantini TW, Hamel MG, et al. Abdominal vascular trauma. Trauma Surg Acute Care Open. 2016;1:e000015. https://doi.org/10.1136/tsaco-2016-000015.
75. Brison D, Ilbeigi P, Sadeghi-Nejad. Reservoir repositioning and successful thrombectomy for deep venous thrombosis secondary to compression of pelvic veins by an inflatable penile prosthesis reservoir. J Sex Med. 2007;4:1185–7.
76. DaJusta DG, Bianco FJ, Ogle A, et al. Deep venous thrombosis due to compression of external iliac vein by the penile prosthesis reservoir. Urology. 2003;61(2):462v–3v.
77. Kelly MP, Franciose RJ, Lloyd GL. Successful salvage reimplantation of penile prosthesis after reservoir erosion into continent urinary reservoir. Urology. 2012;80(5):e63–4.

Chapter 9
The Role of Penile Lengthening Procedures at the Time of Penile Implant Surgery

Mirko Preto and Giulio Garaffa

Introduction

Different medical conditions causing erectile dysfunction (ED) can also lead to a significant loss in penile size. These conditions include ED post radical prostatectomy, radiation and androgen deprivation therapy for prostate cancer, and corporeal fibrosis. The most common causes of corporeal fibrosis are ischemic priapism, penile trauma, previous penile surgery, previous removal of infected PP, and Peyronie's disease (PD) [1–14]. Among PD affected patients, up to 80% report subjective loss of penile length [15]. Quality of life and sexual satisfaction are severely affected by loss of penile length and girth [2, 8, 16].

Penile prosthesis implantation currently represents the gold standard treatment for refractory end-stage ED. Penile prosthesis implantation tends to be associated with good results in terms of patients' satisfaction rates [17]. However, when stratifying patients' satisfaction rates based on the etiology of ED, it is apparent that patients who have lost more penile size are those who are the less satisfied with the outcome of surgery [18–20]. Therefore, patients who have experienced significant loss of penile length should be offered some form of penile length restoration in combination with PP implantation in order to improve satisfaction rates postoperatively [9]. Over the course of the last few decades, several complex techniques aiming to restore penile length loss and to treat end-stage ED have been described.

M. Preto (✉)
A.O.U. Città della Salute e della Scienza di Torino – Clinica Urologica – Presidio Molinette, Torino, Italy

G. Garaffa
The Institute of Urology, University College London Hospitals, London, UK

E. P. Miranda, J. P. Mulhall (eds.), *Penile Implant Surgery*,
https://doi.org/10.1007/978-3-030-82363-4_9

These surgical techniques could be subdivided in to three main groups:

1. Penile prosthesis implantation techniques that maximize corporal length
2. Surgical techniques that determine a real penile shaft lengthening
3. Surgical techniques that improved perceived penile length

Lengthening procedures and concomitant PP implantation (PPI) can be associated with high complication rates, as they are technically quite difficult to perform [21]. Regardless of the type of procedure performed, it is paramount to adequately counsel the patient regarding the realistic outcomes to expect from surgery and the possible risks and benefits associated with each type of technique to allow the patient to take an informed decision on what type of treatment to undergo and to set realistic expectations [21–23].

PPI Procedures That Maximize Corporal Length

Cavernosal Sparing PPI Insertion without Dilatation

The standard PP implantation techniques include the use of Hegar or Brooks dilators to create an intracavernosal tunnel for prosthetic cylinders insertion. Residual erectile tissue could be severely damaged after the dilation leading to higher postoperative pain and potentially to a more extensive cavernosal fibrosis around the cylinders [24].

To minimize disruption of residual cavernosal tissue and to maintain spontaneous penile tumescence during sexual stimulation, various authors have proposed a cavernosal sparing approach that does not involve aggressive corporeal dilatation [25].

In particular, Moncada et al. reported their experience in PP implantation without performing standard corporal dilation. In their series, they measured directly the length of the cavernous body with a Furlow introducer and then inserted the PP. This cavernosal sparing approach has allowed to reduce operative times, as it avoids the unnecessary sequential progressive dilatation of the corpora, to limit postoperative pain, to obtain an higher penile engorgement compared to the standard approach, and to possibly to preserve a longer penile shaft (after 6 months penile length was 10 cm in corporal preservation group vs 8 cm in standard approach group; $p = 0.05$) [24].

Similarly, Zaazaa et al. have reported their results with minimal dilation of the corpora with an 8 FR dilator prior to malleable PP implantation. In his series, patients in the cavernosal sparing group reported significantly higher residual penile tumescence during arousal (89% vs 15%) and a greater postoperative penile girth (11 cm vs 10 cm; $p < 0.001$) compared to patients implanted with the standard dilation approach 1 month after surgery [25].

Subcoronal Incision with Circumferential Penile Degloving

Some conditions that lead to an end-stage ED can be associated with a reduced elasticity of cavernous tissue and overlying tunica albuginea (TA), Buck's fascia, and dartos, thus preventing the physiological expansion of the penis in erection. For this reason, some authors suggest that the classic penoscrotal or infrapubic approaches could lead to less satisfactory results in terms of penile length preservation and/or restoration [1, 9]. Weinberg et al. have therefore proposed a subcoronal approach to proceed with PP in patients where a degree of penile fibrosis is suspected [26].

The subcoronal access therefore allows to perform a complete penile degloving and to eliminate all adhesions between dartos and the underlying Buck's fascia, freeing the shaft completely and allowing it to expand to its maximum capacity before proceeding with the measurement of the corpora cavernosa. This approach has proven effective in determining a penile length gain compared to the infrapubic approach [9, 15, 26–30].

Surgical Techniques That Determine a Real Penile Shaft Lengthening

Penile Prosthesis Implantation with Simultaneous Tunica Albuginea (TA) Incisions

These techniques are particularly indicated in case of acquired penile curvature due to PD and end-stage ED. They aim to restore original penile length by resolving the curvature or deformity at the same time as the PP implantation [31]. In case of penile curvature, additional maneuvers such as Wilson' modeling or Perito's scratch technique [32, 33] allow to safely correct penile curvature in the majority of patients but they do not allow to restore the length lost, mainly because the corporeal measurements are carried out when the contracture is still present. Since postoperative satisfaction rates are strongly associated with penile size, it was hence necessary to develop more effective lengthening strategies that could be offered to patients who were complaining of significant penile size loss. Several procedures reporting relaxing TA incisions and concomitant PPI have been introduced to partially restore the size lost due to underlying pathology with excellent functional outcomes [9].

The first series of patients who underwent TA incision, saphenous vein grafting, and soft silicone penile prosthesis placement was reported by Austoni in 2005. After a mean follow-up period of 5 years, average penile length gain was 1.3 cm (0.8–2 cm), and 95% of patients were fully satisfied with the outcome of surgery [34]. In 2013 Zucchi et al. proposed a modification of Austoni procedure introducing a dovetail TA incision together with bovine pericardial grafting and a soft 8 Fr prosthesis implantation. In their series, an average penile length gain of 2 cm (1.2–2.3 cm) was reported at 6 months follow-up [35]. Although all patients reported an initial temporary partial loss of glans sensitivity, only 17% reported glans paresthesia at the 6-month follow-up visit. Perovic and Djinovic reported similar rates of patient satisfaction (95%) after TA incision, grafting with porcine dermal matrix, and PP implantation. After this procedure, a mean penile length gain of 3.2 cm (2–4.5 cm) was recorded [36]. Recently, the PICS technique (TA incision with self-adhesive collagen fleece grafting and concomitant PP implantation) has been proposed by Hatzichristodoulou et al. [37]. The authors suggested to oversize the length of prosthetic cylinders as penile length will increase after PICS but he did not provide any data about penile length gain after PICS procedure. Still following the principle of TA incisions, Fernandez-Pasqual et al. have described a series of 43 patients that have undergone a multiple incision technique (MIT) and contextual collagen fleece grafting and PP implantation to restore penile length. After a mean follow-up of 21 months, the mean penile length gain reported was 2.5 cm (1–5 cm), and glans hypoesthesia was reported in only 2% of cases 6 months, postoperatively. Overall satisfaction and length restoration satisfaction rates were 90% and 82%, respectively [38].

PPI and Circumferential Grafting or Sliding Technique

Firstly proposed by Rigaud and Berger in 1995 [39], then applied by Sansalone [40] et al., and finally modified by Egydio [41], the circular relaxing incision and concomitant PP implantation may be indicated in case of severe penile shortening and end-stage ED. In this technique the penis is completely disassembled in order to expose the TA extensively enough to allow the surgeon to perform a circumferential incision of the corpora minimizing the insult to the underlying corpora cavernosa. The limiting step to the penile size restoration is the length of the neurovascular bundle, which by definition, does not stretch [9, 41]. The circular incision technique determines one large gap which needs to be grafted to restore TA continuity, improve axial stability, and reduce the risk of hematoma formation [41]. Sansalone et al. reported an average length gain of 2.8 cm (2.2–4.5 cm) with glans hypesthesia in 20% of cases after a median follow-up of 22 months. Overall, 90% of patients were satisfied with cosmetic and functional outcome of surgery [40]. Similarly, after a median follow-up of 18 months, Egydio reported an average increase in length of 3.6 cm (2.5 cm) and patient satisfaction rates of 95.2% in a series of patients that have undergone a modified technique [41].

The sliding technique (ST) firstly described by Rolle in 2012 and then reported on a larger multicentric series in 2016 represented a further modification of the circumferential grafting procedure. In the ST, the TA incision is split into two hemi-circumferential incisions, one ventral and proximal and one dorsal and distal on the corpora cavernosa. These two incisions are connected with two longitudinal lateral incisions which allow the penile shaft to slide when the glans penis is pulled away. Shaft sliding will create two TA defects (one ventral and one dorsal), which will be then grafted prior to PP implantation. The sliding technique resulted in an average length gain of 3.2 cm (2.5–4 cm) and overall 95% of patients were satisfied with their postoperative penile length. Reported complications after ST were penile hematoma in 28.5% of cases, glans hypoesthesia in 3.8%, and PP infection in 7% [30, 42].

The ST was modified by Egydio and Kuehhas, who described the MoST (modified sliding technique). The MoST allows surgeons to avoid the need for grafting materials after simultaneous PPI placement since the TA defects are small enough to avoid the herniation of the cylinders. Hemostasis is achieved with adequate watertight closure of Buck's fascia and with adequate postoperative compression. Like the classical ST, MoST mean length gain was 3.1 cm (2–7 cm), and temporary glans sensitivity reduction was reported in 10% of cases [43].

Penile Prosthesis Implantation and MUST

In 2018, Egydio proposed a further modification of the ST and MoST, the multiple ST (MuST). In this modification, the author proposed the use of multiple pairs of transversal and longitudinal small relaxing incisions, resulting in multiple sliding sections, to restore penile length and girth [9, 44]. Since the TA defects are numerous but small, grafting of the defects is not necessary. Penile length gain reported in MuST series was 3.1 cm (2–7 cm). One case of glans necrosis occurred in a patients where both the neuromuscular bundle and the urethra had been elevated, 5% of cases experienced temporary glans numbness, while 25% of patients developed a small hematoma that resolved spontaneously [44].

Egydio's Tunica Expansion Procedure (TEP): The Last Innovation in Lengthening Strategies

A subsequent evolution of the MUST technique is TEP strategy. The tunica expansion technique allows to restore length and girth lost through an innovative geometrical and mathematical pattern of multiple, staggered, small tunical incisions [45]. The procedure is carried out through a subcoronal incision and complete penile devolving that allow a complete exposure of the corpora cavernosa. The dorsal neurovascular bundle is elevated through two paraurethral incisions. The urethra is left in place since it is not a limiting factor for penile length restoration, due to its intrinsic elasticity, and in order to minimize disruption to the glans blood supply [46, 47]. Egydio also described the intraoperative use of papaverine or alprostadil to stimulate bundle perfusion and minimize glans ischemia [45, 47]. Once the tunica albuginea is released, staggered multiple small incisions are performed in alternate rows, perpendicular to the desired direction of expansion according to the mesh expansion theory [48]. The length, angle, and number of incisions are adjusted according to the type of deformity keeping in mind that larger incisions are associated with an increased risk of tissue healing delay, indentations, and prosthetic cylinder extrusion. By increasing the number of incision, creating smaller defects, a better expansion rate could be achieved without impairing structural resistance of the tunica albuginea and with no need for grafts. The next step consists in a subtunical cavernosal tissue sparing dilation technique and prosthetic cylinders implantation adjusted to the limit of urethra and dorsal neurovascular bundle. Distally, cylinders are fixed to the tunica in order to prevent malpositioning. Glanspexy is performed in case of floppy glans after PP implantation. Buck's fascia is then used to cover the multiple tunical defects and the penis revolved. To support the healing process of the tunica albuginea and to maintain the results obtained in terms of lengthening and girth increase, the cylinders are kept partially inflated for about a month. In his series of 416 patients, Egydio reported a mean penile length gain of 3.3 cm (range 2–6) with good satisfaction outcomes assessed with the IIEF and EDITS questionnaires. Temporary alteration of glans sensitivity and anorgasmia were reported in respectively 3.8% and 7% of cases and resolves spontaneously after 4 months.

Surgical Techniques That Improved Perceived Penile Length

In addition to the previously described surgical strategies, several adjuvant maneuvers are also available to increase perceived penile length. These techniques can be offered in isolation or in combination with the aforementioned techniques to improve the aesthetic outcomes and patients' satisfaction after PP implantation.

Prepubic V-Y Plasty

The V-Y plasty is the most common procedure to produce advancement of penile skin, and it is often indicated in case of previous penile skin loss. It consists in an inverted V-shaped skin flap from the suprapubic area that is then sutured in a Y fashion [49].

Suspensory Ligament Division

Suspensory ligament release is an adjuvant maneuver that can improve perceived penile flaccid length without a real lengthening of the corpora cavernosa. It can be performed in conjunction with suprapubic lipectomy or with a V-Y plasty. This procedure can also be performed at the time of PP implantation surgery [1, 49, 50]. To avoid ligament reattachment and potential penile retraction, some authors have proposed to place a silicone buffer as a spacer (between the pubic bone and the corpora) [49]. Suspensory ligament release is simple, safe, and effective. In particular, Berger et al. reported satisfaction rates of 93%, a median flaccid penile length gain of 2.4 cm (1.4–3.2 cm), and a median erect penile length increase of 1.7 cm (1.1–2.3 cm) [51–53].

Apronectomy or Suprapubic Lipectomy

As previously introduced, the suspensory ligament release can be associated with suprapubic lipectomy especially in the case of buried penis [54]. The combination of these two procedures allows exposing the penile shaft as much as possible, leading to significant cosmetic and functional improvements [55]. This procedure can be performed in isolation NR in combination with the PPI [50, 56]. In severe cases, more complex reconstructions such as panniculectomy, Z-plasty, and split-thickness skin grafting of the penile shaft are required to obtain an adequate exposure of the penis [57, 58].

Ventral Phalloplasty (VP) or Scrotoplasty

Ventral phalloplasty is indicated to correct webbed penis and can be performed in isolation or in combination with PP surgery [57]. Ventral phalloplasty consists in a wedge-like skin excision of the penoscrotal web and the creation of a new more proximal penoscrotal junction. Ventral phalloplasty has shown to be safe and effective, as an increased perceived penile length was reported in 86% of cases and satisfaction rate reached 98% [59–61].

Discussion and Conclusion

In case of severe penile shortening and end-stage ED, patients are better served with PP implantation and concomitant size restoration strategies to improve functional and satisfaction outcomes. These strategies are not without risks since neurovascular mobilization could lead to glans hypoesthesia or to glans necrosis in up to 20% and 2% of cases, respectively [9]. Since using these techniques, PP infection rates are slightly higher (about 7%) than in traditional penile prosthesis implantation in virgin cases [9, 43, 44, 62], an adequate preoperative counseling addressing risks, benefits, and realistic outcomes of each procedure is mandatory in order to allow the patient to make an informed decision and to manage unrealistic expectations [22].

Preoperative evaluation of penile length and associated deformities is useful for planning the right lengthening procedure and surgical strategy.

Despite the higher risk of complications when compared to PP traditional implantation in a virgin case, available data reported high level of postoperative satisfaction among patients who underwent lengthening procedures (range 77%–100%). On the other hand, there is a high rate of heterogeneity among the different studies in terms of sample size, lack of control groups, pre- and postoperative evaluation tools, and timing that makes difficult to compare different results and to obtain a definitive conclusion about each surgical strategy.

References

1. Tran H, Goldfarb R, Ackerman A, Valenzuela RJ. Penile lengthening, girth, and size preservation at the time of penile prosthesis insertion. Sex Med Rev. 2017;5(3):403–12.
2. Smith JF, Walsh TJ, Conti SL, et al. Risk factors for emotional and relationship problems in Peyronie's disease. J Sex Med. 2008;5:2179–84.
3. Egydio PH, Kuehhas FE. Penile lengthening and widening without grafting according to a modified "sliding" technique. BJU Int. 2015;116:965–72.
4. Dillon BE, Chama NB, Honig SC. Penile size and penile enlargement surgery: a review. Int J Impot Res. 2008;20:519–29.
5. Haliloglu A, Baltaci S, Yaman O. Penile length changes in men treated with androgen suppression plus radiation therapy for local or locally advanced prostate cancer. J Urol. 2007;177:128–30.
6. Park KK, Lee SH, Chung BH. The effects of long-term androgen deprivation therapy on penile length in patients with prostate cancer: a single-center, prospective, open-label, observational study. J Sex Med. 2011;8:3214–9.
7. Whelan P, Levine LA. Additional procedures performed at time of penile prosthesis implantation: a review of current literature. Int J Impot Res. 2020;32(1):89–98.
8. Kueronya V, Miernik A, Stupar S, et al. International multi-centre psychometric evaluation of patient-reported outcome data for the treatment of Peyronie's disease. BJU Int. 2015;115(5):822–8.
9. Gaffney CD, Pagano MJ, Weinberg AC, et al. Lengthening strategies for Peyronie's disease. Transl Androl Urol. 2016;5(3):351–62.
10. Reddy AG, Alzweri LM, Gabrielson AT, et al. Role of penile prosthesis in priapism: a review. World J Mens Health. 2018;36(1):4–14.
11. Munding MD, Wessells HB, Dalkin BL. Pilot study of changes in stretched penile length 3 months after radical retropubic prostatectomy. Urology. 2001;58(4):567–9.
12. Akin Y, Sahiner IF, Usta MF. The impact of diabetes mellitus on penile length in men undergoing inflatable penile prosthesis implantation. Turk J Urol. 2013;39:161–4.
13. Kadono Y, Machioka K, Nakashima K, et al. Changes in penile length after radical prostatectomy: investigation of the underlying anatomical mechanism. BJU Int. 2017;120:293–9.
14. Frey A, Pederson C, Lindberg H, et al. Prevalence and predicting factors for commonly neglected sexual side effects to external-beam radiation therapy for prostate cancer. J Sex Med. 2017;14:558–65.
15. Deveci S, Martin D, Parker M, et al. Penile length alterations following penile prosthesis surgery. Eur Urol. 2007;51:1128–31.
16. Lever J, Frederick DA, Peplau LA. Does size matter? Men's and women's views on penis size across the lifespan. Psychol Men Masc. 2006;7:129–43.
17. Montorsi F, Rigatti P, Carmignani G, et al. AMS three-piece inflatable implants for erectile dysfunction: a long-term multi-institutional study in 200 consecutive patients. Eur Urol. 2000;37:50.
18. Wang R, Howard GE, Hoang A, et al. Prospective and long-term evaluation of erect penile length obtained with inflatable penile prosthesis to that induced by intracavernosal injection. Asian J Androl. 2009;11:411–5.
19. Osterberg EC, Maganty A, Ramasamy R, et al. Pharmacologically induced erect penile length and stretched penile length are both good predictors of post-inflatable prosthesis penile length. Int J Impot Res. 2014;26:128–31.
20. Sellers T, Dineen M, Salem EA, et al. Vacuum preparation, optimization of cylinder length and postoperative daily inflation reduces complaints of shortened penile length following implantation of inflatable penile prosthesis. Adv Sex Med. 2013;3:14–8.
21. Barrett-harlow B, Clavell-hernandez J, Wang R. New developments in surgical treatment for penile size preservation in Peyronie's disease. Sex Med Rev. 2019;7:156–66.

22. Hatzichristodoulou G, Osmonov D, Kübler H, Hellstrom WJG, Yafi FA. Contemporary review of grafting techniques for the surgical treatment of Peyronie's disease. Sex Med Rev. 2017;5:544–52.
23. Hatzichristodoulou G. Grafting techniques for Peyronie's disease. Transl Androl Urol. 2016;5:334–41.
24. Moncada I, Martinez-Salamanca JI, Jara J, et al. Inflatable penile prosthesis implantation without corporeal dilation: a cavernous tissue sparing technique. J Urol. 2010;183:1123–6.
25. Zaazaa A, Mostafa T. Spontaneous penile tumescence by sparing cavernous tissue in the course of malleable penile prosthesis implantation. J Sex Med. 2019;16:474–8.
26. Weinberg AC, Pagano MJ, Deibert CM, et al. Sub-coronal inflatable penile prosthesis placement with modified no-touch technique: a step-by-step approach with outcomes. J Sex Med. 2016;13:270–6.
27. Yavuz U, Ciftci S, Ustuner M, et al. Surgical treatment of erectile dysfunction and Peyronie's disease using malleable prosthesis. Urol J. 2015;12:2428–33.
28. Safarinejad MR. Re: Surgical treatment of erectile dysfunction and Peyronie's disease using malleable prosthesis. Urol J. 2015;12:2434–5.
29. Yafi FA, Hatzichristodoulou G, DeLay KJ, et al. Review of management options for patients with atypical Peyronie's disease. Sex Med Rev. 2017;5:211–21.
30. Rolle L, Falcone M, Ceruti C, et al. A prospective multicentric international study on the surgical outcomes and patients' satisfaction rates of the "sliding" technique for end-stage Peyronie's disease with severe shortening of the penis and erectile dysfunction. BJU Int. 2016;117:814–20.
31. Do F, Matter C, Kozacioglu Z, Degirmenci T, Gunlusoy B, Kara C, et al. Effect of tunical defect size after Peyronie's plaque excision on postoperative erectile. Urology. 2012;80:1051–5.
32. Wilson SK, Delk JR. A new treatment for Peyronie's disease: modeling the penis over an inflatable penile prosthesis. J Urol. 1994;152:1121–3.
33. Perito P, Wilson SK. The Peyronie's plaque "scratch": an adjunct to modeling. J Sex Med. 2013;10:1194–7.
34. Austoni E, Colombo F, Romanò AL, Guarneri A, Kartalas Gou-mas I, Cazzaniga A. Soft prosthesis implant and relaxing albugineal incision with saphenous grafting for surgical therapy of Peyronie's disease: a 5-year experience and long-term follow-up on 145 operated patients. Eur Urol. 2005;47:223–9.
35. Zucchi A, Silvani M, Pecoraro S. Corporoplasty with small soft axial prostheses (VIRILIS I®) and bovine pericardial graft (HYDRIX®) in Peyronie's disease. Asian J Androl. 2013;15:275–9.
36. Perovic SV, Djinovic RP. Current surgical management of severe Peyronie's disease. Arch Esp Urol. 2010;63(9):755–70.
37. Hatzichristodoulou G. The PICS technique: a novel approach for residual curvature correction during penile prosthesis implantation in patients with severe Peyronie's disease using the collagen fleece TachoSil. J Sex Med. 2018;15:416–21.
38. Fernández-Pascual E, Gonzalez-García FJ, Rodríguez-Monsalve M, et al. Surgical technique for complex cases of Peyronie's disease with implantation of penile prosthesis, multiple corporeal incisions, and grafting with collagen fleece. J Sex Med. 2019;16(2):323–32.
39. Rigaud G, Berger RE. Corrective procedures for penile shortening due to Peyronie's disease. J Urol. 1995;153:368–70.
40. Sansalone S, Garaffa G, Djinovic R, Egydio PH, Vespasiani P, Miano R, et al. Simultaneous penile lengthening and penile prosthesis implantation in patients with Peyronie's disease, refractory erectile dysfunction, and severe penile shortening. J Sex Med. 2012;9:316–21.
41. Egydio PH, Kuehhas FE, Sansalone S. Penile length and girth restoration in severe Peyronie's disease using circular and longitudinal grafting. BJU Int. 2013;111(4 Pt B):E213–9.
42. Rolle L, Ceruti C, Timpano M, Sedigh O, Destefanis P, Galletto E, et al. A new, innovative, lengthening surgical procedure for Peyronie's disease by penile prosthesis implantation with double dorsal-ventral patch graft: the "sliding technique". J Sex Med. 2012;9:2389–95.

43. Egydio PH, Kuehhas FE, Valenzuela RJ. Modified Sliding Technique (MoST) for penile lengthening with insertion of inflatable penile prosthesis. J Sex Med. 2015;12(5):1100–4.
44. Egydio PH, Kuehhas FE. The Multiple-Slit Technique (MUST) for penile length and girth restoration. J Sex Med. 2018;15(2):261–9.
45. Egydio PH. An innovative strategy for non-grafting penile enlargement: a novel paradigm for tunica expansion procedures [published online ahead of print, 2020 Jul 4]. J Sex Med. 2020:S1743-6095(20)30646-9.
46. García Gómez B, Romero Otero J, Díez Sicilia L, Jiménez Alcaide E, García-Cruz E, Rodríguez AA. Ischemic gangrene of the glans following penile prosthesis implantation. Case Rep Urol. 2013;323574:2013.
47. Wilson SK, Mora-Estaves C, Egydio P, Ralph D, Habous M, Love C, et al. Glans necrosis following penile prosthesis implantation: prevention and treatment suggestions. Urology. 2017;107:1448.
48. Vandeput JJ, Tanner JC, Boswick J. Implementation of parameters in the expansion ratio of mesh skin grafts. Plast Reconstr Surg. 1997;100:653–6.
49. Srinivas B, Vasan S, Mohammed S. Penile lengthening procedure with V-Y advancement flap and an interposing silicone sheath: a novel methodology. Indian J Urol. 2012;28:340–2.
50. Baumgarten AS, Beilan JA, Shah BB, et al. Suprapubic fat pad excision with simultaneous placement of inflatable penile prosthesis. J Sex Med. 2019;16:333–7.
51. Li CY, Kayes O, Kell PD, et al. Penile suspensory ligament division for penile augmentation: indications and results. Eur Urol. 2006;49:729–33.
52. Shaeer O, Shaeer K, El-Sebaie A. Minimizing the losses in penile lengthening: "V-Y half-skin half-fat advancement flap" and "T-closure" combined with severing the suspensory ligament. J Sex Med. 2006;3:155–60.
53. Borges F, Hakim L, Kline C. Surgical technique to maintain penile length after insertion of an inflatable penile prosthesis via infrapubic approach. J Sex Med. 2006;3:550–3.
54. Ce H, Vorstman B, Teasley D, Winslow B. Hidden penis release: adjunctive suprapubic lipectomy. Ann Plast Surg. 1987;19:131–4.
55. Shaeer O. Supersizing the penis following penile prosthesis implantation. J Sex Med. 2010;7:2608–16.
56. Vollstedt A, Gross MS, Antonini G, et al. The infrapubic surgical approach for inflatable penile prosthesis placement. Transl Androl Urol. 2017;6:620–7.
57. Pestana IA, Greenfield JM, Walsh M, et al. Management of "buried" penis in adulthood: an overview. Plast Reconstr Surg. 2009;124:1186–95.
58. Adham M, Teimourian B, Mosca P. Buried penis release in adults with suction lipectomy and abdominoplasty. Plast Reconstr Surg. 2000;106:840–4.
59. Miranda-Sousa A, Keating M, Moreira S, Baker M, Carrion R. Concomitant ventral phalloplasty during penile implant surgery: a novel procedure that optimizes patient satisfaction and their perception of phallic length after penile implant surgery. J Sex Med. 2007;4:1494–9.
60. Caso JR, Myers MD, Wiegand L, et al. Phalloplasty and penile implant surgery. Curr Urol Rep. 2009;10:475–7.
61. Gupta NK, Sulaver R, Welliver C, Kottwitz M, Frederick L, Dynda D, et al. Scrotoplasty at time of penile implant is at high risk for dehiscence in diabetics. J Sex Med. 2019;16:602–8.
62. Chung E. Penile reconstructive surgery in Peyronie disease: challenges in restoring normal penis size, shape, and function. World J Mens Health. 2018;36

Chapter 10
Implant Surgery in Patient with a Neophallus

Gideon A. Blecher, Nim Christopher, and David J. Ralph

Rationale for Prostheses in Phalloplasty

Whilst phalloplasty ensures a cosmetically acceptable organ, many patients who undergo this procedure will want a functional phallus as well. Voiding in a standing position is a goal of many phalloplasty patients and either single- or multistaged urethral incorporation will enable this aspect of function. Although multiple procedures are required to get to this point, particularly in the gender subpopulation, a significant milestone of phalloplasty is the placement of a penile prosthesis, which thus enables erectile and sexual capacity. Ideally, such a device should appear perfectly natural whilst flaccid and achieve excellent rigidity when required. It should also be made of affordable inert material, be easily activated, inserted and exchanged. There have been several developments which have improved these qualities over the past years, although none yet is perfectly ideal.

Phalloplasty Techniques

There are a variety of options for tissue transfer for phalloplasty. Local and pedicled flaps have been described, and we suggest the review by Hage et al. [1] for excellent descriptions of many of these techniques, including single and tubularised

G. A. Blecher (✉)
The Alfred Hospital, Melbourne, VIC, Australia

Department of Surgery, Monash University, Melbourne, VIC, Australia
e-mail: gideon.blecher@monash.edu.au

N. Christopher · D. J. Ralph
University College London Hospitals & St Peter's Andrology, London, UK
e-mail: david@andrology.co.uk

E. P. Miranda, J. P. Mulhall (eds.), *Penile Implant Surgery*,
https://doi.org/10.1007/978-3-030-82363-4_10

abdominal flaps, scrotal and groin flaps as well a free flaps from the thigh, gracilis, rectus abdominis, forearm and latissimus dorsi. Whilst each of these has their advantages, considerations for choice include patient factors and tissue availability and viability, cosmetic appearance, hair-bearing nature, morbidity of donor site, vascular supply, sensory quality, ability for orgasmic function and complexity of surgical technique.

History of Prostheses in Phalloplasty

Some authors have suggested that no stiffener is required for phalloplasty, but rather, scarring and oedema alone may suffice [2, 3]. The development of a device to improve rigidity further was based on the baculum: a structure made of cartilage which assists in mammalian erection [4].

The first description of phalloplasty used tubularised skin grafts and rib cartilage for rigidity [5]. However rib cartilage does not produce natural flaccidity and the erection and may become displaced or distorted over time. The length may also be insufficient. Whilst autologous materials may incur less infection risk, alternatives such as bone seemed promising but tend to resorb over time [6]. An osteocutaneous radial flap has been described with reasonable success, although early bone fracture was also reported [7].

Synthetic devices were introduced over half a century ago – these acrylic devices unfortunately, and unsurprisingly, led to a significant inflammatory response [8]. A solution to this problem was devised by Mukherjee, who described a skin-lined pouch which was incorporated in the phalloplasty, into which a removable prosthesis could be inserted when required [9].

As an alternative to full phalloplasty, whilst not providing function other than aesthetic and some sexual applicability, a simple option involves a titanium bone anchor, to which a penile episthesis is attached when needed [10]. The contrast to this is a full phalloplasty, innervated for tactile and erogenous sensation, with urethra for voiding function, and a penile implant for sexual purposes.

The first description of such an inflatable prosthesis as we recognise today, into a transgender phalloplasty, was in 1978 [11]. Whilst initial high failure rates were described, more encouraging results were subsequently reported [12, 13]. Several contemporary series of both gender and genetic male cohorts have been published and will be explored later in this chapter [14–20].

Timing for Placement of Prostheses

Within surgical practice, there is the urge and desire to make complicated surgeries simpler and more efficient. Thus there is the drive to minimise the number of procedures required to create a functional phallus. This is also the case where related surgeries may already have taken place, in the genetic cis-male patients, for example, partial or total penectomy for carcinoma or penile curvature correction in epispadias. In gender patients, other surgeries including mastectomy or facial operations, as well as hysterectomy/oophorectomy, may already have taken place. This further adds to the desire to minimise phalloplasty creation. However, to date, the complete phallic reconstruction requires multiple stages. Although performing fewer number of stages increases efficiency, an increase in surgical complications may arise.

These steps for total phallic reconstruction currently include phallus creation, glans-sculpting and penile implantation. In trans-gender clients, a urethral anastomosis, vaginectomy (with hysterectomy/oophorectomy if not already performed), scrotoplasty, testicular prosthesis and management of the clitoris are additional components which need consideration.

Whilst some phalloplasty techniques such as the osteocutaneous flap have their erectile component already embedded, most other flaps require penile implants. The phallus therefore needs to be created as a first stage, and due to the higher stakes at play, it is wise to consider this as a solitary step. Once other steps have been concluded and their complications addressed (tissue ischaemia/necrosis, urethral fistula or stricture, vaginectomy related collections, scar contracture, etc.), penile prosthesis can be performed.

Penile Implant: Surgical Technique

The technique for penile implant varies slightly depending on whether the patient is cis- or trans-male. Whilst the distal (phallic) part of the procedure is similar, the proximal placement of the prosthesis is quite different, based on the lack of anatomical corpora cavernosa in trans-males.

General anaesthetic and intravenous antibiotics are administered. The patient is placed in a supine position with the legs slightly apart and appropriate topical surgical antiseptic applied. A 14F urethral catheter is inserted – for trans-males, an introducer of occasionally a flexible cystoscope is required to navigate the cavity just distal to the urethra-neourethral anastomosis. Occasionally for obese patients, surgical access may be easier in the lithotomy position.

Approach: Cis-males

A transverse incision is made 2 cm below the phallo-scrotal junction (Fig. 10.1). The corpora cavernosal stumps are identified (Fig. 10.2). If a spacer (shortened semi-rigid implant or rear tip extender) was previously inserted, identifying these residual corpora is significantly easier. The spacers should be removed and the corpora irrigated with antibiotic solution. The proximal corporal length should be dilated as required and then measured with a Furlow.

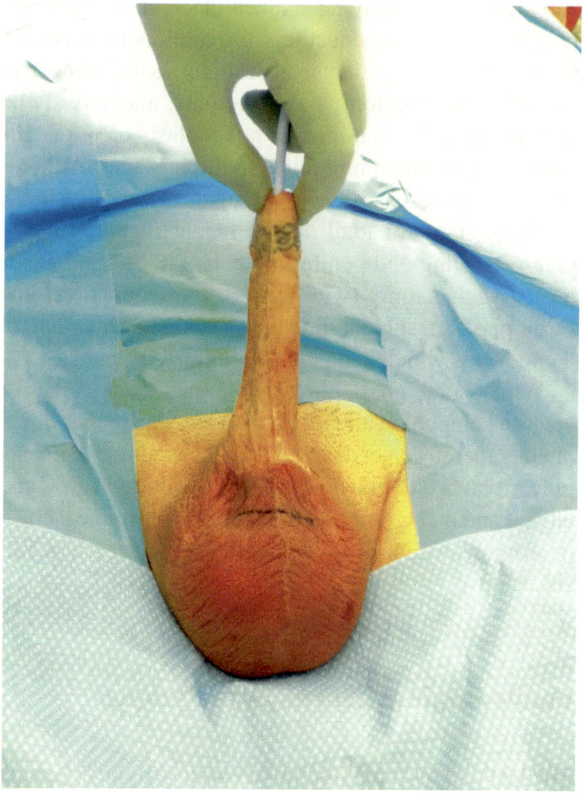

Fig. 10.1 Penoscrotal approach for genetic male

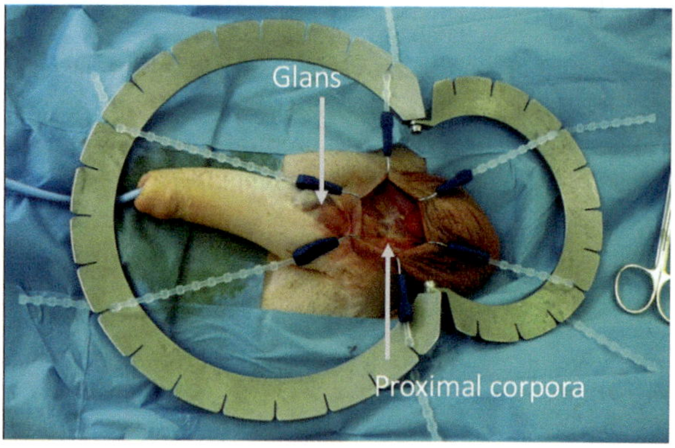

Fig. 10.2 Penoscrotal incision for genetic male

Approach: Trans-males

The phallus and pubis can be accessed in a variety of ways. An infrapubic (cephalad) approach works well particularly when the vascular supply arises inferolaterally, for example, in a pedicled anterolateral thigh flap phalloplasty or any free flap phalloplasty connected to the superficial femoral artery.

When the vascular pedicle enters from the supero-lateral aspect (e.g. from the inferior epigastric artery), it may suit the surgeon to perform incisions in the groin crease (Fig. 10.3), between the scrotum and medial border of the thigh. This approach affords excellent visualisation of the anterior aspect of the pubis.

A final option when there is no urethra is a ventral incision through the phallus/neoscrotum.

Pubis Dissection and Proximal Fixation: Trans-males

Due to the absence of anatomical corpora, the proximal aspects of the prostheses will need to be secured *onto* the pubis. The pubic periosteum therefore needs to be identified either uni- or bilaterally. A self-retaining retractor, along with a Langenbeck retractor, facilitates the view and dissection superficial to the periosteum. Staying superficial to the fascia prevents pain and bleeding. The dissection is continued across the midline (in case of single cylinder insertion). For dual cylinders, the pubis on both sides needs to be dissected, via a contralateral incision.

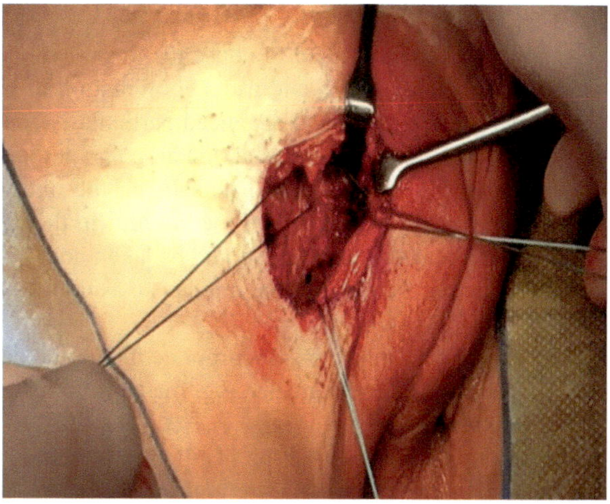

Fig. 10.3 Lateral approach and pubic fixation sutures for trans-male

Avoidance of dissecting caudal to the pubic symphysis will keep the surgeon away from a large venous plexus, the clitoral nerve and the native urethra.

Several options are available to secure the proximal end of the penile prosthesis.

If the cylinder(s) is simply inserted and left in place, a fibrous capsule will ultimately form and keep the device in place. Unfortunately, this results in cylinder dislocation and instability during sexual intercourse. Alternatively, the rear tip or rear tip extender of the cylinder can be sutured to the pubis. Whilst this provides somewhat more security, hinging and instability of the prosthesis may occur. To provide the best stability, a non-absorbable sock is secured to the anterior surface of the pubis. The penile implant is housed within the sock providing better stability.

Three heavy, non-absorbable anchoring sutures are placed in a triangle arrangement (Fig. 10.3). These are placed unilaterally for a single cylinder or bilaterally for dual cylinder insertion. To improve prosthetic stability, the surgeon should ensure adequate distance between the upper and lower sutures. The lower lateral suture affects the angle of the erect phallus and hence the stability during tumescence. The position of the implant relative to the phallus is determined by the upper lateral and medial sutures. The surgeon should avoid placing sutures in the adductor tendon which can lead to chronic pain. It is important not to inadvertently anchor the device to the adductor tendon as this causes a lot of pain.

As an alternative to the above described methods of proximal fixation, another alternative is to drill a well in the cephalic portion of the pubis, thus providing a shallow hole to house the rear tip of the cylinder [21].

Phallus Dilatation

A space needs to be created to house the distal cylinders of the implant. To create this space, the surgeon should use a combination of blunt dissection, and scissors can be carefully opened and advanced particularly in regions of fibrosis. Typically this can occur at the phallo-scrotal junction and at the neo-coronal sulcus.

The space should be created dorsally in the midline (if one cylinder is being placed) or dorsally either side of the urethra (in the case of dual cylinders). Hegar dilators can then be used. Care should be taken not to dilate all the way through and ensure that some fat protects the implant so as to prevent device erosion (Figs. 10.4 and 10.5).

If a non-absorbable cap is incorporated, then the dilation should be at least one size larger than the cap diameter, e.g. for 16-mm-wide Dacron™ Caps, we suggest dilating to Hegar 18.

Antibiotic solution should be instilled into the neo-corporal spaces, which also excludes urethral injury. If a urethral injury occurs, the prosthesis should not be placed. Rather, the urethra is repaired and the penile implant deferred.

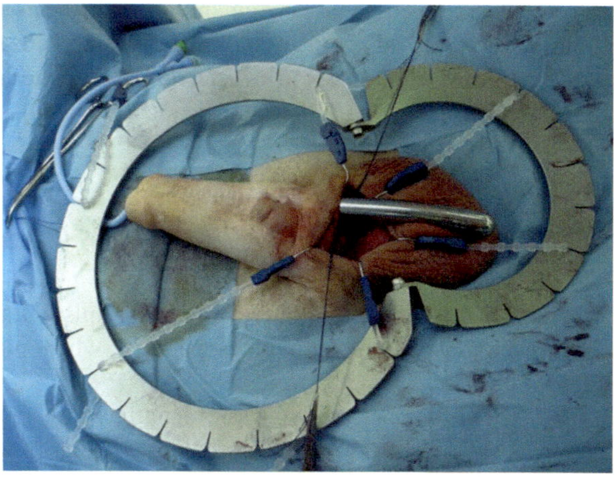

Fig. 10.4 Dilatation of corporal space – genetic male

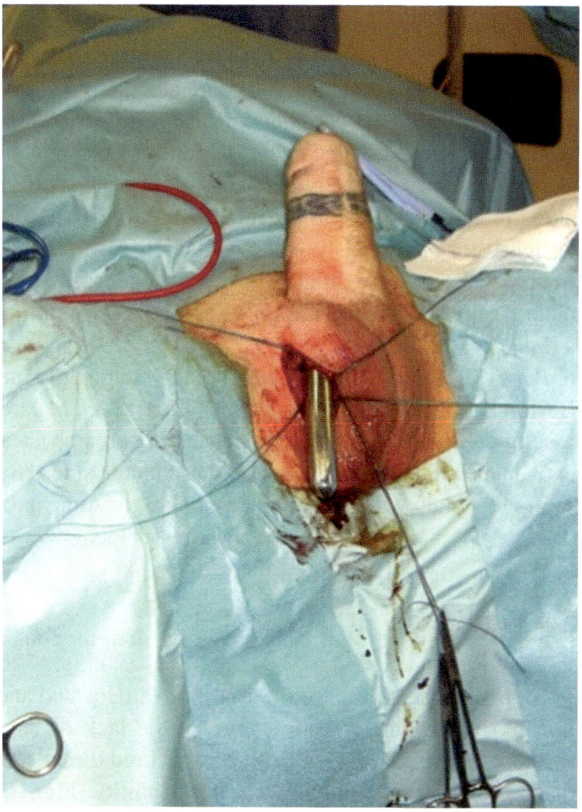

Fig. 10.5 Corporal dilatation for trans-male

Neo-corporal length measurement is made from the most caudal anchoring suture point to the mid glans of the partially stretched phallus in the proposed erect position. A non-disposable Furlow can be used, or alternatively, the disposable measuring tool from the AMS™ accessory kit works well.

Choosing a Prosthesis and the Number of Cylinders

Several prosthetics are currently available. Whilst surgeon experience may play a role, several aspects should be considered when placing an implant within a neophallus.

The size of the phallus, in terms of length, width and glans size, will play a role. The longer the phallus, the greater the requirement for increased axial rigidity. The wider the phallus, the heavier it will be and thus will also accommodate two, as opposed to one cylinder. The neo-glans may not be large enough to house two cylinders, and when placing dual cylinders, the volume of the phallus increases significantly; a bulky and wide phallus may not be appealing to some patients. To increase stability, ideally rear tip extenders are avoided.

Anecdotally, most patients will fit a single, and a third of patients will accommodate dual cylinder placement. The authors feel that an inflatable Coloplast Titan® provides slightly more rigidity yet is slightly more prominent during flaccidity compared to a Boston Scientific AMS 700CX™. In 2016, an implant was specifically designed for phalloplasty – the inflatable ZSI 475 FTM (Zephyr Surgical Implants, Switzerland). It has a single but wide cylinder, a distal glans shape and a proximal plate designed for securing onto the pubis. The pump is oval shaped to replicate a testis.

As an alternative to inflatable implants, semi-rigid implants (Coloplast Genesis®, Boston Scientific Spectra™, Zephyr ZSI 100 FTM) are simple to insert, and in the case of complication (infection or pending erosion), a single cylinder can be easily explanted without affecting the contralateral side. However, the appearance of a semi-erect state will remain unacceptable for some patients.

Sock and Cap Formation

In cis-males, the native proximal corpora are located and are ideal for proximal fixation. For trans-gender patients, given the lack of anatomical corpora, whilst the cylinders can remain free-floating or secured directly with sutures, the authors feel that a proximal sock provides the best stability (Fig. 10.6).

Various synthetic materials have been used, including Gore-Tex, Prolene® Mesh, Vicryl-Pro® Mesh. Dacron vascular graft results in appropriate fibrosis and is therefore well suited. The original description by Hage included a full cylinder

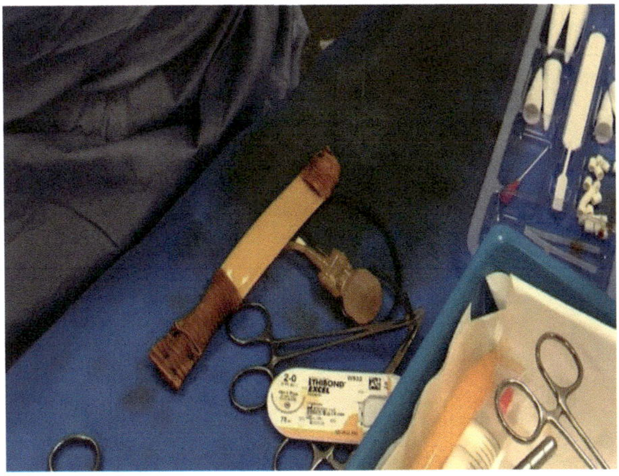

Fig. 10.6 Sock and cap formation for trans-male

synthetic sheath [1]. However, by performing a limited sheath, i.e. sock and cap only, the surgery is easier to perform and the phallus remains softer. Furthermore, it would be reasonable to assume that the more synthetic material used, the higher the infection rate may become. In our experience, a full sheath is required during placement of a semi-rigid device, to prevent displacement.

To fashion a proximal sock, Dacron or Gore-Tex [22] can be used. A 6 cm length of vascular graft is cut and the base folded over itself and secured with sutures. To enable the tubing to exit the sock, a small incision can be made antero-medially.

The distal cap, as described by Jordan et al. [13], aims to minimise the risk of distal erosion. To create a cap, a 3–4 cm length of vascular graft is fashioned and the distal two corners are trimmed to create a rounded end. A continuous suture closes off the tip. A traction suture should be placed through the cap, through the pre-manufactured holes in the tips on the implant and then back through the internal surface of the cap to the external aspect. These sutures can then be loaded onto a Keith needle when required to facilitate implant placement into the dilated spaces.

Insertion of the Implant

For the distal cylinder, a Furlow is used with the Keith needle and pusher, to advance the needle through the distal tip of the phallus. Inflation of the device should occur to check its position (Fig. 10.7). The external component of the suture is cut once the device is completely implanted. The proximal cylinders should be inserted prior.

In trans-males, the pre-placed pelvic anchoring sutures are placed through the sock and each sequentially tied in place. For cis-males, the cylinders are inserted into the proximal corporal stumps. If an inflatable device is used, then the pump is placed into the scrotum or neoscrotum.

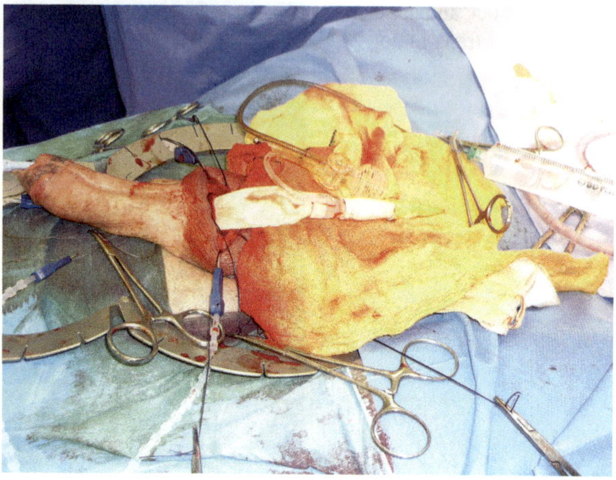

Fig. 10.7 Placement of inflatable implant for genetic male

Reservoirs can be placed in a retropubic, extraperitoneal or ectopic location. The location ultimately is dependent on the presence and location of a vascular pedicle as well as the surgeon's preference. If the vascular pedicle arises from femoral or inferior epigastric arteries, ipsilateral space of Retzius should ideally be avoided as it risks injury. Similarly, blind ectopic placement posterior to the rectus sheath may injure vascular pedicle. An anterior extraperitoneal approach provides access to the iliac fossa/paracolic gutter. Tubing should be placed deep to the rectus sheath and exits lateral to the superficial inguinal ring avoiding any vascular pedicles as well as the ilioinguinal nerve. Tubing can be tunnelled subcutaneously if the patient has a moderate amount of adipose tissue. Closure of tissues should occur in layers. Whilst drains can be used to potentially reduce infection [13], the authors of this chapter feel drains should only be placed when clinically required.

Post-operative Care

Despite a lack of published evidence, we suggest the use of post-operative antibiotic administration for 5–7 days. The urethral catheter should be removed on day 1 post-op. In the case of inflatable penile implants, the device should be left semi-inflated for a week to promote pseudo-capsular formation around a larger volume. If there are concerns regarding ischaemia, the device should be deflated. The implant can start to be cycled at 2 weeks or when the patient is comfortable enough to do so. At 6 weeks, the implant can be utilised for sexual purposes. A schedule of regular inflation of the implant is recommended for 20–30 min daily for at least 1 month to help ensure that the pseudo-capsule matures in a straight position (Figs. 10.8 and 10.9).

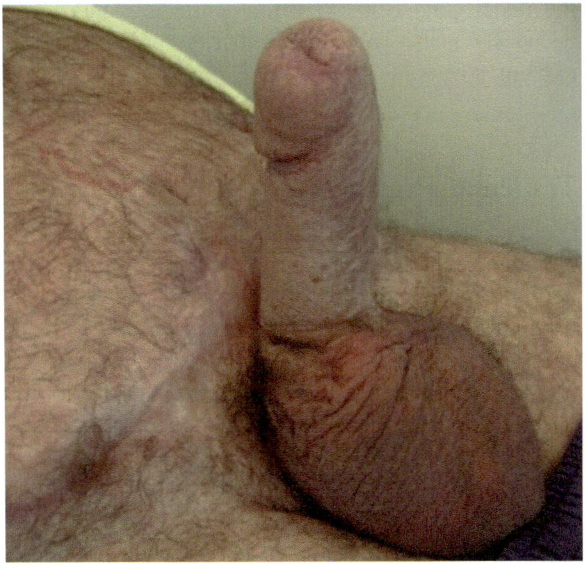

Fig. 10.8 End result – genetic male

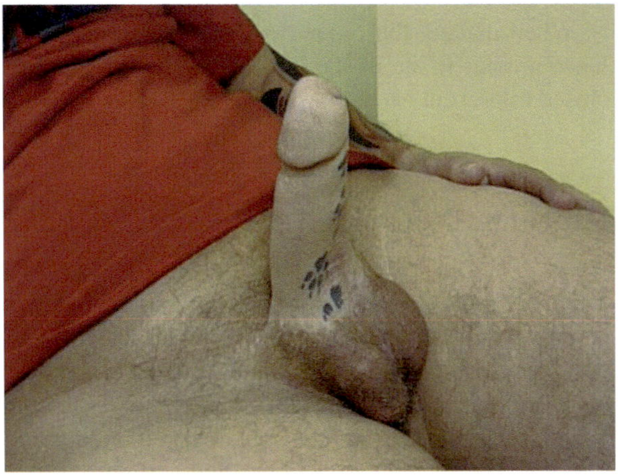

Fig. 10.9 End result – trans-male

Future Outlook

A novel recent advance is the incorporation of a semi-automated device, controllable via a mobile phone [23]. It is not only personal electronic equipment which has been used as a replacement for a manual pump. A nickel-titanium prosthesis has been investigated and using an external magnetic wand, activates a change in shape of the subcutaneously implanted alloy [24]. Infections and erosions remain a relatively common complication; to address this, bioengineered tissues, such as acellular matrix from donor tunica *albuginea*, may play a role [25]. Despite the fact that the underlying technology for penile implants has not changed significantly in decades, it is inevitable that further research and development in this area will yield exciting advances.

Testicular Prosthesis

For transgender patients, the pump for an inflatable prosthesis will fill one hemi-neoscrotum. For the contralateral side, a testicular prosthesis can be placed. The original description utilising vitallium was in 1939 [26]. Several options exist nowadays and include both silicone- and saline-filled devices. For a small/tight neoscrotum, one can consider either tissue expanders prior to prosthesis placement [22] or a self-expanding ellipsoid tissue expander (Osmed GMBH, Germany). These *increase* their volume from 1.1 to 10 ml. Choosing a size is surgeon and patient *dependent* but will often be dictated by the capacity of the neoscrotum. There is no data in the literature regarding these implants in transgender cohorts; however, it would *not be* unreasonable to *presume that* certain complications, such as infection, haematoma, erosion or discomfort/tethering, would be similar to non-trans populations [27, 28].

When placing these devices, the implant should be placed superficially in the loose areolar tissue of the labia majora. The neck of the dilated space should be closed to prevent caudal migration.

Patient Satisfaction

There are multiple studies of penile implants in phalloplasty in the literature, many of which have small patient numbers (Tables 10.1 and 10.2). The largest series of trans-gender phalloplasty outcomes involved 247 patients [29]. Following inflatable penile implants, with a median of 20 months follow-up, patients completed a non-validated questionnaire. 77% of patients reported an ability to participate in penetrative intercourse, with functional and cosmetic satisfaction rates of 88%. Other studies have concluded penetrative intercourse ability in 23–86% [29–33]. A report of ten trans-males who underwent phalloplasty demonstrated that following psychological interview, 80% were able to orgasm during sex [34].

The penile implant data for phalloplasty in cis-males is exceedingly limited.

Ralph et al. reported on 108 men (history of bladder exstrophy-epispadias complex, penile cancer, micropenis, trauma): 76% were able to achieve orgasm, whilst 76% would have the operation again and 90% would recommend phalloplasty to a friend [35]. However, outcomes from the penile implants were not discussed. Young et al. reported on a small cohort ($n = 12$) of cis-males (trauma and bladder exstrophy cohort) who underwent total phallic reconstruction. Satisfaction scores of 5/10, orgasm rate 6/10, intercourse satisfaction 10.5/15 and subjective quality of life

Table 10.1 Studies of penile prostheses in trans-gender phalloplasty

Year	Author	Number of transgender clients (total in study)	Implant type (number cylinders)	Duration of follow-up	Complication					Sexual function
					Infection	Erosion	Mechanical failure	Malposition/ migration	Other	
1994	Jordan	3 (8)	Duraphase [1]	Up to 3 years	2/4	–	–	–		Sexually active – synergist device x1
			Uniflate 1000 [1] x3							Difficult sexual activity x2
1995	Alter	8 (13 total)	Duraphase [8]	Minimum 6 months	4/14	0	1	–	–	–
			Uniflate [2]							
			AMS700CX [1]							
1999	Zielinski	127 (47 implants)	Silicone rod [41]						19 (40%) total complication	
			Polypropylene [6]							
2005	Bettocchi	85	Dynaflex [9]		–	6	–	–	–	
			Malleable [8]							
2007	Krueger	105	AMS 650 malleable [1]	–	2/105	2/105	7/105	3/105	3/105	–
			AMS Dynaflex [1]							
			AMS 700CXM [2]							

(continued)

Table 10.1 (continued)

Year	Author	Number of transgender clients (total in study)	Implant type (number cylinders)	Duration of follow-up	Complication					Sexual function
					Infection	Erosion	Mechanical failure	Malposition/ migration	Other	
2008	Leriche	38 (56)	Prototype	Mean 110 month	11 (29%) *(some were mechanical failure)	–	–	–	Exchange 8 (21%)	18 (51%) satisfactory sexual function
			Ambicor						Explant 3 (8%)	
			AMS 600							
			AMS 700S							
2010	Hoebeke	129 (189 implants)	15 Dynaflex [1]	Mean 56 months	1 (6.7%)	0 (0%)	8 (6%)	2 (13%)	2 (13%) leakage	–
			69 AMS CX/ CXM	Mean 42 months	9 (13%)	7 (10%)	11 (8.5%)	14 (20%)	12 (17.6%) leakage	
			(1)x37						1 (1.4%) other	
			(2)x13							
			47 Ambicor	Mean 12 months	9 (15%)	5 (8.5%)	0 (0%)	7 (11.9%)	1 (12.5%) leakage	
			(1)x22							
			(2)x25							
			8 Coloplast [2]	Mean 22 months	1 (12.5%)	0 (0%)	2 (1.6%)	1 (12.5%)	1 (12.5%) other	
			AMS CX InhibiZone	Mean 28 months	2 (5.9%)	3 (8.8%)	4 (3.1%)	3 (8.8%)		
			(1)x13				Overall Infection/ erosion 18 (13.8%)	Overall Mechanical failure 40 (30.8%)	3 (8.8%) leakage	
			[2] x4							

2014	Terrier	14	–	–	1/14	1/14	21% *includes malposition			79% satisfied with current sexual life *includes all aspects of phalloplasty
2015	Segal	2 (9 total)	AMS 700CX (–)	Mean 9.6 months	1 (33%)	2 (66%) erosion				–
			Semi-rigid (–)							
			AMS700CXR (–)							
2015	Zuckerman	15 (31 total)	Semi-rigid (–) x21	Mean 59.7 months	3 (9.7%)	2 (6%)	1 (3%)	1 (3%)		Sexually active 81%
			AMS700CX/ CXR							
			Coloplast Titan							
			[1] 5%							
			[2] 95%							
2016	Neuville	62 (95 total)	Ambicor (–)	Mean 4 years	8 (8.4%)	4 (4.2%) erosion	10 (10.5%)	12 (12.6%) malposition	–	
			Ambicor with graft (–)							
2017	Cohen	8	IPP	Mean 49 months	5/10 (50%)	–	2/10 (20%)	3/10 (30%)	–	–

(continued)

Table 10.1 (continued)

Year	Author	Number of transgender clients (total in study)	Implant type (number cylinders)	Duration of follow-up	Complication					Sexual function
					Infection	Erosion	Mechanical failure	Malposition/ migration	Other	
2018	Falcone	247	AMS700 CX/ CXM/R	Median 20 months	21 (8.5%)		38 (15.4%)		48 (19.4%) dissatisfaction	97 (77%) engaged in penetrative sexual intercourse
			Coloplast Titan							97 (88%) fully satisfied with function
			Ambicor							
			[1] x 39							
			[2] x 208							
2019	Neuville	20	ZSI 475 FtM	Mean 8.9 months	1 (4.7%)	–	2 (9.5%)	1 (4.7%)	2 (9.5%)	12 (85.7%) engaged in regular penetrative intercourse
2019	Van der Sluis	32 (45 implants)	AMS Dynaflex 13	Mean 4.6 years	5 (15.6%)	5 of initial (11.1%)	5 (11.1%)	5 (11.1%)	1 (2.2%) pain	–
			AMS Ambicor 3			17.8% of all implants				
			AMS Spectra 2							
			Coloplast Genesis 14							

2019	Djordjevic	129 (61 implants)	IPP 22 Malleable 39	Mean 43 months (for $n = 129$, specific follow-up for implants not mentioned)	2 (3%)		2			14/61 (23%) engaged in penetrative intercourse
2020	Pigot	25	ZSI 100 FtM	Mean 6.3 months	3 (12%)	4 (16%) (Protrusion)	–	1 (4%)	3 (8%)	13/25 (52%) or 13/14 (93%) remaining implants, engaged in penetrative intercourse
2020	Verla	46	ZSI 475 FtM	Median 12 months	5 (11%)	2 (4.3%)	2 (4.3%)	1 (2.2%)		–

Table 10.2 Studies of penile prostheses in genetic male phalloplasty

Year	Author	Number of patients (total in study)	Implant type (number cylinders)	Duration of follow-up	Complication					Sexual function
					Infection	Erosion	Mechanical failure	Malposition/ migration	Other	
2019	Ralph	108		Mean 78.5 months	–	–	–	–	–	76% able to achieve orgasm
2017	Young	12		Mean 8 months [5–41]	–	3 (33.3%)	–	1	–	SQOL 60/100 IIEF-OS 5/10

60/100 were reported [20]. In the same study, IIEF erectile function domain scores of 26/30 were reported, with intercourse satisfaction domain scores of 10.5/15. This study also reported erosion rates of 33%, with one patient requiring replacement of the implant due to pain.

Implant Survival

A significant source of morbidity arises from complications related to the penile implant. Several advances have improved the mechanical reliability of inflatable implants including multilayer woven fabrics, kink-resistant tubing and other reinforcements. Parylene reduces silicone friction and improved 3-year revision rates for the AMS700 series devices from 78.6% to 87.4% [36]. To improve tensile strength, silicone was subsequently exchanged with Bioflex polyurethane, in Coloplast Mentor inflatable implants [37].

In order to appreciate implant survival, it is worthwhile considering the non-phalloplasty context. Implant survival rates at 5, 10 and 15 years of 85%, 68% and 57%, respectively, were reported for the AMS 700CXTM device [38]. Contemporary data estimates mechanical failure rates for AMS 700TM and Coloplast Titan® inflatable implants at 87–91% at 5 years [39]. Clearly, malleable devices are not prone to mechanical failure – studies have demonstrated absence of mechanical failure at 5.7 and 11.7 years [40, 41].

Whilst these numbers are comforting, implant survival in phalloplasty is significantly lower, with failure rates approximating 15% at a very early 20 months [15]. Cylinder rupture (69%), cylinder aneurysm (19%) and rupture of the tubing between the cylinder and the pump (12%) are the most common reason for mechanical failure. At 5 years, survival rates of 78% were described in the Falcone study, with overall median survival of implants ranging from 4.2 to 4.9 years in other studies [15, 42, 43].

Infection rates for implants in phalloplasty are also relatively high. In the largest study, infection rates were 8.5% (median 20 month follow-up) and in other studies, up to 10%, with revision rates of 23% at 4–5 years [31]. Infection rates in contemporary studies have reached as high as 50% [44].

Erosion may occur in non-phalloplasty populations. However, both distal erosion and proximal migration are much more common in phalloplasty, due to lack of anatomical corpora. Proximal migration occurs in 3–20% in contemporary studies [2, 16, 31, 33, 42–44]. Distal erosion rates are again higher than in non-phalloplasty cohorts – distal caps help to mitigate this risk which approaches 4–18% at 4–5 years [16, 31, 43].

Summary

Multiple advances in phalloplasty technique, as well as penile implants and their incorporation into phalloplasty, have enabled many patients to attain both a cosmetic and functional phallus. Satisfaction rates are reasonably high. The standard penile implants have been somewhat 'forced' into the phalloplasty resulting in seeming ever-present complications. Two phalloplasty implants have been recently developed, and we remain excited for further significant technological developments which are required to ensure the morbidity of penile implants becomes comparable to the non-phalloplasty cohort.

Disclosures
- GB: Advisory Board Consultant for Coloplast
- NC: Innovations Advisory Board Member for Coloplast
- DJR: Consultant for Coloplast, Advisory board Boston Scientific

Key Points
- Whilst significant developments have occurred over the last century, the inflatable hydraulic prosthesis remains the best tool in aiming for the ideal phalloplasty erectile device.
- Penile implantation should occur as a last stage of phalloplasty, once other complications of surgery have been dealt with and stabilised.
- Key differences in surgical placement include absence of corpora, scarring within the shaft, proximal pubic fixation and distal sock formation, scarring and vascular pedicle considerations for incision and reservoir placement.
- Prosthesis options include semi-rigid devices and inflatable two- or three-piece devices.
- Complications are higher in phalloplasty cohorts, including infection, mechanical failure, erosion and malposition/migration.

References

1. Hage J, Bloem J, Bouman F. Obtaining rigidity in the neophallus of female-to-male transsexuals: a review of the literature. Ann Plast Surg. 1993;30(4):327–33.
2. Krueger M, Yekani SAH, Hundt GV, Daverio PJ. Use of erectile prostheses in patients with free forearm flap phalloplasty. Int J Transgend. 2007;10(1):19–22.
3. Morales PA, O'Connor JJ Jr, Hotchkiss RS. Plastic reconstructive surgery after total loss of the penis. Am J Surg. 1956;92(3):403–8.
4. Theodore Bergman R, Howard AH, Barnes RW. Plastic reconstruction of the penis. J Urol. 1948;59(6):1174–82.
5. Bogoras N. Uber die voile plastische Wiederherstellung eines zum Koitus fahigen Penis (Peniplastica totalis). Zentralbl Chir. 1936;22:1271–6.
6. Munawar A. Surgical treatment of the male genitalia. J Int Coll Surg. 1957;27:352.

7. Fang R, Kao Y, Ma S, Lin J. Phalloplasty in female-to-male transsexuals using free radial osteocutaneous flap: a series of 22 cases. Br J Plast Surg. 1999;52(3):217–22.
8. Goodwin WE, Scott WW. Phalloplasty. J Urol. 1952;68(6):903–8.
9. Mukherjee GD. Use of groin and mid-thigh flap in reconstruction of penis with penile and perineal urethra and a dorsal skin-lined socket for a removable prosthesis. Ann Plast Surg. 1986;16(3):235–41.
10. Selvaggi G, Branemark R, Elander A, Liden M, Stalfors J. Titanium-bone-anchored penile epithesis: preoperative planning and immediate postoperative results. J Plast Surg Hand Surg. 2015;49(1):40–4.
11. Puckett CL, Montie JE. Construction of male genitalia in the transsexual, using a tubed groin flap for the penis and a hydraulic inflation device. Plast Reconstr Surg. 1978;61(4):523–30.
12. Levine LA, Zachary LS, Gottlieb LJ. Prosthesis placement after total phallic reconstruction. J Urol. 1993;149(3):593–8.
13. Jordan GH, Alter GJ, Gilbert DA, Horton CE, Devine CJ Jr. Penile prosthesis implantation in total phalloplasty. J Urol. 1994;152(2):410–4.
14. Hoebeke P, De Cuypere G, Ceulemans P, Monstrey S. Obtaining rigidity in total phalloplasty: experience with 35 patients. J Urol. 2003;169(1):221–3.
15. Falcone M, Garaffa G, Gillo A, Dente D, Christopher AN, Ralph DJ. Outcomes of inflatable penile prosthesis insertion in 247 patients completing female to male gender reassignment surgery. BJU Int. 2018;121(1):139–44.
16. van der Sluis WB, Pigot GL, Al-Tamimi M, Ronkes BL, de Haseth KB, Özer M, et al. A retrospective cohort study on surgical outcomes of penile prosthesis implantation surgery in transgender men after phalloplasty. Urology. 2019;132:195–201.
17. Stojanovic B, Bizic M, Kojovic V, Pusica S, Bencic M, Djordjevic M. MP04-15 Phalloplasty followed by penile prosthesis insertion in female to male transsexuals. J Urol. 2019;201(Supplement 4):e36–e.
18. Nimal Christopher A, Garaffa G, Ralph D. PD44-03 Outcomes of 764 inflatable penile prostheses in 547 female-to-male transsexuals undergoing phalloplasty. J Urol. 2019;201(Supplement 4):e821–e2.
19. Ralph DJ, Falcone M, Anfosso M, Gontero P, Nim Christopher A, Ralph O. MP04-14 Total phallic reconstruction in the genetic male: a single centre analysis. J Urol. 2019;201(Supplement 4):e35–e6.
20. Young EE, Friedlander D, Lue K, Anele UA, Khurgin JL, Bivalacqua TJ, et al. Sexual function and quality of life before and after penile prosthesis implantation following radial forearm flap phalloplasty. Urology. 2017;104:204–8.
21. Large MC, Gottlieb LJ, Wille MA, DeWolfe M, Bales GT. Novel technique for proximal anchoring of penile prostheses in female-to-male transsexual. Urology. 2009;74(2):419–21.
22. Alter GJ, Gilbert DA, Schlossberg SM, Jordan GN. Prosthetic implantation after phallic construction. Microsurgery. 1995;16(5):322–4.
23. Robles-Torres JI, Gómez-Guerra L, Ramos-Cuevas D, Sánchez-Uresti A, Gutiérrez-González A. PD40-04 Semiautomatic inflatable electronic penile implant prototype. J Urol. 2018;199(4S):e804–e5.
24. Le B, McVary K, McKenna K, Colombo A. A novel thermal-activated shape memory penile prosthesis: comparative mechanical testing. Urology. 2017;99:136–41.
25. Garcia M, Banie L, Lin G. 071 A novel biological device to secure and protect neophallus penile prosthesis cylinders and the neourethra following phalloplasty: acellular matrix of intact penile tunica made from human penis specimens following vaginoplasty. J Sex Med. 2017;14(2):e35.
26. Girsdansky JNH. Use of a vitallium testicular implant. Am J Surg. 1941;53(3):514.
27. Marshall S. Potential problems with testicular prostheses. Urology. 1986;28(5):388–90.
28. Turek PJ, Master VA. Testicular Prosthesis Study G. Safety and effectiveness of a new saline filled testicular prosthesis. J Urol. 2004;172(4 Pt 1):1427–30.

29. Pigot GL, Sigurjónsson H, Ronkes B, Al-Tamimi M, van der Sluis WB. Surgical experience and outcomes of implantation of the ZSI 100 FtM malleable penile implant in transgender men after phalloplasty. J Sex Med. 2020;17(1):152–8.
30. Leriche A, Timsit M-O, Morel-Journel N, Bouillot A, Dembele D, Ruffion A. Long-term outcome of forearm flee-flap phalloplasty in the treatment of transsexualism. BJU Int. 2008;101(10):1297–300.
31. Zuckerman JM, Smentkowski K, Gilbert D, Storme O, Jordan G, Virasoro R, et al. Penile prosthesis implantation in patients with a history of total phallic construction. J Sex Med. 2015;12(12):2485–91.
32. Djordjevic ML, Bencic M, Kojovic V, Stojanovic B, Bizic M, Kojic S, et al. Musculocutaneous latissimus dorsi flap for phalloplasty in female to male gender affirmation surgery. World J Urol. 2019;37(4):631–7.
33. Neuville P, Morel-Journel N, Cabelguenne D, Ruffion A, Paparel P, Terrier J-E. First outcomes of the ZSI 475 FtM, a specific prosthesis designed for phalloplasty. J Sex Med. 2019;16(2):316–22.
34. Callens N, De Cuypere G, T'Sjoen G, Monstrey S, Lumen N, Van Laecke E, et al. Sexual quality of life after total phalloplasty in men with penile deficiency: an exploratory study. World J Urol. 2015;33(1):137–43.
35. Ralph DJ, Falcone M, Anfosso M, Gontero P, Christopher AN, Ralph O. Total phallic reconstruction in the genetic male: a single Centre analysis. Eur Urol Suppl. 2019;18(1):e510.
36. Salem EA, Wilson SK, Neeb A, Delk JR, Cleves MA. Mechanical reliability of AMS 700 CX improved by parylene coating. J Sex Med. 2009;6(9):2615–20.
37. Merrill DC. Mentor inflatable penile prosthesis: clinical experience in 52 patients. Br J Urol. 1984;56(5):512–5.
38. Wilson SK, Delk JR, Salem EA, Cleves MA. Long-term survival of inflatable penile prostheses: single surgical group experience with 2,384 first-time implants spanning two decades. J Sex Med. 2007;4(4, Part 1):1074–9.
39. Chung E, Solomon M, DeYoung L, Brock GB. Comparison between AMS 700™ CX and Coloplast™ titan inflatable penile prosthesis for Peyronie's disease treatment and remodeling: clinical outcomes and patient satisfaction. J Sex Med. 2013;10(11):2855–60.
40. Kim YD, Yang SO, Lee JK, Jung TY, Shim HB. Usefulness of a malleable penile prosthesis in patients with a spinal cord injury. Int J Urol. 2008;15(10):919–23.
41. Ferguson KH, Cespedes RD. Prospective long-term results and quality-of-life assessment after Dura-II penile prosthesis placement. Urology. 2003;61(2):437–41.
42. Hoebeke PB, Decaestecker K, Beysens M, Opdenakker Y, Lumen N, Monstrey SM. Erectile implants in female-to-male transsexuals: our experience in 129 patients. Eur Urol. 2010;57(2):334–41.
43. Neuville P, Morel-Journel N, Maucourt-Boulch D, Ruffion A, Paparel P, Terrier J-E. Surgical outcomes of erectile implants after phalloplasty: retrospective analysis of 95 procedures. J Sex Med. 2016;13(11):1758–64.
44. Cohen AJ, Bhanvadia RR, Pariser JJ, Hatcher DM, Gottlieb LJ, Bales GT. Novel technique for proximal bone anchoring of penile prosthesis after radial forearm free flap neophallus. Urology. 2017;105:2–5.

Chapter 11
The Approach to Prevention and Management of Device Extrusion and Erosion

Jonathan Clavell-Hernández and Run Wang

Acronyms

ECT	Extracapsular tunneling
IPP	Inflatable penile prosthesis
MPP	Malleable penile prosthesis
NVB	Neurovascular bundle
PTFE	Polytetrafluorethylene

Introduction

The inflatable penile prosthesis (IPP) is one of the most reliable medical devices currently available with over 95% 5-year survival, 80% 10-year survival, 70% 15-year survival, and 50% 20-year survival rate [1, 2]. IPPs have been proven to be so reliable that some experts suggest that penile prosthesis revisions are required more for nonmechanical reasons than mechanical complications [3, 4]. Moreover, reported revision surgeries for IPP placement is more commonly required for either

J. Clavell-Hernández (✉)
St Joseph Medical Center, Houston, TX, USA

McGovern Medical School at Houston, University of Texas Health Science Center, Houston, TX, USA

R. Wang
McGovern Medical School at Houston, University of Texas Health Science Center, Houston, TX, USA

University of Texas MD Anderson Cancer Center, Houston, TX, USA
e-mail: run.wang@uth.tmc.edu

E. P. Miranda, J. P. Mulhall (eds.), *Penile Implant Surgery*,
https://doi.org/10.1007/978-3-030-82363-4_11

cosmetic problems or erosion as opposed to mechanical failure [5]. Even though complication rates for either infectious or non-infectious reasons are low, every surgeon should be prepared and know how to troubleshoot these obstacles.

Two challenging complications for surgeons are impending erosion and complete erosion which can cause cosmetic deformities and lead to patient dissatisfaction, device infection, and subsequent removal. Erosion can occur from any portion of the implant which includes the distal or proximal cylinders, the reservoir, and/or the prosthetic pump. Most experts consider an eroded device to the exterior to be infected given its exposure and contact with the outer skin or urine from the urethral tract. Moreover, a device requiring explantation after erosion may lead to significant corporal fibrosis and scarring of the penile tissue which will render subsequent implantation extremely difficult. The goal of this chapter is to present ways to avoid and work through erosion-related complications in order to increase and maintain patient satisfaction. Given more than half of iatrogenic complications occur during corporal dilation of the corpora cavernosa [3], we will also provide a brief overview of this critical step to prevent cylinder erosion.

Corporal Dilation

We believe the process of corporal dilation starts in the preoperative setting. All patients who are being offered a penile prosthesis should have a proper history and physical examination which include assessment of risks for corporal fibrosis such as previous priapism or penile infection, history of Peyronie's disease, penile curvature or palpable plaques on examination, and history of abdominal surgery and/or retropubic space scarring.

Intraoperatively, regardless of which approach the surgeon decides to use for implantation, the corpora cavernosa should be accessible and visible without any overlying tissues. Moreover, corporotomies should be properly sized. A corporotomy that is too small can cause difficulty during both dilation and cylinder placement, while a corporotomy that is too large can cause an incompletely closed corporotomy which can increase the risk of bleeding or hematoma. When the surgeon is going to dilate distally, dilators should always be angled dorsolaterally to avoid injury to the urethra. On the other hand, proximal dilation should be performed taking into consideration that the proximal crura travel laterally.

In the setting of corporal fibrosis, dilation of the corpora has been reported to be a challenging step for the delayed occurrence of complications [3]. Corporal crossover occurs when one of the cylinders crosses the midline and both cylinders end up within the same corporal body either proximally or distally. This occurs due to the fenestrated weakness within the corporal septum which lends itself to violation during instrumentation. Indicators for corporal crossover include unequal corporal measurements, difficulty with placement of the second cylinder, misalignment of the urethral catheter off midline, and an unequal erection upon cylinder inflation. In the intraoperative setting, this is usually remedied by removing both cylinders, placing a dilator in the common cavity that received the crossover, and re-dilating the opposite cavity making sure to dilate laterally. The Furlow needle introducer device is then passed to place the first cylinder while maintaining the dilator in the "crossover" side. Finally, the dilator is removed and the Furlow is passed on the side originally holding both cylinders to place the second cylinder. When not corrected, crossover may also result in penile deformity and development of a fibrous capsule around the implant that can lead to persistent postoperative pain and device extrusion.

Impending Cylinder Erosion

Impending cylinder erosion, also described as extrusion in scientific literature, occurs when the prosthetic cylinder has worked its way against or through a weakened tunica albuginea and is pressing under the skin (Fig. 11.1a,b), the glans penis, or impinging upon the urethral meatus (Fig. 11.1c). Increasing factors for this occurrence include aggressive dilation, placement of a cylinder into a very narrow corporal cavity, or chronic mechanical pressure from the cylinder [6, 7]. Distal cylinder ends with impending erosion most commonly occur in the lateral or ventral aspects of the distal penile shaft and can be easily palpated immediately under the skin. Hsu et al. reported that the distal corporal tunica albuginea is thinner than the tunica in the penile shaft, particularly on the ventral aspect where most IPPs tend to extrude. This was evidenced in cadaver studies which showed lack of outer longitudinal collagen layers in the distal penile tunica albuginea. The authors also reported that intravenous pillars coursing laterally have an important role in maintaining the shape of the corpora cavernosum toward the distal end of the penile shaft [8]. Tissue compromise in these areas may suggest an anatomic and physical foundation for

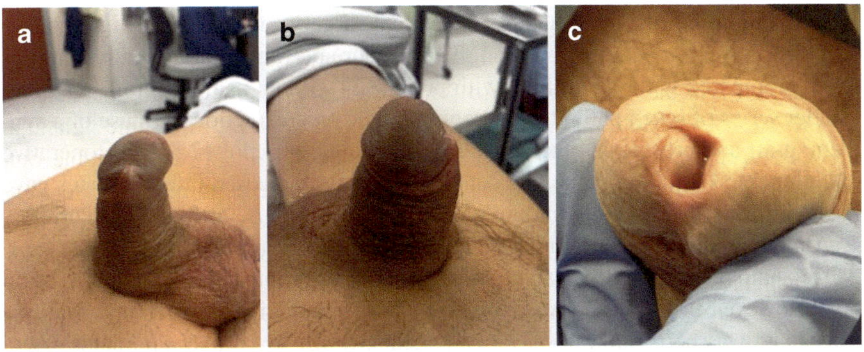

Fig. 11.1 (**a**, **b**) Lateral extrusion with impending erosion. (J. Clavell) **c**. Impending distal erosion into the urethral meatus. (Courtesy: Dr. R Carrion)

this process. Experts believe that previous infection, oversizing of prosthetic cylinders, and/or vigorous lateral dilation with the use of small (size 6–8) Hegar or Brooks dilators can cause "microperforations" that can lead to device extrusion [3].

Distal extrusion and erosion are unusual with a reported incidence ranging from 1.2% to 8.0% [9–11]. Although malleable penile prostheses (MPPs) are known to constantly exert pressure to the tunica albuginea, it is important to note that comparative series have not found a higher complication rate of erosion or extrusion for MPPs when compared to IPPs [9, 10]. One of the larger series of reported cases was recently published by Fuentes et al. Their retrospective series analyzed 797 patients who underwent IPP placement of which 26 (3%) cases had impending or complete cylinder erosion. Most common locations of extrusion were distal lateral (46.2%) and distal urethra (34.6%), although other locations included glanular (7.7%), mid shaft (7.7%), and coronal sulcus (3.8%). Reported risk factors included corporal fibrosis, diabetes, history of additional prior implant surgery, and prolonged device inflation. Mean time from initial placement to extrusion repair surgery was 8.4 years (median 5.5 years). Seventeen patients (65.4%) underwent successful repair or device replacement, and 34.6% had prosthesis removal [11].

Repairs with Distal Counter-incision

When dealing with these cases, it is important that the surgeon determines whether the impending erosion is secondary to an underlying infection and distinguish between urethral/skin extrusion and frank/complete erosion. Impending erosions with underlying infection are characterized by the presence of redness, induration, or slight drainage.

Historically, surgeons attempted to manage impending distal erosions using different techniques with or without grafting [12–20]. In 1998, Smith et al. [15] reported management of impending distal erosions with polytetrafluorethylene (PTFE) distal windsock graft. However, Knoll and Furlow [16] presented 30 patients with cavernosal fibrosis who had penile implant surgery and reported a higher infection rate of 30% on patients who had the procedure performed along with synthetic grafts, compared with 5% in men with prosthesis without use of a graft [17]. In a smaller series of seven patients undergoing penile reconstruction with use of a synthetic graft and prosthesis placement, Jordan et al. reported a 42.8% postoperative infection rate [18]. Ever since, the concern related to increased infection rates gave rise to efforts to manage impending erosions without the use of foreign material.

Alter et al. described a technique that utilized a flap of prefabricated tunica vaginalis to help reconstruct the distal tunica albuginea after impending cylinder erosion [19]. However, their method was based on a limited experience which involved two stages and was performed in only two patients. In the first stage, the rectus fascia was grafted onto the testes' external tunica vaginalis. The second stage was performed 2 weeks later, during which the prefabricated tunica vaginalis flap was transposed to the distal corpora to replace and strengthen the weakened tunica albuginea. Their flap also served as tissue padding between the cylinder and outer tissues.

A more commonly used approach was described by Mulcahy who proposed a distal corporoplasty that uses native tissue to provide padding over the threatening cylinder tip. His technique involved a distal corporotomy to expose the fibrotic sheath around the prosthesis [20, 21]. The fibrotic sheath is then incised, and a new plane of dissection is developed with the use of Metzenbaum scissors and dilators behind the sheath distally (Fig. 11.2). With the use of a Keith needle and a Furlow introducer, the cylinder is directed once again into the new cavity. The cylinder is then secured in proper position with the back wall of the original through fibrotic capsule sheath and the tunica albuginea of the corporotomy for closure (Fig. 11.2b). If the cylinder is impinging on the glans or urethra, an additional step would be necessary. The distal "abnormal" tract of the capsule can be closed with a purse string using nonabsorbable suture prior to redirecting the cylinder into the new cavity [22] (Fig. 11.3).

Carson and Noh compared distal corporoplasty to windsock graft utilization on their experience with 28 patients presenting with impending extrusion [23]. Mulcahy's distal corporoplasty was performed in 18 men while 10 patients underwent repair with Gore-Tex windsock. Of these men, 44.4% who underwent corporoplasty and 60% of the windsock repair group also required glans fixation for glans hypermobility. There were no infections or extrusion recurrence among men who underwent distal corporoplasty while one patient in the windsock repair group had a postoperative infection. Moreover, two patients who underwent windsock repair had postoperative recurrence of extrusion, 6 and 18 months after windsock repair, respectively. Even though functional outcomes were similar among both groups,

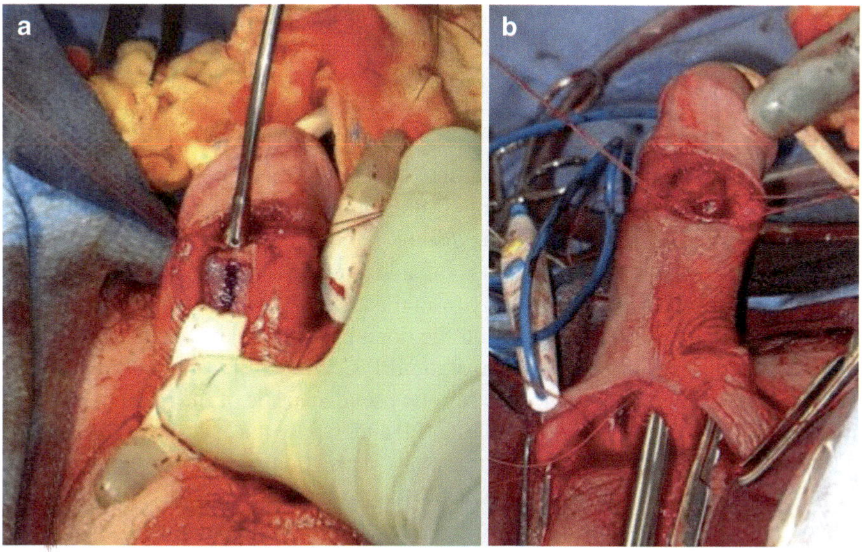

Fig. 11.2 Distal corporoplasty. (**a**) A distal counter-incision is made and a new intracorporal channel is created posterior to the pseudocapsule. (**b**) The dilator is then navigated into the new and true intracorporal channel where the IPP cylinder will be placed. (Courtesy: Dr. R Carrion, MD)

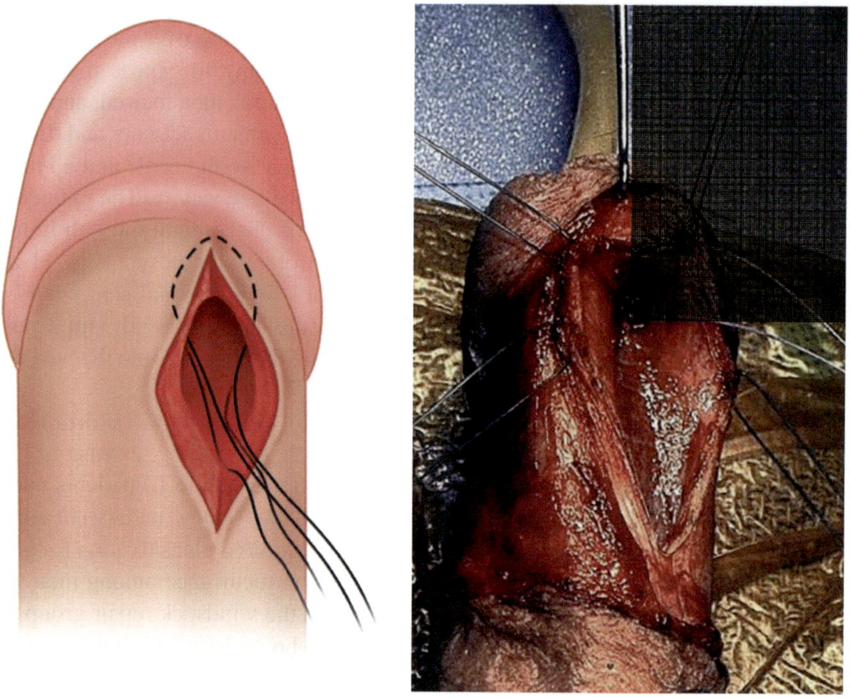

Fig. 11.3 Purse string suture is performed with nonabsorbable suture prior to incising the back wall of the capsule to prevent urethra or glans impingement. (Courtesy: Dr. SK Wilson)

patients undergoing distal corporoplasty had less operative time when compared to windsock repair (mean 52.8 min vs 89.6 min, respectively). The authors concluded that distal corporoplasty was an overall superior method because of fewer complications and reduced surgical time.

In an effort to simplify and shorten the procedure, Shindel et al. proposed a different approach for the management of impending distal erosions using a transglanular incision with reseating of the distal tip of the IPP [24]. Once the impending extrusion is identified, the prosthesis is inflated, and the tip of the cylinder is pushed to the middle of the hemi-glans, away from the area of extrusion. An approximately 1–1.5 cm vertical incision is made on the dorsum of the glans penis lateral to the urethral meatus and immediately above the IPP's cylinder tip using cutting electrocautery current (Fig. 11.4). Once the fibrotic pseudocapsule of the implant is identified, this is incised to reveal the tip of the IPP and expose the eyehole of the cylinder where the original pull-through suture was placed. A nonabsorbable 3-0 suture (Ti-Cron, Covidien, Mansfield, MA, USA) is inserted through the eyehole of the device and secured to the underside of the capsule contralateral to the area of impending erosion. Additional sutures are placed through the solid polymer tip of the distal implant to further secure the implant and minimize migration. Finally, the glans tissue is closed in multiple layers using 5-0 synthetic absorbable monofilament sutures (Fig. 11.4).

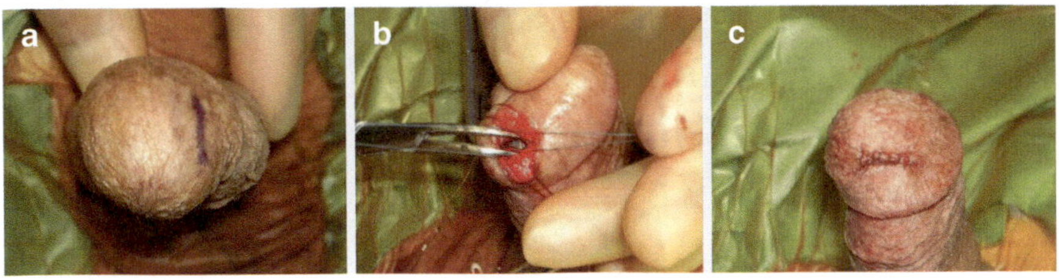

Fig. 11.4 Transglanular repair. (**a**) Vertical incision made on the dorsum of the glans penis. (**b**) Distal pseudocapsule is incised to reveal the tip of the penile prosthesis in order to expose the eyehole of the cylinder. (**c**) Closure of the incision. (Courtesy: Dr. T Lue, UCSF)

Their series consisted of six patients with mean age of 56 years. Mean operative time for the transglanular repair was 25 min [24]. Two of the six patients required repeat revision surgery. The authors recognized particular challenges using this approach for the management of impending cylinder erosion. Visualization can be challenging when working in a small space in combination with brisk bleeding from the highly vascular glans penis. Even though none of their patients complained of decreased penile sensation or bother from the permanent sutures, there remains a theoretical concern for reduced penile sensitivity when operating through the glans penis. In order to minimize this potential complication, the authors advocate for a longitudinal incision in the glans (Fig. 11.4a) that is less likely to disrupt nerves and also tends to reduce the risk of severing sensory nerves.

In 2017, Antonini and colleagues described a surgical technique which combines concepts of Mulcahy's distal corporoplasty and Shindel et al.'s transglanular repair. This novel technique involves a distal corporal anchoring stitch which is placed through a subcoronal corporotomy [25]. Similar to Mulcahy's corporoplasty, this approach comprises a lateral, longitudinal, and subcoronal incision of 1 cm on the side where the "extruded" cylinder should be positioned. A transverse corporotomy incision of the tunica albuginea and underlying pseudocapsule is made and the distal aspect of the affected cylinder is delivered. A 4-0 PDS suture is then placed through the distal cylinder ring and a new, properly positioned intracorporal channel is created using Metzenbaum scissors and Hegar or Brooks dilators. The previously placed 4-0 PDS suture is passed through the distal end of the new channel using a Keith needle and Furlow (Fig. 11.5). Finally, a small cruciate incision is made on the glans, at the location of the anchor stitch (Fig. 11.5c), the suture is tied down, and the knot is buried in the glans tissue which creates a fibrotic process that fixes the prosthesis to the glans. The cruciate incision in the glans is closed with Dermabond (Ethicon, Cincinnati, OH, USA). In their series of 53 patients, 14 had distal crossover while 39 had lateral extrusion. There were no reported intraoperative complications and mean OR time was 69 min. After a median follow-up of 46.8 months, satisfaction rate was high and there were no reported infections, wound healing defects, or altered sensation. Although two patients (3.8%) reported recurrence of lateral herniation, none of the prostheses required replacement because of mechanical failure, infection, or extrusion.

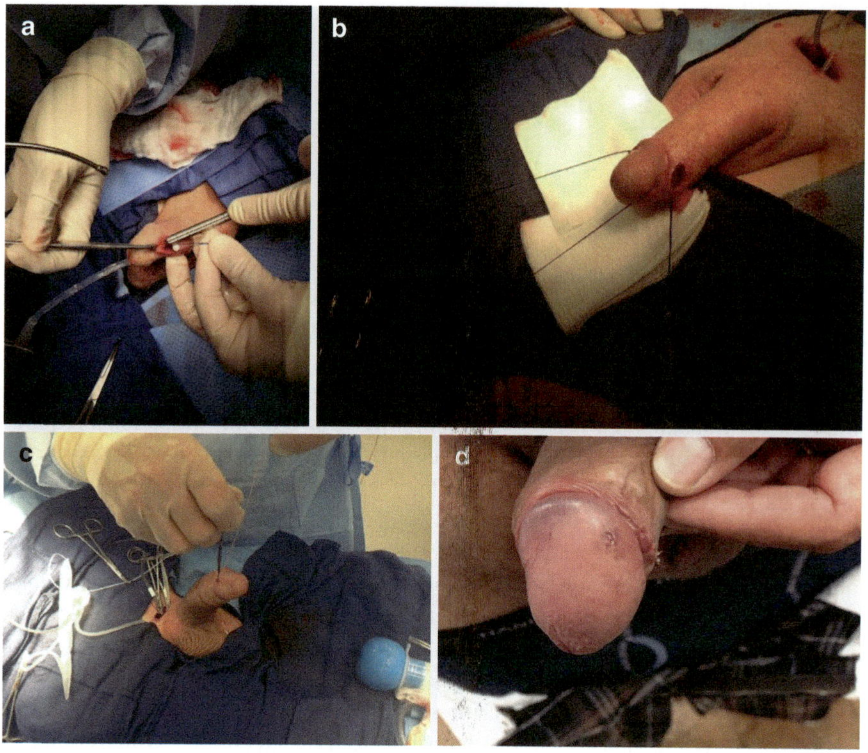

Fig. 11.5 Distal anchoring stitch. (**a**) Lateral subcoronal incision on the side of extrusion. Notice the new PDS suture that will be re-passed through the new corporotomy channel. (**b**) Suture is passed and cylinder is noted in proper position. (**c**) Cruciate incision is made parallel to the suture. (**d**) Photograph of the incision several weeks after the procedure. (Courtesy: Dr. P Perito)

Repairs Without Counter-incision

In order to minimize surgical dissection and avoid counter-incisions in the glans or distal corpora, Karpman et al. reported a simplified technique using a distal biologic cap (DBC) for the management of impending distal erosions (Fig. 11.6) [26]. Prior to the surgery, the authors advocate for a preoperative cystoscopy evaluation of the urethra to ensure there is no evidence of microperforations or visible cylinders. This procedure is performed via a standard penoscrotal or infrapubic approach for IPP surgery. A piece of biologic acellular matrix at a minimum dimension of 4 cm in length and 2 cm in width is used to cover the distal tip of the penile prosthesis. A Keith needle is deployed through the midpoint of a cadaveric dermis or pericardium graft, although an autologous graft may be used if commercially distributed grafts are not available. Then the 3-cm segment is folded over the apex of the implant giving an approximately 1.5 cm coverage of the distal implant. The lateral edges of the graft are then oversewn with 4-0 Vicryl suture. In order to prevent damage of the inflatable cylinder, sewing should be performed with an instrument clamping the

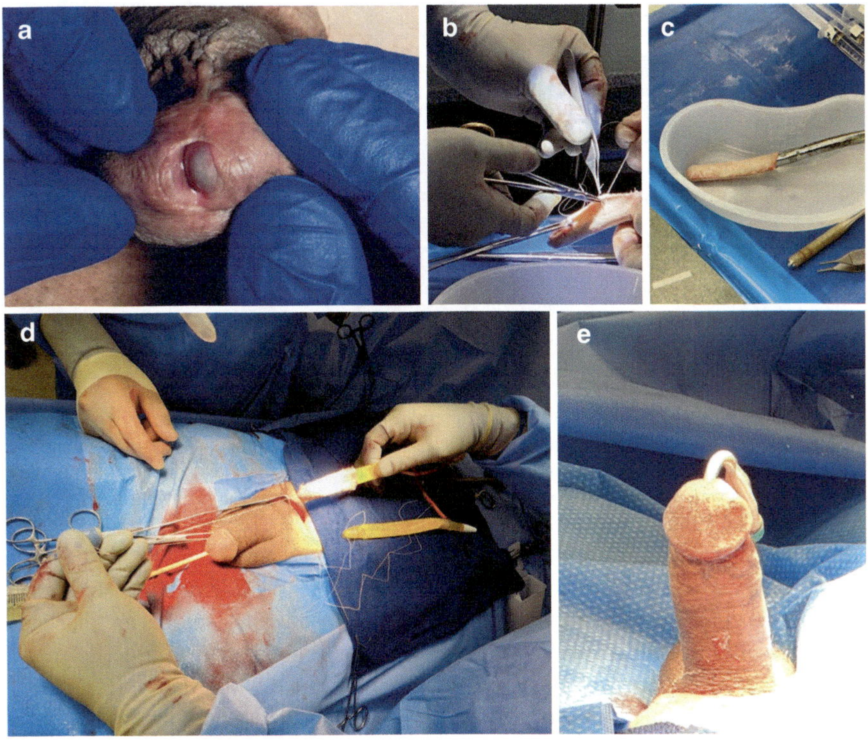

Fig. 11.6 Distal biologic cap. (**a**) Prosthetic tip extrusion into the urethral meatus. (**b**, **c**) Biologic graft is sewn over a Hegar dilator. (**d**) Once formed, the biologic cap is placed over the distal tip of the cylinder. (**e**) Final result without signs of extrusion. (Courtesy: Dr. E Karpman)

lateral border of the graft or over a 12/13 Hegar dilator (Fig. 11.6a). Any graft redundancy can be trimmed accordingly, and the DBC can be placed over the distal cylinder tip (Fig. 11.6d). The remainder of the surgery is then carried out in a standard fashion. As long as the DBC is made to contour the tip of the implant, it will remain covering the apex of the cylinder after the cylinder is pulled through the corporotomy to sit under the glans. After an average follow-up of 5.5 months (3–8 months), all patients undergoing IPP replacement with DBC were functional without evidence of recurrent impending erosion.

Some patients with impending erosion present with concomitant infection or device malfunction that requires explantation and reimplantation of a new device. In these salvage cases, prosthetic cylinders can be inserted into the cavernous tissue surrounding the surgical capsule. This "proximal extracapsular tunneling (ECT)" was most recently described by Clavell-Hernandez [27]. Via a penoscrotal or infrapubic approach, a proximal corporotomy is superficially cut through the tunica albuginea until the surgeon is able to identify the anterior wall of the surgical capsule surrounding the prosthetic implant. The capsule is incised, all prosthetic components are explanted, and the tissues are thoroughly irrigated. The posterior wall of

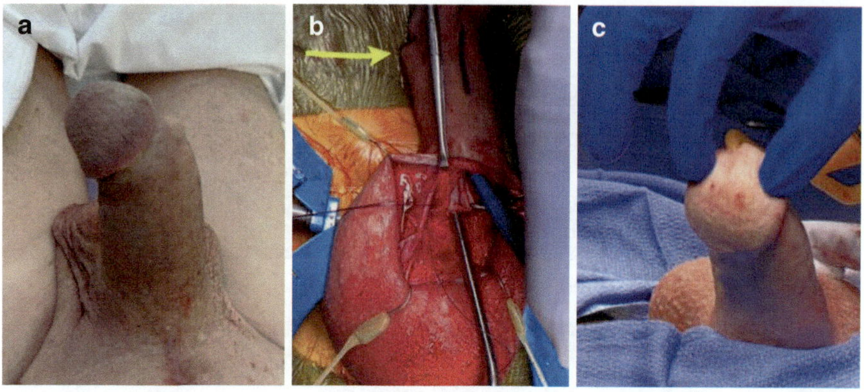

Fig. 11.7 Extracapsular implantation. (**a**) Lateral extrusion of right cylinder tip. (**b**) Dilation through the extracapsular space posterior to the pseudocapsule for new cylinder placement. The blue dilator demarcates the previous pseudocapsular space while the metal dilator is in the new extracapsular space. Notice the tip of the blue dilator that identifies area of extrusion (yellow arrow). (**c**) Final result with proper bilateral cylinder placement

the surgical capsule is identified and incised with either a blade or sharp scissors to identify the corporal sinusoidal tissue behind the capsule. Stay sutures are placed at the edges of both the capsule and corporotomy and pulled apart in order to reveal the extracapsular space which is subsequently developed with dilation (Fig. 11.7). The girth of the penile prosthesis compresses the capsule and obliterates the intracapsular space. This way, prosthesis replacement in the extracapsular sinusoidal space could potentially decrease reinfection rate [28].

Clavell-Hernandez recently published his series of six patients undergoing proximal ECT [27]. Reason for use of the ECT technique was three impending erosions, one severe glans hypermobility, one delayed proximal crossover, and one proximal cylinder aneurysm. After a mean follow-up of 6.6 months, all men were doing well without recurrence of IPP malposition, malfunction, or device infection. Studies describing techniques for impending cylinder erosion are summarized in Table 11.1.

Complete Cylinder Erosion

Complete distal erosion can occur medially into the urethral meatus, laterally through the distal shaft and less commonly through the glans penis. Cylinders that are oversized by either length or girth may wield extraneous pressure on the corporal tissue which may lead to "wear and tear" through the exterior. Experience has shown that this is more common in the presence of semirigid MPPs where the cylinder tips are harder and cannot recess proximally [6].

Most urethral injuries are recognized intraoperatively. When subtle, these can go unrecognized, and over time, a fistula connection between the urethral lumen and

Table 11.1 Studies describing techniques for the management of impending cylinder erosion

Author	Year	Study Population	Surgical Technique	Outcomes	Comments
Seftel et al. [13]	1992	1	PTFE graft	0% infection rate	Polytetrafluorethylene tube graft as a circumferential neotunica
Knoll and Furlow [16].	1992	30	PTFE graft	30% infection rate	All patients had corporal fibrosis
Levine et al. [14]	1993	4	PTFE graft	0% infection rate	All four cases underwent total phallic reconstruction
Jordan et al. [18]	1994	8	PTFE graft	42.8% infection rate	Included a variety of patients with total phalloplasty for either trauma or GRS
Alter et al. [19]	1995	2	Prefabricated tunica vaginalis flap	0% infection rate	Required 2 stage surgery
Smith et al. [15]	1998	5	PTFE windsock graft	0% infection rate	Mean OR time 111 min
Mulcahy [12]	1999	14	DC	0% infection rate	4 patients (29%) were noted to have an infection during the repair surgery, which were salvaged
Carson and Noh [23]	2002	28	DC ($n = 18$)	0% infection (DC)	DC: Mean OR time 53 min, no extrusion recurrence
			PTFE windsock ($n = 10$)	10% infection (PTFE)	PTFE: Mean OR time 90 min, 20% extrusion recurrence
Shindel et al. [24]	2010	6	Transglanular repair	0% infection rate	Mean OR time 25 min. No reported decreased sensation
				33.3% revision rate	
Antonini et al. [25]	2017	53	DC with anchoring stitch	0% infection,	Mean OR time 69 min. 3.8% lateral herniation recurrence
				0% extrusion recurrence	
Shaeer et al. [28]	2019	18	Extracapsular tunneling	5.6% reinfection rate	All cases were salvage procedures for IPP infection and were reimplanted in the extracapsular space with MPP
					Mean OR time for creation of extracapsular space: 10 min

(continued)

Table 11.1 (continued)

Author	Year	Study Population	Surgical Technique	Outcomes	Comments
Karpman et al. [26]	2020	4	Distal biologic cap	0% infection	Average follow-up 5.5 months
				0% extrusion recurrence	
Clavell-Hernandez et al. [27]	2021	6	Extracapsular tunneling	0% infection	Average follow-up 6.6 months. Cases for which procedure done included impending erosion [3], flail penis [1], proximal crossover [1], and cylinder aneurysm [1]
				0% extrusion recurrence	

C distal corporoplasty, *GRS* gender-reaffirming surgery, *IPP* inflatable penile prosthesis, *MPP* malleable penile prosthesis, *OR* operating room, *PTFE* polytetrafluoroethylene

the injured corpora can occur which leads to a delayed urethral perforation. These patients typically present with glans hyperemia, dysuria, urinary obstruction, prosthesis infection, or a visible implant through the urethral meatus (Fig. 11.8) [6]. Risk factors include frequently instrumented urethras by either clean intermittent catheterization or indwelling catheters and patients with decreased distal penile sensation such as those with spinal cord injury, diabetes, or history of radiation.

Management of Complete Erosion

Salvage procedures for patients presenting with IPP infection are common in the scientific literature. These usually involve variations of Mulcahy's technique of removing all device components, thoroughly washing out the component spaces with antiseptic solutions and replacing a new implant in the same setting [20]. When the device completely erodes through the skin or urethra, salvage with replacement is not a feasible option since the procedure will lack a closed system that can be thoroughly irrigated. Nevertheless, there are ways to salvage the procedure depending on where the erosion occurred. If the cylinder eroded laterally through the skin, the surgeon may remove all foreign parts, wash the wound thoroughly, and perform a distal corporoplasty on the side of the erosion as previously discussed [12, 25]. After proper repair of the previous injury site, both cylinders may be replaced. However, experience has shown limited success with this approach, and some believe it is more prudent to replace only one cylinder on the non-eroded corpora and return at a later date to replace the second cylinder [6].

When a cylinder erodes through the urethra, as opposed to the lateral skin, the site of erosion is inaccessible for proper closure, and a cylinder should not be replaced in that corporal body. If an IPP was originally placed, all components should be removed, and all cavities should be thoroughly washed with antiseptic

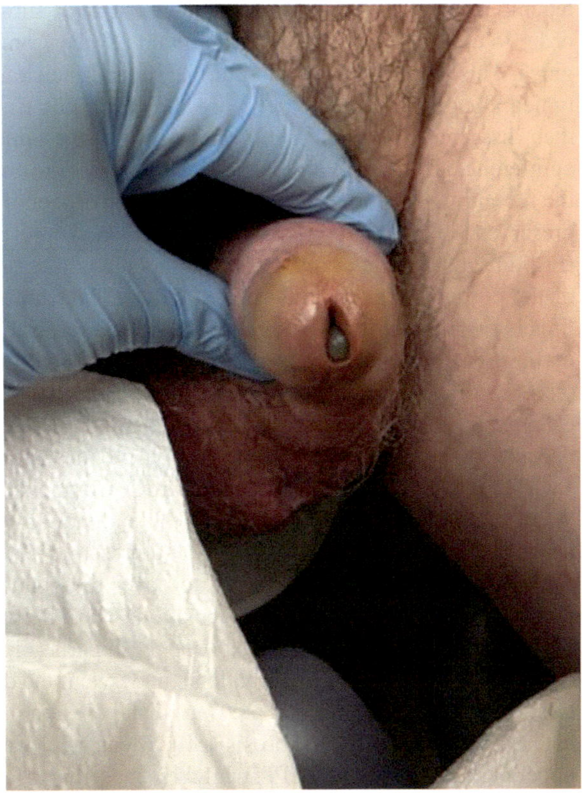

Fig. 11.8 Urethral erosion

solutions. A salvage procedure may be performed with only a single cylinder placed on the corporal cavity opposite to the erosion side [6, 29]. If the patient originally had a MPP and only one rod eroded into the distal urethra, the offending cylinder should be removed. However, the contralateral rod may be left in place since its pseudocapsule anatomically isolates it from the contaminated side [6, 30].

Delayed Replacement After Complete Distal Erosion

Delayed penile prosthesis placement after cylinder erosion is a challenge for many surgeons. The amount of corporal fibrosis that follows an eroded implant and the loss of integrity of the tunica albuginea increases the risk of perforation, erosion recurrence, and infection. To address this concern, Egydio and Kuehhas described their technique of distal penile shaft reconstruction with reinforcement which they called "the double-windsocks technique." [31] This technique is based on a modification of the windsock developed by Carson and Noh [23]. The double-windsocks technique involves a circumcision incision with subsequent penile degloving in order to elevate the neurovascular bundle (NVB) from the underlying tunica albuginea. This is followed by longitudinal, lateral incisions at 3 and 9 o'clock into the tunica albuginea in order to expose the cavernous tissue. The cavernous tissue is then dissected from the dorsolateral aspect of the tunica albuginea around the circumference, from the 3 o'clock to the 9 o'clock position. This dissection allows for the remaining cavernous tissue on the ventral aspect of the corpora cavernosa to be preserved, which subsequently supports and prevents injury to the urethra (Fig. 11.9a). It is important that the surgeon continues dissection up to the distal tip of the corpora to guarantee glans stability. This can be done with the use of two fingers or dilators. Prior to creation of the neocorpora, the surgeon must assess for urethral perforation. If urethral perforation is noted, the authors propose primary repair with absorbable suture and advocate for keeping a suprapubic cystostomy catheter for 3–4 weeks to ensure a better urethral healing process. After this, two neocorporas are formed from a polypropylene mesh graft for MPPs or a polypropylene/PTFE composite patch mesh (Bard® Composix™ mesh [Bard Davol Inc., Warwick, RI, USA]) for IPPs. The mesh is divided by an artificial septum created using nonabsorbable mononylon 3-0 sutures to prevent crossover. Once created, these "neocorporas" are then used to cover the penile implant and help stabilize both cylinders in a symmetrical position. The NVB and Buck's fascia are then replaced and used to cover the exposed mesh parts (Fig. 11.9).

In their series, a total of 69 patients underwent the double-windsock reconstruction, of which 45 patients had previous distal erosion of the tunica albuginea and 24 had unspecified corporal fibrosis [30]. Mean age was 56 years, and 57 patients underwent repair with a MPP while 12 chose an IPP. After a mean follow-up of 22.5 months (range 6–48 months), satisfaction rate was 88.4%. There were no reported cases that exhibited device extrusion, postoperative infection, or skin dehiscence. Neuropraxia occurred in five cases (3.4%) which resolved within 6 months. Seventeen patients (24.6%) endorsed delayed orgasms but they regained orgasmic ability within 4 months [31]. For surgeons who are concerned about the use of synthetic graft material, we believe the concept behind the "double-windsocks" technique could theoretically be performed using biologic tissues similar to that reported by Karpman et al. [26] instead of polypropylene mesh. However, this has not been verified in the available scientific literature.

Erosion of Prosthetic Reservoir

In a cadaver study, Henry and colleagues showed that the urinary bladder may be as close as 2 cm to the inguinal ring when full, while 6.75 cm when decompressed [32]. Therefore, the best way to avoid a bladder injury or erosion is to ensure that the bladder is empty prior to implantation of the reservoir. Various case reports have

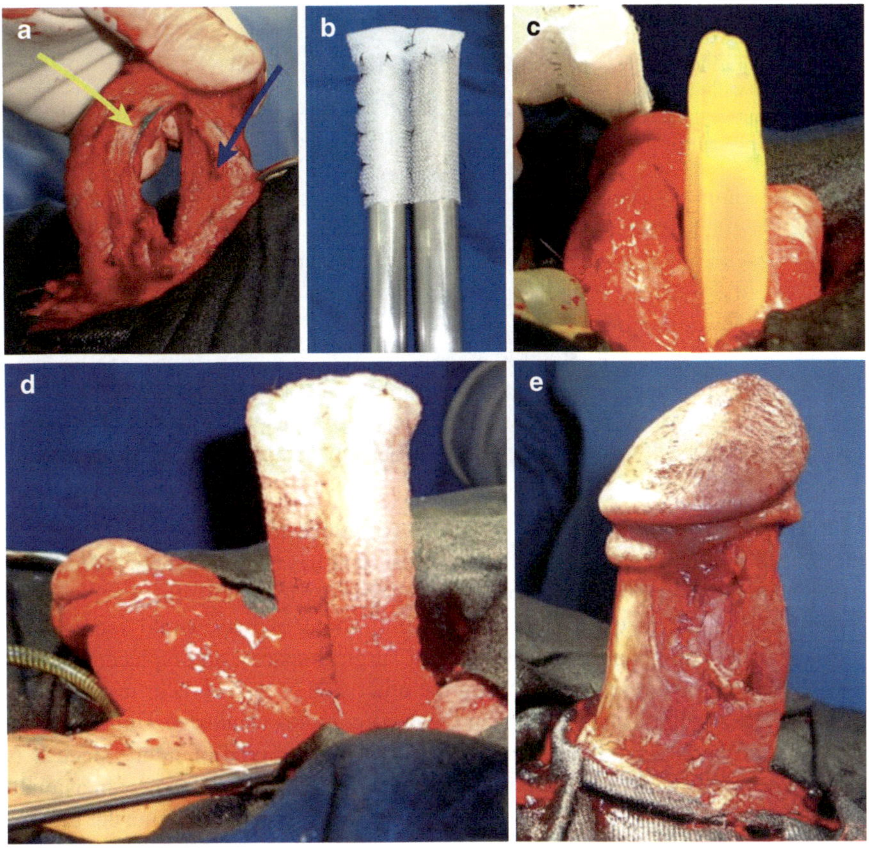

Fig. 11.9 Double windsock technique. (**a**) Dissection of bilateral corporas through lateral incisions. Notice the ventral aspect of the corpora (yellow arrow) and dorsal corpora (blue arrow). (**b**) Preparation of "neocorporas" over Hegar dilators. (**c**, **d**) Placement of IPP into neocorporas. (**e**) Re-approximation of Buck's fascia and neurovascular bundle prior to closure. (Courtesy: Dr. P. Egydio)

been published on patients with bladder perforation and/or erosion [33–38]. The largest series was reported by Furlow and Goldwasser who found erosion of the reservoir in a total of eight patients, six cases into the bladder and two cases into an ileal conduit (0.4%) [33]. Risk factors for visceral erosion include prior pelvic surgery and radiation. Patients with bladder erosion usually present with either gross hematuria or irritative voiding symptoms (Fig. 11.10) [33, 34]. Injury is confirmed with a cystoscopy or an imaging study, and depending on the extent of injury, the bladder defect should be repaired or a Foley catheter/suprapubic tube should be left in place until the bladder injury is healed.

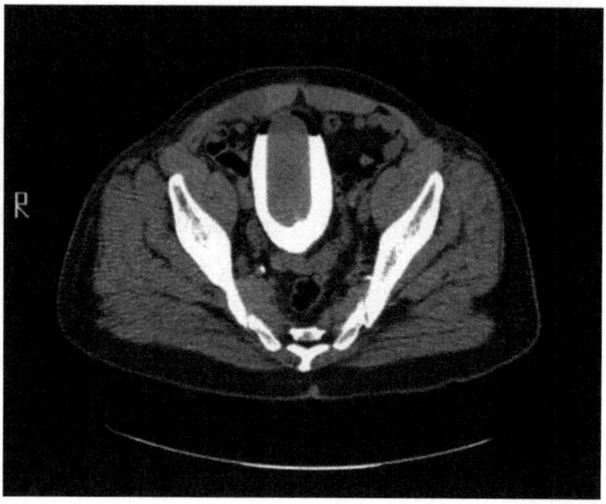

Fig. 11.10 Erosion of prosthetic reservoir within bladder which is noted as a filling defect within the bladder. (Courtesy: Dr. R Carrion, USF Health)

Intraoperatively, management of a bladder injury may be addressed without removal of the penile prosthesis. If the IPP reservoir has eroded into the bladder, the surgeon must perform a suprapubic incision in order to remove the reservoir and repair the bladder laceration. In this setting, some experts would recommend removal of all components, irrigation of all surgical spaces, and replacement of a new device with the reservoir placed in the other side of the pelvis or in an ectopic location. Bowel injury, on the other hand, is more complex to manage. Unfortunately, there are no studies of the proper management of this type of injury since it is extremely rare. Mulcahy recommends extension of the incision or a new incision to visualize the injury, resection of the involved bowel part, and anastomosing the two bowel segments, while repositioning the reservoir elsewhere with copious wound irrigation [6].

Pump-Related Erosion

Erosion of the prosthetic pump occurs as a result of infection in most occasions and manifests as pump fixation with eventual breaking through the skin with purulent discharge [22, 39]. However, there are times when pump erosion may also result from not having enough Dartos tissue covering the pump during closure. When combined with excess friction, this can cause the pump and or its tubing to erode through the groin or scrotal skin without necessarily having gross signs of infection (Fig. 11.11) [40]. Traditionally, these patients would require removal of the entire device, but there are a few cases that have been successfully managed with removal and replacement of the pump alone with good success [40, 41].

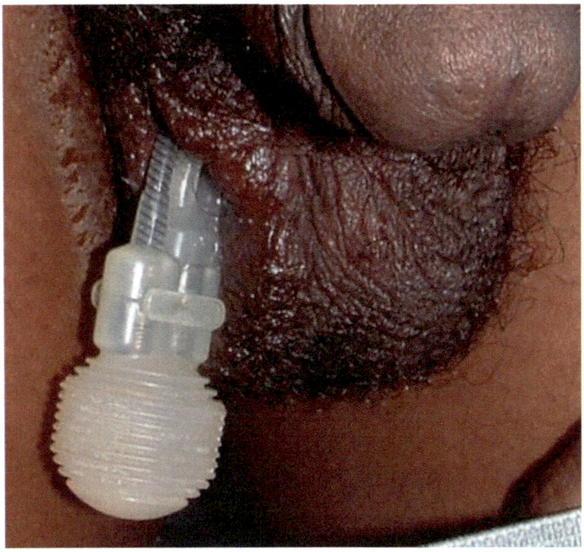

Fig. 11.11 Pump erosion without gross signs of infection. (Courtesy: Dr. R. Carrion, USF Health)

Conclusion

Although rare, penile prosthesis extrusion and erosion are challenging complications that may require complex maneuvers by the prosthetic surgeon. Techniques such as the distal corporoplasty, transglanular repair, and "distal anchoring stitch" which are performed through a distal incision may be offered for patients not requiring IPP removal and replacement. For those requiring an explantation with reimplantation, a "distal biologic cap" and "proximal ECT" techniques are alternative options that avoid a counter-incision and hence, patient discomfort and subsequent complications. Patients presenting with erosion-related issues should be aware of the risks associated to these procedures including reinfection. Most importantly, it is critically important for implant surgeons to be familiar with the different maneuvers to avoid complete erosion in order to maintain patient satisfaction.

References

1. Ziegelmann M, Kohler TS, Baile GC, et al. Surgical selection and counseling. Transl Androl Urol. 2017;6(4):609–19.
2. Chierigo F, Capogrosso P, Deho F, et al. Long-term follow-up after penile prosthesis implantation-survival and quality of life outcomes. J Sex Med. 2019;16(11):1827–33.
3. Henry GD, Laborde E. A review of surgical techniques for impending distal erosion and intra-operative penile implant complications: part 2 of a three-part review series on penile prosthetic surgery. J Sex Med. 2012;9:927–36.
4. Henry GD, Wilson SK, Delk JRII, Carson CC, Silverstein A, et al. Penile prosthesis cultures during revision surgery: a multicenter study. J Urol. 2004;172:153–6.

5. Henry GD, Wilson SK. Updates in inflatable penile prostheses. Urol Clin North Am. 2007;34:535–47, vi
6. Mulcahy JJ. The prevention and management of noninfectious complications of penile implants. Sex Med Rev. 2015;3:203–13.
7. Stember DS, Kohler TS, Morey AF. Management of perforation injuries during and following penile prosthesis surgery. J Sex Med. 2015;12(suppl 7):456–61.
8. Hsu GL, Brock G, Martinez-Pineiro L, et al. Anatomy and strength of the tunica albuginea: its relevance to penile prosthesis extrusion. J Urol. 1994;151:1205–8.
9. Minervi A, Ralph DJ, Pryor JP. Outcome of penile prosthesis implantation for treating erectile dysfunction: experience with 504 procedures. BJU Int. 2005;97:129–33.
10. Carson CC, Mulcahy JJ, Govier FE. Efficacy, safety, and patient satisfaction outcomes of the AMS 700CX inflatable penile prosthesis: results of a long-term multicenter study. J Urol. 2000;164:376–80.
11. Fuentes JL, Yi YA, Davenport MT, et al. Long-term sequelae of inflatable penile prosthesis: clinical characteristics of patients who developed distal cylinder tip extrusion. Transl Androl Urol. 2020;9(1):38–42.
12. Mulcahy JJ. Distal corporoplasty for lateral extrusion of penile prosthesis cylinders. J Urol. 1999;161:193–5.
13. Seftel AD, Oates RD, Goldstein I. Use of polytetrafluorethylene tube graft as a circumferential neotunica during placement of a penile prosthesis. J Urol. 1992;148:1531–3.
14. Levine LA, Zachary LS, Gottlieb LJ. Prosthesis placement after total phallic reconstruction. J Urol. 1993;149:593–8.
15. Smith CP, Kraus SR, Boone TB. Management of impending penile prosthesis erosion with a polytetrafluoroethylene distal wind sock graft. J Urol. 1998;160(6 Ptl):2037–40.
16. Knoll LD, Furlow WL. Corporeal reconstruction and prosthetic implantation for impotence associated with non-dilatable corporeal cavernosal fibrosis. Acta Urol Belg. 1992;60(1):15–25.
17. Knoll LD, Furlow WL, Benson RC, et al. Management of nondilatable cavernous fibrosis with the use of a downsized inflatable penile prosthesis. J Urol. 1995;153:366–7.
18. Jordan GH, Alter GJ, Gilbert DA, et al. Penile prosthesis implantation in total phalloplasty. J Urol. 1994;152:410–3.
19. Alter GJ, Greisman J, Werthman PE, et al. Use of a prefabricated tunica vaginalis fascia flap to reconstruct the tunica albuginea after recurrent penile prosthesis extrusion. J Urol. 1998;159:128–32.
20. Brant MD, Ludlow JK, Mulcahy JJ. The prosthesis salvage operation: immediate replacement of the infected penile prosthesis. J Urol. 1996;155:155–7.
21. Carson CC, Mulcahy JJ, Govier FE. Efficacy, safety, and patient satisfaction outcomes of the AMS 700CX inflatable penile prosthesis: results of a long-term multicenter study. AMS 700CX Study Group. J Urol. 2000;164(2):376–80.
22. Clavell-Hernandez J, Carrion R, Wang R. Management of non-infectious complications during and after penile prosthesis placement. In: Martins FE, Kulkarni SB, Kohler TS, editors. Textbook of male genitourethral reconstruction. Cham: Springer; 2020. p. 623–47.
23. Carson CC, Noh CH. Distal penile prosthesis extrusion: treatment with distal corporoplasty or Gortex windsock reinforcement. Int J Impot Red. 2002;14:81–4.
24. Shindel AW, Brant WO, Mwamukona K, et al. Transglanular repair of impending penile prosthetic cylinder extrusion. J Sex Med. 2010;7:2884–90.
25. Antonini G, Busetto GM, Del Giudice F, et al. Distal corporal anchoring stitch: a technique to address distal corporal crossovers and impending lateral extrusions of a penile prosthesis. J Sex Med. 2017;14:767–73.
26. Karpman E, DiGiorgio L, Carrion RE. Distal biologic cap for impending distal erosion. J Sex Med. 2020;17:551–5.
27. Clavell-Hernandez J. Proximal extracapsular tunneling: a simple technique for the management of impending cylinder erosion and complications related to corporal dilation. Sex Med. 2021; E.pub ahead of print https://doi.org/10.1016/j.esxm.2021.100379

28. Shaeer O, Shaeer K, AbdelRahman IFS. Salvage and extracapsular implantation for penile prosthesis infection or extrusion. J Sex Med. 2019;16:755–9.
29. Suarez-Sarmiento AJ, Perito P, Brennan M, et al. Delayed distal urethral perforation in patients with inflatable penile prosthesis surgery: A retrospective study of etiology and management. Presented at 19th annual SMSNA Meeting. Miami, FL, USA. Nov 8–11, 2018. Abstract 282.
30. Gross MS, Phillips EA, Balen A, et al. The malleable implant salvage technique: infection outcomes after Mulcahy salvage procedure and replacement of infected inflatable penile prosthesis with malleable prosthesis. J Urol. 2016;195:694–8.
31. Egydio PH, Kuehhas FE. Distal penile shaft reconstruction and reinforcement: the "double-windsocks" technique. J Sex Med. 2013;10:2571–8.
32. Henry G, Hsiao W, Karpman E, et al. A guide for inflatable penile prosthesis reservoir placement: pertinent anatomic measurements of the retropubic space. J Sex Med. 2014;11:273–8.
33. Furlow WL, Goldwasser B. Salvage of the eroded inflatable penile prosthesis: a new concept. J Urol. 1987;138:312.
34. Kramer AC, Chason JK, Kusakabe A. Report of two cases of bladder perforation caused by reservoir of inflatable penile prosthesis. J Sex Med. 2009;6:2064–7.
35. Dupont MC, Hochman HI. Erosion of an inflatable penile prosthesis reservoir into the bladder, presenting as bladder calculi. J Urol. 1988;129:367–8.
36. Eldefrawy A, Kava BR. An unusual complication during inflatable penile prosthesis implantation. Urology. 2010;76:847.
37. Brusky J, Dikranin A, Aboseif S. Retrieval of inflatable penile prosthesis reservoir from the bladder. Int J Impot Res. 2005;17:302–3.
38. Fitch WP 3rd, Roddy T. Erosion of inflatable penile prosthesis reservoir into bladder. J Urol. 1986;136:1080.
39. Talib RA, Shamsodini A, Salem EA, et al. Isolated pump erosion of an inflatable penile prosthesis through the scrotum in a diabetic patient. Arch Ital di Urol e Androl. 2013;85:1.
40. Morales A. Tubing erosion of an inflatable penile prosthesis long after implantation. Sex Med. 2014;2:103–6.
41. Köhler TS, Gupta NK, Wilson SK. Wilson's pearls, perils, and pitfalls of penile prosthesis surgery. Fort Smith: Calvert McBride Publishers; 2018. p. 127–8.

Chapter 12
Management of Long-Term Complications of Penile Implant Surgery

Daniar Osmonov and Ahmed M. Ragheb

The "Sticky" Pump

History

With the improving rates in surgery-related complications ever since the implantation of the first IPP [1], manufacturers have been focusing their efforts on improving IPP versatility and reliability [2–5]. Large series studies have shown that the majority of IPP revision surgeries were due to mechanical failure [6, 7] with almost half of these failures being attributed to pump malfunction [8]. In parallel to enhancements in implant designs and material, famous manufacturers have developed sophisticated control valve pumps that allow easy inflation and deflation of the cylinders while preventing autoinflation caused by increased intra-abdominal pressure. Examples are the two most widely used pumps today are the Momentary Squeeze (MP) pump by American Medical Systems (AMS; Minnetonka, MN, USA) in their 700 series IPP and the One-Touch Release (OTR) pump by Coloplast (Minneapolis, MN) in their Titan series. Both pumps are similar in allowing complete deflation of the implant upon briefly squeezing a release valve situated above the pump. However, despite their successful utilization by millions of patients around the

D. Osmonov (✉)
University Medical Center Schleswig Holstein, Kiel, Germany
e-mail: daniar.osmonov@uksh.de

A. M. Ragheb
Department of Urology, Beni-Suef University, Beni Suef, Egypt

Bedaya Fertility & IVF Hospitals, Cairo, Egypt

IHUN, Cairo, Egypt
e-mail: ahmed.ragheb@med.bsu.edu.eg

E. P. Miranda, J. P. Mulhall (eds.), *Penile Implant Surgery*,
https://doi.org/10.1007/978-3-030-82363-4_12

world, rarely could they also share in a common phenomenon related to the control valve mechanisms known as stiction [9]. By definition, that is when the pump fails in the absence of fluid loss from the implant tubing system.

The Problem

The terms "stiction syndrome," "sticky pump," "pump stickiness," and lately "pseudomalfunction" are all synonyms to the same problem [10, 11]. Although IPP pump stickiness is a rare form of transient pump malfunction, it may be troublesome for both the patient and the surgeon during the postoperative follow-up period. The patient complains of inability to inflate the implant cylinders especially after prolonged periods of inactivity. Hence, this costs the surgeon a significant increase in the number of postoperative teaching sessions required for the patient to properly operate the device. It may also be recurrent and may present early or late. An idle pump for at least 6 weeks is the common factor in most of the cases [10]. According to the laws of mechanical engineering, a prolonged period of valve inactivity was hypothesized to generate static friction or stiction between the active components of the valve control systems leading to increased resistance to their mobility [10]. Pump valves become fixed in the deflated position rendering the pump bulb incompressible or in some cases hard to decompress, thus preventing fluid circulation and cylinder inflation.

Differential Diagnosis

The surgeon must differentiate this type of transient failure from other types of persistent pump malfunction as those caused by a disruption in the hydraulic loop of the implant. Presentations may vary according to the nature of the defect. Sometimes the pump may fail to inflate the implant despite repeated compressions in addition to hearing a characteristic sound of turbulence upon squeezing. This denotes acute fluid leakage. However, in cases of needle punctures or minute tears, the pump may fail to decompress with diminution of the quality of erection over months to years. Nevertheless, the only remedy for the latter two conditions would be revision and replacement.

Another cause of sticky pump that may require revision without replacement is when the pump becomes surrounded by a hindering thick inflammatory capsule. In these cases both inflation and deflation may become impossible (Fig. 12.1). It is hypothesized that missed lacerations to the tunica vaginalis may cause fluid to leak, causing a dense inflammatory reaction around the pump. The only way the pump regains its function is by excising this thick capsule and releasing the pump (Fig. 12.2).

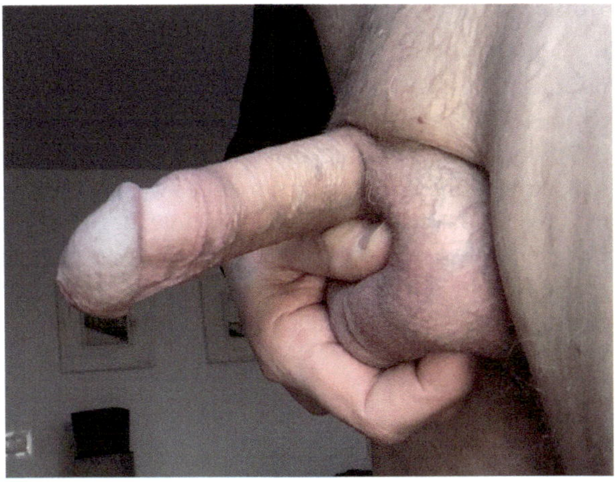

Fig. 12.1 Patient unable to palpate and deflate the implant (Osmonov®)

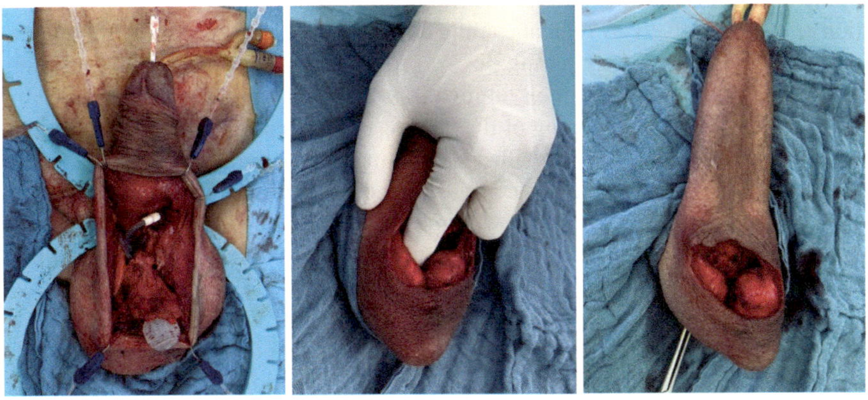

Fig. 12.2 Pump surrounded by dense scar tissue. (left) Placing pump in most dependent area after scar release. (middle) Pump made easy to palpate after scar removal. (right) (Osmonov®)

Studies

To our knowledge, two studies on IPP pumps have addressed this complication [10, 11]. Garber and his group were the first to refer to this problem as a "pseudomalfunction" in their study on 550 patients whom were implanted by a single surgeon with the Coloplast Titan IPP One-Touch Release pump (Coloplast Corp, Minneapolis, MN, USA). Forty-three patients returned complaining of a "hard-to-squeeze" pump. Only 2.5% were able to overcome this recurrent problem on their own by applying firm pressure, while the rest required the surgeon's assistance. Upon examination, it was obvious that this was caused by a fixed inflate-deflate valve disk in the deflate position. Firm pressure to the pump bulb was able to shift the valve disk to the inflate position and allow proper inflation. In conclusion, all patients were managed conservatively [11]. In a later study on over 300 patients receiving the AMS 700 series (AMS; Minnetonka, MN, USA) IPP, a total of 10 patients presented with difficulty activating the Momentary Squeeze pump after a prolonged period of at least 6 weeks during which the IPP was not cycled.

Although they revised the initial four patients with pump mobilization and replacement, the last six patients (60%) were successfully managed nonoperatively by forced deflation in the office. Therefore, the investigators concluded in both studies that the phenomenon of pump stiction was to be treated conservatively whenever possible. They also recommended against prolonged periods of pump inactivity by daily cycling to prevent recurrence of such a complication in the future.

Management

Pump stiction may be prevented as early as intraoperatively during device preparation or postoperatively by regular cycling of the device. Intraoperative valve lubrication can be achieved early during device preparation simply by forcibly injecting 20 mL of saline into the reservoir tubing of the pump and repeating until you see the pump jump or hear the popping of the control valve inside. Another way is by rapidly and forcibly squeezing the bulb and deflating several times until the pump pops. Both techniques are complemented by device cycling several times to ensure adequate pump lubrication. As a rule, you must always conclude cycling by applying one bulb compression to engage the pump valve in the standby position which makes it easy for the next use.

Several maneuvers have been introduced to treat sticky pumps conservatively negating the need for revision, provided leakage was excluded. All these approaches are based on the idea of stiction compensation either by forcible deflation for the one-way MS valve or by forcible inflation for the OTR pump. The "forced deflation" procedure is achieved by compressing both implant cylinders with one hand proximally while depressing the pump deflation button with the other hand. This causes the fluid to overcome the static friction at the points of contact of the valve [10]. For the OTR pump, several solutions have been suggested by the manufacturer. The first maneuver is to ensure the straightening of the tubing and compress the pump while pulling down on it. The second is to use both hands to stabilize and rapidly press the deflate button repeatedly while compressing the pump bulb in succession whether gently or firmly. Pump activation may be deferred if the patient is in the early postoperative period (less than 6 weeks) or if in pain while advising regular hot baths to decrease scrotal pain and edema around the pump. Finally, the surgeon may resort to pump release under sedation or anesthesia if all the previous measures fail.

As maintenance, all patients are advised to cycle their devices routinely daily afterward to prevent stiction recurrence. Not necessarily completely but enough to ensure adequate pump valve lubrication.

SST Deformity: What Is True, What Is a Myth?

Definition and Cause

SST stands for supersonic transporter, which accurately describes a rare yet troublesome glans penis deformity post penile prosthesis implantation (PPI) resembling the nose of the famous Concorde aircraft. In other words, it represents a drooping glans, which is hypermobile despite a fully erect penis. An SST deformity is also the ventral variant of the floppy glans syndrome (FGS). Such a deformity may be a false SST due to an improper implant cylinder length or position or a true SST that is hypermobility of the glans despite proper implantation (Fig. 12.1). The latter usually is a result of the lack of natural intrinsic granular support over the distal corpora despite proper implant sizing and positioning [12]. Too short implants causing an SST deformity may arise early postoperative as a result of inadequate sizing or later on due to inadequate proximal corporal dilation or proximal implant migration via an unrecognized crural perforation. Penile tissue expansion induced overtime by the implant itself may also lead to the same picture.

Incidence

Data on the true incidence of the SST deformity, in general, remain scarce and controversial. A couple of studies recorded laxity at the glanulo-cavernous junction post-PPI requiring repair in 8.5–10% of the cases [13] opposed to less than 5% in another report [14]. Nevertheless, the false SST subtype was reported in 0.2–0.9% of PPI cases. Wilson recalled correcting only six true-SST deformities in over 11,000 patients which were more noticeable among uncircumcised men. Undersized cylinders were responsible for the vast majority of SST cases in his view [15] (Fig. 12.3).

The Problem

The SST deformity, although rare, can be a troublesome complication for the patient from both cosmesis and functionality standpoints. A drooping glans renders penetrative sex uncomfortable or painful to both partners due to buckling [6] or loss of the natural cushioning effect of the glans at the tip of the penile shaft [16].

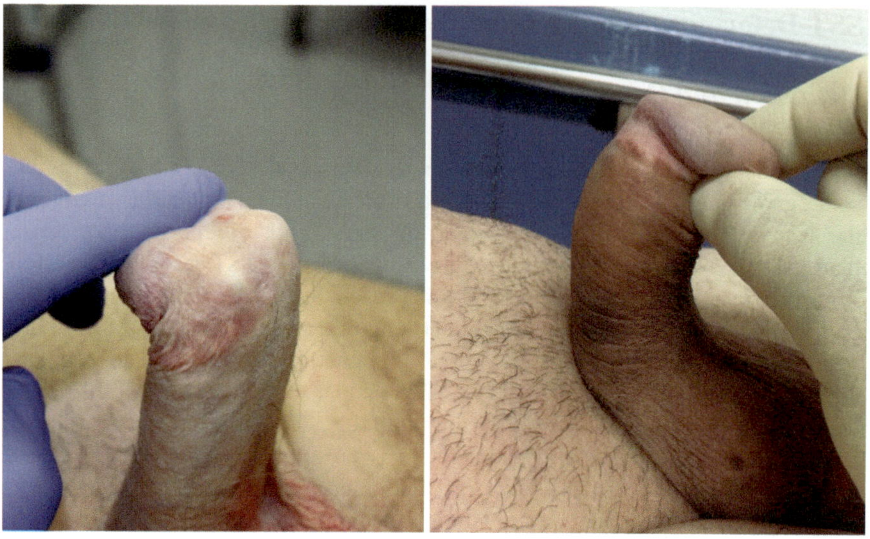

Fig. 12.3 Two variants of the floppy glans syndrome; false SST deformity which is due to either undersized or mispositioned cylinders (left) and true SST deformity which is due to glans hypermobility despite proper cylinder implantation (right) (Osmonov®)

Differential Diagnosis

A false SST deformity can be easily delineated from true glans hypermobility by simply pulling on the shaft skin of the erect penis toward the pelvis. In the case of an undersized implant, the glans will retreat and settle on the tip of the two cylinders, thus abolishing the SST picture. In contrast, a true hypermobile glans will persist to be floppy since the implant is properly sized. The type of FGS dictates the line of management (Fig. 12.2).

Management

The ideal management of an SST deformity begins with an accurate delineation of the SST subtype. Nevertheless, the treatment approach for both types remains an area of debate. Treatment options range from sole observation to medications to finally surgery. Wilson advocates a "wait and see" approach in case the implant was properly sized. Healing together with scar and capsule formation around the cylinder tips 3 months postoperative seemed to resolve the problem in most cases [15]. Other, under-supported, conservative options reported were oral PDE5 inhibitors, intraurethral prostaglandin injections, novel glans bulking agents as Durasphere®, or utilizing a vacuum device [13] (Fig. 12.4).

When it comes to surgical intervention, replacing an undersized implant with a properly sized one after a mini washout to avoid the 10% increased infection risk is the procedure of choice [17] (Fig. 12.5). However, for a true SST several

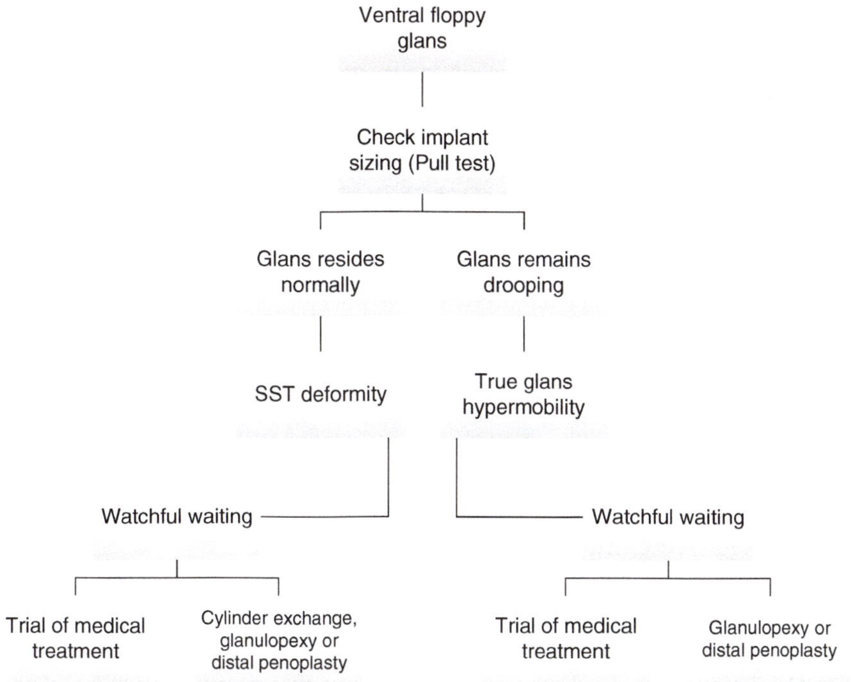

Fig. 12.4 Ventral FGS management algorithm

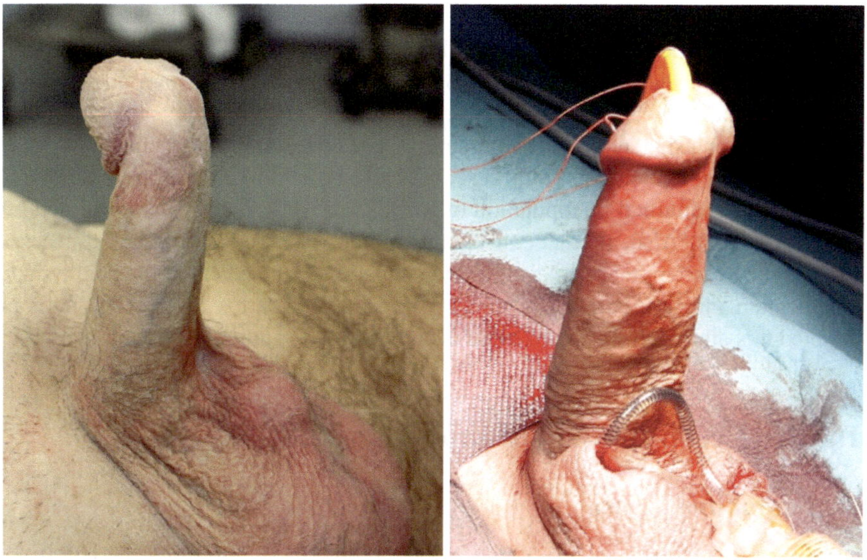

Fig. 12.5 False SST deformity due to undersized or mispositioned cylinders (left) fixed by properly sized cylinder replacement (right) (Osmonov®)

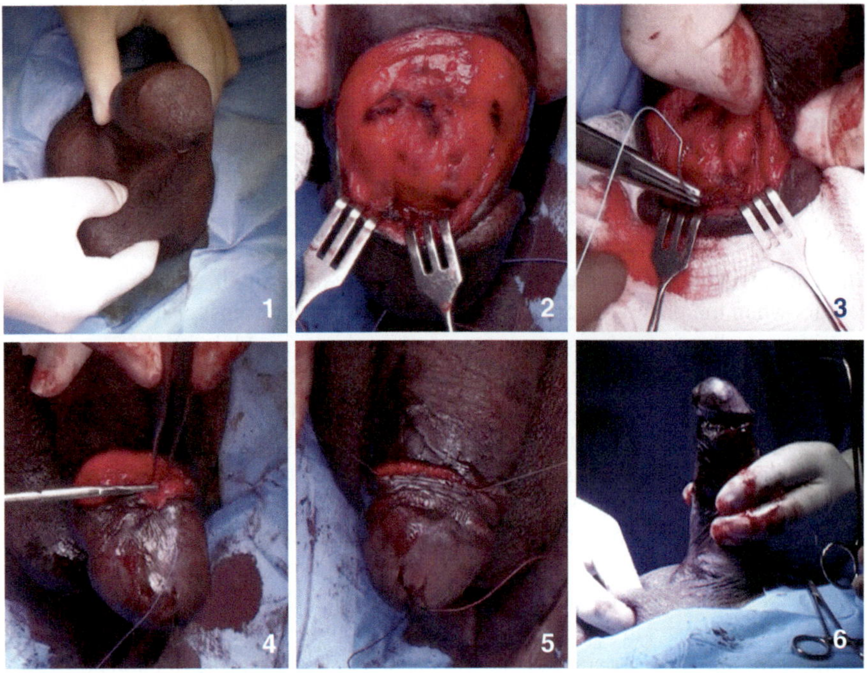

Fig. 12.6 Example of a glanulopexy (in steps): (1) Preoperative picture of true SST. (2) Dorsal hemisubcoronal incision and anchoring suture markings. (3) Deep fixation sutures between glans and corporal tips. (4) Superficial reinforcing sutures. (5) Closure. (6) Postoperative picture (Osmonov®)

glanulopexy and penoplasty techniques have been proposed (Fig. 12.6). Ball used a silk suture to fix the glans distally to Buck's fascia proximally via a dorsal semi-circumcisional incision [18]. Later, variable modifications of the same "glanular hitch" concept using nonabsorbable sutures became popular with favorable outcomes and nil complications [16]. This could also be achieved through smaller incisions and with minimal manipulation of Buck's fascia as recently demonstrated by Ziegelmann [13]. Also, another concept of penoplasty proved to be equally successful. Glanular realignment was achieved via plication of the layers of the penile shaft whether the tunica albuginea or simply the skin and dartos layers. The authors adopted this approach aiming to avoid accidental needle injury of the implant [19].

Delayed Urethral Injury or Erosion

Definition and Cause

A delayed urethral injury or erosion can occur at any time post-implantation, in any type of patient, and without any predictive factors. Iatrogenic urethral injuries PPI can be subtle and missed during surgery. Eventually, a fistulous tract develops

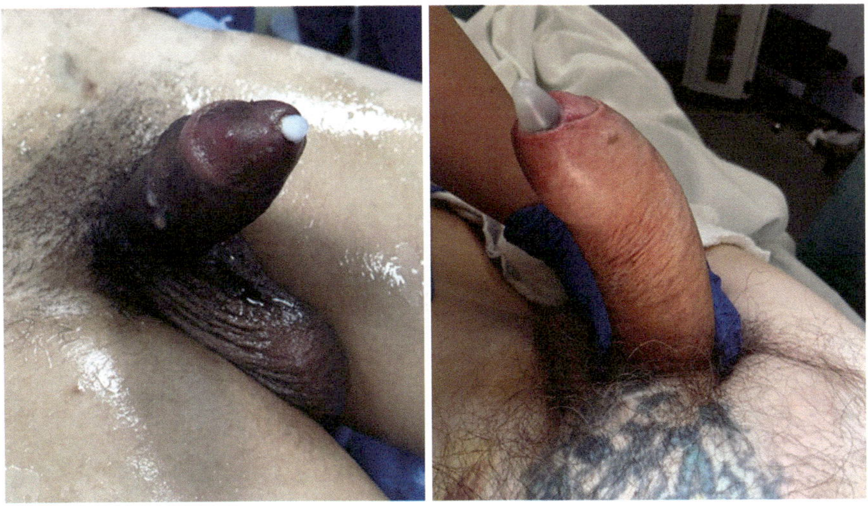

Fig. 12.7 Semirigid rod protruding through the meatus associated by a concomitant infection after eroding through the urethra weeks following PPI (left) (Ragheb®). Inflatable cylinder protruding 8 years after surgery (right) (Osmonov®)

between the injured corpora and the urethral lumen. It may present weeks to years following a PPI as new-onset hematuria whether gross or microscopic, glans hyperemia, burning micturition, device infection, or erosion of the implant into the urethra [20, 21] (Fig. 12.7). The primary risk factor for such a complication is the anatomical configuration of the urethra, especially at its distal part. The region around the fossa navicularis is the weakest and most compressed by the corpora cavernosa [22]. Aggressive corporal dilation, faulty cylinder positioning, or implant oversizing may predispose to delayed urethral erosion (Fig. 12.8). Also a missed urethral tear during a modeling maneuver may also be the trigger before the cylinder finds its way through the urethra and eventually out of the meatus (Fig. 12.9). Less often can the pendulous urethra be the site of injury thus a corpora-urethral fistula. Bleeding at the meatus would be the first sign upon implant inflation. It is worthy to mention that delayed injury of the urinary bladder caused by reservoir erosion may also present with hematuria. A cystoscopy will aid in such a differential diagnosis.

Other potential causes of delayed urethral erosion are repeated catheterization post-implantation by clean intermittent catheterization, an indwelling catheter, or regular cystoscopy. Chronic friction against the tips of the prosthesis may facilitate cylinder erosion into the urethra. Compromised distal penile sensation in certain populations such as diabetics, paraplegics, and irradiated patients may also predispose delayed urethral erosion and cylinder extrusion [23].

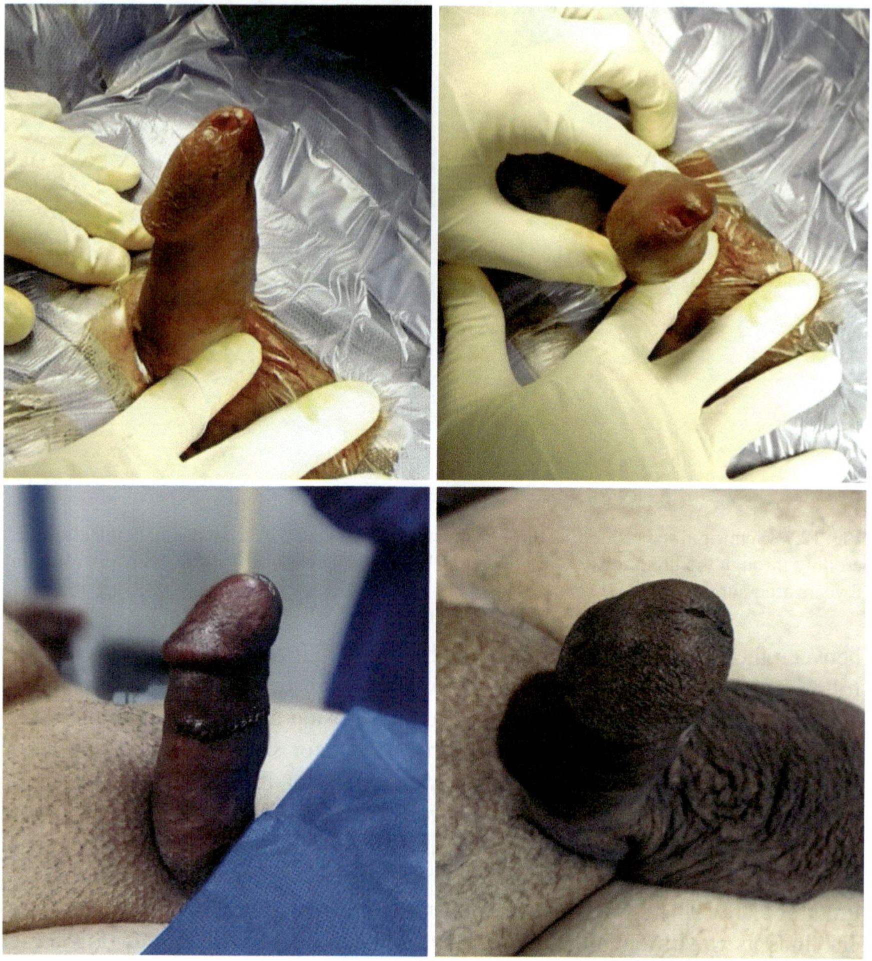

Fig. 12.8 Pictures of oversized protruding rods after faulty corporal dilation and oversizing by an inexperienced surgeon (top row). Postoperative pictures after realignment combined with bilateral distal corporoplasty and rod length resizing via hemisubcoronal incision (bottom row) (Ragheb®)

Prevention

The risk of urethral perforation or injury during implantation surgery should be avoided by following certain precautions and safety rules during the procedure. It starts with early anticipation of potentially challenging cases such as revised implants which are commonly associated with fibrotic corpora. It is also mandatory that the surgeon properly plans his procedure and have the necessary experience and instruments required particularly for expected cases of difficult dilation [20]. During all steps of the procedure, the urethra must always be identified and protected. This is achieved primarily by adequate exposure and catheterization. During corporal

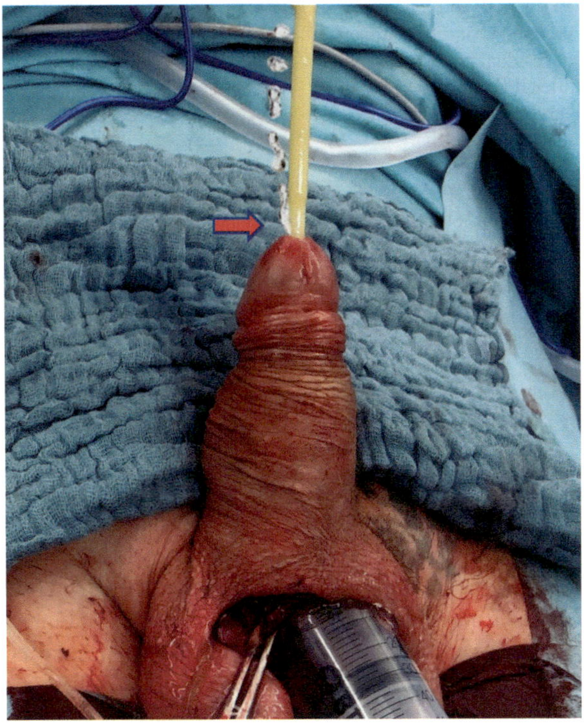

Fig. 12.9 Positive water check denotes urethral tear (Osmonov®)

dilation, the urethra is secured away using the non-dominant hand while maintaining dilation in the lateral and dorsal direction away from the thinnest, weakest, and closest part of the tunica albuginea to the urethra [24]. The fossa navicularis may also be protected specifically by squeezing the glans for increased stability while advancing dilators in a controlled manner [25].

Another maneuver to prevent urethral compromise during modeling for residual curvature after PPI is to apply the bending hand on the penile shaft rather than the glans while firmly supporting the corporotomies with the opposing hand [17, 26] (Fig. 12.4).

Switching to a perineal urethrostomy or a suprapubic tube for men requiring clean intermittent catheterization was found to obviate the risk of urethral erosion especially when utilizing the inflatable types of implants [22] (Fig. 12.10).

Management

When cylinder erosion through the urethra has been diagnosed, management varies according to the presence or absence of signs of infection. The presence of erythema, pain, or discharge will demand total device explantation with delayed revision as opposed to noninfected cases. A cylinder that has eroded into the urethra is

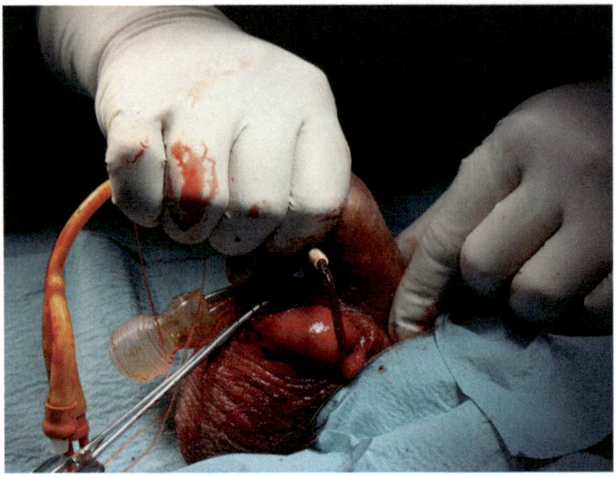

Fig. 12.10 Intraoperative modeling for the treatment of residual penile curvature after IPP implantation. The surgeon's bending hand must be at the shaft, not the glans, to avoid the risk of a distal urethral perforation (Osmonov®)

to be considered contaminated [21]. Nevertheless, in the absence of overt signs of infection, sole removal of the offending cylinder with thorough salvage washout and installing a urethral catheter for 3 days is a justified option. Often leaving in a single cylinder may be adequate for satisfactory sexual intercourse. Tubing that has been cut in the inflatable types is sealed off by special end caps or via Hemaclips®. Otherwise, the offending cylinder is replaced either 6–8 weeks later or immediately as a salvage procedure. For IPP salvage cases, some recommend implanting a single malleable rod in the intact corpora or bilaterally if the defect was repairable. Sole explantation of the extruding rod while leaving in its isolated counterpart suffices when salvaging a malleable case. With adequate patient counseling, the single rod may be satisfactory negating the need for a future reimplantation procedure. As a rule, corporal defects may be left to heal spontaneously if small and the patient opted not to immediately replace the eroding cylinder. In contrast, if the defect was large or an immediate replacement was planned, the injury would be primarily repaired leaving in a urethral catheter for a few days [27]. Men with compromised wound healing may need a more reinforced reconstruction approach for the urethro-cavernosal defect either by using a dermal graft or by simply double-breasted closure [28].

Glans Denervation or Devascularization

Definition and Cause of Glans Devascularization

Glans ischemia and necrosis is a rare and underreported, yet dreadful, complication post-PPI related to both malleable or the inflatable types. A typical presentation is a dusky glans on the first postoperative day following PPI, which may be associated with blisters (Fig. 12.11). Anatomically, the glans penis is supplied by a rich anastomotic network of end arteries derived from the terminal branches of the dorsal penile artery as well as tributaries from the bulbourethral artery [29]. Correspondingly, glans ischemia would more likely require a systemic pathogenesis to occur rather than a local cause. Hence, the same predisposing factors to peripheral vascular disease have been identified for this unusual complication. The majority of cases include diabetes mellitus as the common denominator, smoking, metabolic syndrome, chronic renal failure, end-stage atherosclerosis, as well as previous irradiation and implant revision cases [30]. Over 90% of compromised glanular blood supply was attributed to novel surgical approaches that have gained popularity starting from the mere subcoronal incision to ancillary techniques needed as penile shaft degloving, neurovascular bundle or urethral mobilization, and penile lengthening procedures (Fig. 12.12). A simple hematoma collection under the subcoronal incision against the tough intracorporal components and combined with a pressure wrap

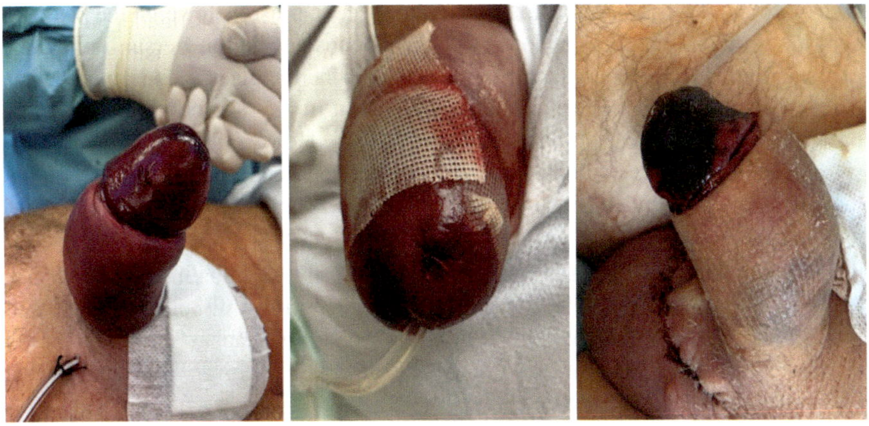

Fig. 12.11 Variants of dusky or blistered glans on the first postoperative day (Osmonov®)

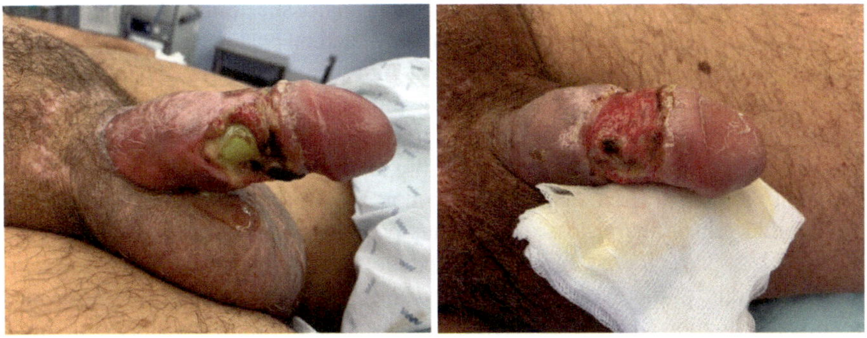

Fig. 12.12 A complicated penile lengthening (sliding) procedure (left). Spontaneous reepithelialization and healing 6 weeks after device removal (Osmonov®)

might explain the immediate postoperative glans ischemia and necrosis [31]. Penile pressure bandages were the cause in nearly 70% of predisposed patients. Interestingly, with no evidence of severe arterial insufficiency on performing a pre-operative penile duplex in these patients, one could not predict such a complication [31].

Management

Due to the scarcity of reported glans necrosis cases, a management protocol remains to be established. Treating a case of glans necrosis post-PPI remains a dilemma. Deciding whether to conserve or intervene depends mainly on the clinical picture and the surgeon's personal opinion. The first crucial step is to differentiate between a dry gangrene picture due to ischemia that may allow less emergent intervention and wet gangrene with an infection that contradicts conservative treatment [32]. In case of opting for conservative treatment, the surgeon must then weigh the pros and cons of watchful waiting in hopes of spontaneous resolution versus immediate explantation. During observation of a suspected ischemic glans with implant left in place, the authors recommend instant debridement of any necrotic area to prevent bacterial invasion and gangrene development [33]. However, if systemic or local signs of infection were evident from the start (wet gangrene), immediate removal of the implant would be the treatment of choice accompanied by debriding of the necrotic areas to the extent of partial amputation if necessary [34].

A noninfected ischemic glans failing to resolve while observing the implant will eventually result in an extruding implant or a necrotic glans (dry gangrene) requiring prompt debridement and tissue loss (Fig. 12.13). In contrast, emergent implant removal once in doubt reverses glans ischemia, thus allowing spontaneous reepithelialization and healing without complications.

Wilson et al. advise surgeons to avoid extensive IPP adjunctive surgical approaches in patients with a high risk of peripheral vascular. Moreover, dealing with signs of glans necrosis postoperatively in these particular patients should be in a more assertive manner to avoid inevitable glans tissue loss and disfigurement. Hence, once a glans appears suspicious or congested on postoperative day 1, immediate implant removal to prevent subsequent glans necrosis is crucial [31]. Although the reports on granular hypoesthesia following PPI are very rare, yet injury of the penile dorsal nerve injury or its branches in the neuromuscular bundle is a dreaded complication during PPI surgery especially via the infrapubic approach due to the proximity of the operative field to the dorsal nerve. This will consequently result in irreversible sensorineural loss of the glans penis which in turn devastates sexual function [35, 36]. The risk of decreased penile sensation increases following revision cases due to the associated distorted anatomy [37]. In contrast to previous reports of litigation cases for decreased penile sensation following successful infrapubic IPP surgeries, the majority of recent reports appear to be promising. Using a glans/elbow biothesiometer to compare pre-IPP implantation glans sensation in 62 patients who underwent IPP surgery via the classic penoscrotal approach to that

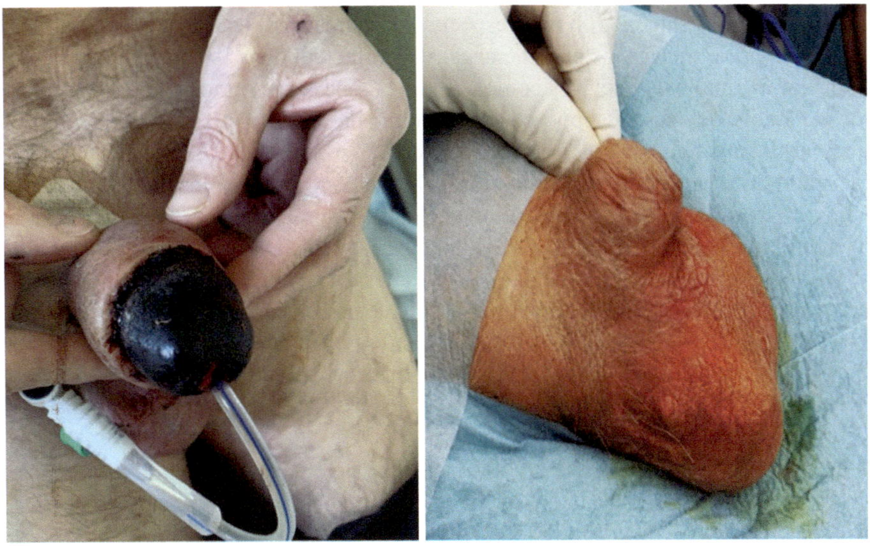

Fig. 12.13 Development of dry gangrene after 2 weeks of expectant management (left). Glanular tissue loss 3 weeks postoperative (right) (Osmonov®)

6 weeks and 6 months post-implantation revealed no change in sensation [38]. In a comparison of the penoscrotal approach with the infrapubic approach in 65 men, penile sensitivity to vibration after IPP implantation was similarly not affected upon resuming normal sexual activity. The authors recommended the utilization of optical magnification for clear identification of the dorsal nerve when using the infrapubic approach. A review published the same year of 22 studies comparing the infrapubic to the penoscrotal approach for IPP placement did not report a single case of glans hypoesthesia after IPP placement regardless of the approach [39]. Nevertheless, a retrospective study including 126 virgin IPP implantations reported 11 cases of altered penile sensations. However, the majority were related to those implanted via a penoscrotal incision (nine patients) compared to the infrapubic approach (two patients) [40]. In conclusion, despite the exceedingly rare incidence of penile sensory loss following PPI via the infrapubic approach, careful dissection of the neurovascular bundle remains critical to ensure intact penile sensation.

Penile Shortening

Introduction

With the wide utilization of the modern three-piece inflatable penile prostheses, penile girth rarely becomes an issue after PPI surgery. Instead, because of patients' unrealistic post-PPI expectations and their comparison to their predysfunction erect penile length, loss of penile length is the common complaint [41]. Subsequently, patient post-PPI satisfaction rates especially for those associating their masculinity to the length of their penis become negatively affected [42]. This is seen more common among malleable devices compared to IPP ones. The uniform and solid nature of malleable devices, as opposed to the inflatable one, forces wise implanters to incline toward choosing a more "comfortable" size to avoid subsequent chronic pain and pressure erosion complications. On the contrary, the pliable nature of IPPs allows oversizing during implantation depending on the tissue-expanding nature of penile tissues. Hence, IPPs are more likely to allow penile size preservation or gain. Nevertheless, even after oversizing the cylinders, several patients still complain of length loss post-IPP implantation [43–47]. The loss of penile length may be objective or subjective. Unrealistic expectations and myths surrounding penile prosthesis surgery are the primary causes of patient and partner dissatisfaction post-PPI [43].

Etiology

Excluding intentional downsizing as in the case for malleable devices, the causes behind post-PPI penile length loss may be classified into false (subjective) and true (objective) causes. Treatment-refractory ED patients likely have had a long history of dysfunction leading to inaccurate recollection of their true erect length. Moreover, these men often suffer from obesity which compromises their perceived penile lengths [41]. On the other hand, true causes arise from conditions known to be the primary cause or associated with ED. They may include tunical scarring as in Peyronie's disease, loss of glanular engorgement, and corporal tissue fibrosis or loss by ischemia or denervation following priapism or prostate cancer treatments [48–51].

Incidence

One of the earlier reports documented post-PPI shortening in 60 out of 200 men who had received the AMS three-piece IPP [44]. Deveci and his group compared stretched flaccid penile lengths before implantation to penile lengths 1 and 6 months postoperative in 56 patients. Although they found no statistically significant difference in objective penile length after the surgery compared to preoperative measurements, 72% reported a subjective loss of length and were less satisfied [43].

The first study to objectively show a significant decrease in erect penile length after IPP implantation demonstrated an average decrease of 0.7 cm. However, in this study, they used preoperative ICI-induced erect penile length for comparison [45]. By utilizing both preoperative pharmacologically induced and stretched penile lengths, another study showed a median loss of 0.5 cm, which was only perceived, in 43% of the men [46]. Contradicting results were reported by another group years later. Xie et al. observed a statistically significant increase in penile length and girth after IPP surgery in 62 patients. Hence they considered PPI to be a penile size preserving surgery [38]. To further confirm their results, Habous and his group reported an overall gain in penile length and girth of 0.36 cm and 1.04 cm, respectively, for both malleable and inflatable implantations with the latter being superior in size gain. They preferred to use preoperative stretched penile length opposed ICI-induced measurements to avoid residual erectile function as a confounding factor [52]. Despite increases in penile circumference and width after implanting the AMS 700™ LGX (AMS, Minneapolis, MN, USA) by Wallen et al., a statistically significant length loss was observed in stretched penile length. The authors attributed it to healing fibrotic changes, lack of granular tumescence, erectile tissue hypoxia and atrophy, capsular contraction, or a combination of them all. They recommended early maximum inflation and cycling of the devices as a means of overcoming this phenomenon.

Strategies to Preserve Length

In parallel to the major advancements in penile implant technology by manufacturers, serious implanters continue to innovate new techniques to optimize patient satisfaction. Among these approaches are strategies to maintain or enhance penile length after PPI surgery. These approaches can be adopted at the three different stages of surgery: preoperative, intraoperative, or later on postoperative (Table 12.1).

By applying 2–4 h of daily external traction therapy in the preoperative period, Levine et al. were able to gain a mean of 1.5 cm in stretched penile length [53]. Similarly, stretching the penis months via vacuum devices before PPI surgery

Table 12.1 Approaches to optimize post-PPI penile length classified according to perioperative stage

Before surgery	Penile stretching techniques
	Relying on an experienced surgeon
	Prompt PPI once indicated
During surgery	Penile degloving via the subcoronal approach
	Using inflatable versus malleable implant
	Aggressive length measuring techniques
	Using size-expanding implant
	Oversizing cylinder length
	Cavernous tissue-preserving dilation
	Augmentation corporoplasty
	Ventral phalloplasty
	Suspensory ligament division
	Suprapubic lipectomy
After surgery	Glans augmentation using fillers
	Using glans-engorging medications (oral/local)
	Second stage size enhancement techniques
	PPI revision with larger cylinders

allowed longer IPP placements during surgery [54, 55]. Choosing a center of excellence surgeon as well as immediate to early PPI when indicated, especially in cases with expected corporal fibrosis, e.g., refractory ischemic priapism, were also strategies found to have a positive impact on the size of implant used [56, 57].

Apart from the tissue-expanding capability of oversized IPPs as opposed to malleable implants, several new aggressive length measuring techniques have succeeded in adding length to the penis. Adding an extra cm proximally and distally on corporal measurement when in doubt of reaching the far ends of the corpora was suggested [58]. When coupling the new length measurement technique with consistent and maximal postoperative device cycling for 2 years, 77% of the men perceived an increased or maintained penile length [59]. Another beneficial intraoperative strategy is to avoid unnecessary corporeal dilation in virgin cases. The volume of residual intact cavernosal tissue appeared to be directly proportional to postoperative penile length at 6 months [60].

Penile degloving via the subcoronal approach was found to allow maximal relaxation of dartos fascia tethering to the tunica albuginea caused by longstanding ED and corporal fibrosis. Penile lengths increased by 0.6 cm on average in a single surgeon series of 200 patients following the subcoronal approach [61] (Fig. 12.14).

More aggressive and complex approaches requiring specialized training and experience were introduced to provide more length gain during PPI surgery. Augmentation corporoplasty by circumferential tunical incision and grafting, namely, the sliding technique, resulted in a length enhancement reaching up to

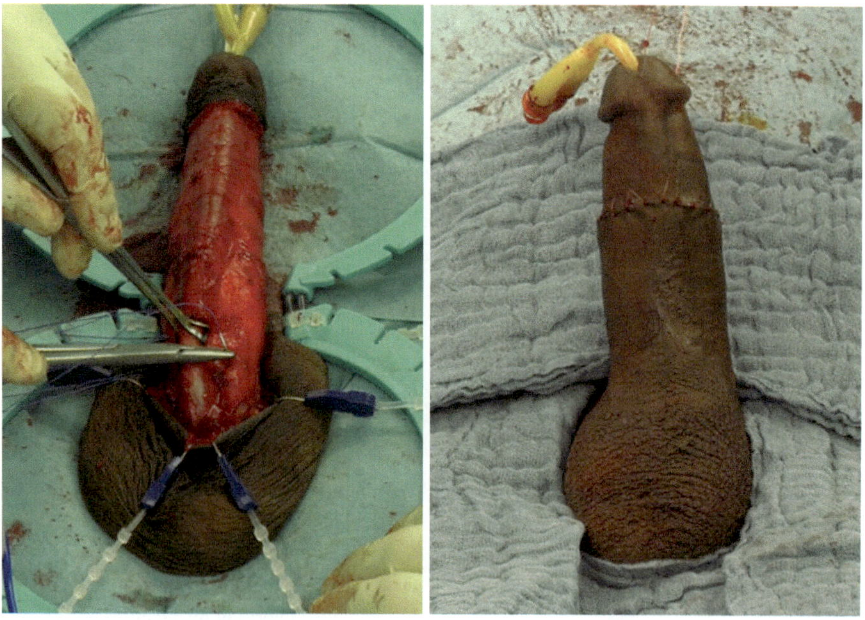

Fig. 12.14 The subcoronal degloving incision for IPP implantation allows unrestricted exposure of the corpora cavernosa (left). Appearance after closure (right) (Osmonov® and Ragheb®)

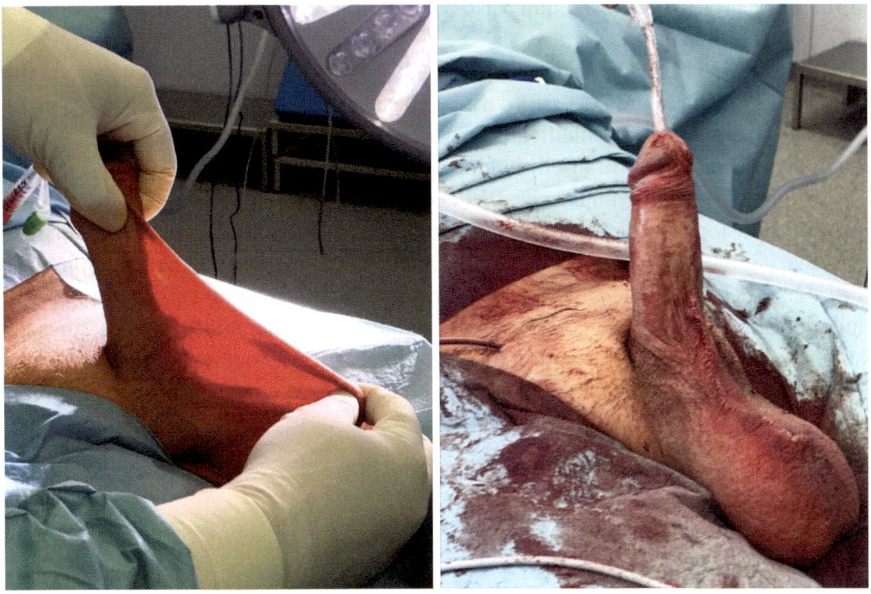

Fig. 12.15 Ventral phalloplasty (scrotoplasty) is achieved by excising the penoscrotal web (dashed line) demonstrated by transillumination (left). Postoperative appearance (right) (Osmonov®)

3.6 cm in some studies [62–65]. Less aggressive techniques as the modified sliding and multiple slice techniques were later introduced as upgrades of the former technique in an attempt to provide the same benefit with a lower risk of complications [66–68].

In addition to these penile lengthening techniques, less sophisticated ancillary techniques can be used to increased perceived penile length. These may be done either during PPI or later on as separate procedures if needed. Excising the penoscrotal web (Fig. 12.15) or incising the penile suspensory ligament combined with an inverted V-Y skin plasty or suprapubic lipectomy after implant insertion are valid options for penile length enhancement but with inconclusive data to date [69–73]. Glans augmentation using fillers or dermal fat has also been described with variable results regarding penile sensitivity [74, 75].

Another option is the use of expanding penile implants as the AMS 700 Ultrex (American Medical Systems, Minnetonka, MN, USA), recently upgraded to the AMS 700™ LGX (AMS, Minneapolis, MN, USA) which provided up to 2 cm of penile length expansion ever since it was first introduced in 1990 [41]. Similar implants are also capable of stretching fibrotic corpora in cases of neglected priapism or previous corporal infection. If these cases were to be revised after several months of usage, the explanted cylinders would be substituted with wider and often longer ones [76]. In contrast, a recent study of the same device reported a slight decrease in stretched penile length despite significant increases in penile circumference and width with early device cycling and daily maximal inflation [77]. Hence, further research would be required to validate the true effect of the AMS 700™ LGX on penile length.

The absence of glans tumescence post-PPI is a common cause for perceiving penile length loss in the post-PPI period. These cases can be successfully managed by using glans-engorging medications whether orally by phosphodiesterase inhibitors [78] or locally by intraurethral alprostadil [79].

In conclusion, men undergoing PPI should be thoroughly counseled on their expected postoperative penile size. Documenting preoperative penile dimensions and sharing them with the patient is crucial for improving patient satisfaction post-PPI. Besides all strategies mentioned to enhance perceived penile size, simply refining the surgical approach will always remain fundamental for optimizing the surgery. Afterward, the surgeon may choose the suitable size-enhancing approach according to need [48].

Chronic Pain Syndrome

Definition and Cause

Although modern implants and techniques have resulted in high patient satisfaction rates, post-implantation chronic pain is not uncommon in some cases. However, rarely does it lead to device removal [80]. Occasionally, patients may complain of post-PPI pain around any of the implanted components (cylinders/rods, reservoir, or pump) that may persist from weeks to years after surgery (Fig. 12.16). Hence, the pain may be penile, scrotal, or even pelvic. Pain following PPI surgery is considered to be chronic if persists beyond 6 weeks postoperative and in other reports for more than 2 months [81, 82]. The pathophysiology of chronic penile and scrotal pain remains poorly understood [80]. Nonetheless, the fact that the genital area is highly sensitive due to its rich cutaneous nerve supply may explain the lower pain threshold following PPI surgery compared to other surgeries in the proximity. Moreover, neuropathy associated with the majority of diabetic patients undergoing this particular surgery may also result in more severe and persistent pain compared to non-diabetic patients. Chronic pelvic pain is another form of persistent pain following PPI surgery.

Differential Diagnosis

Chronic pain following PPI surgery has been attributed to different causes in previous studies. The list includes subclinical infection, faulty sizing or positioning of the prosthesis, diabetic neuropathy, and autoimmune rejection of the device [80]. The buckling of oversized inflatable cylinders has also been reported to be a cause of

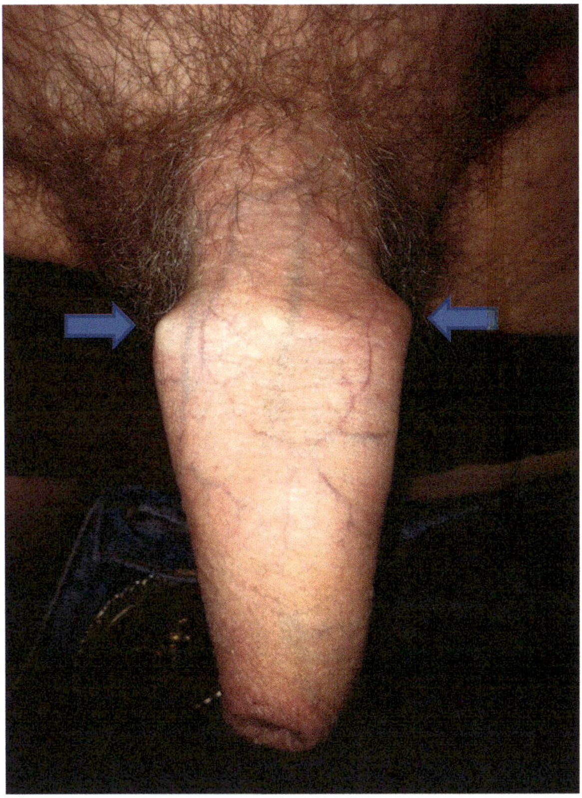

Fig. 12.16 Dog ear deformity which may cause stitching pain at the angle points (arrows). Pain usually subsides with capsule formation (Osmonov®)

prolonged penile pain after prosthesis implantation [82]. The surgeon must carefully differentiate the cause for the persistent pain and address accordingly.

Management

Treating chronic pain after PPI surgery may be as easy as just reassurance and watchful waiting allowing the tincture of time to solve the problem. However, in other cases, medical or surgical intervention may be mandatory. In an early case report of persistent pain after PPI, Krauss successfully used a series of four lidocaine injections to cure penile pain lasting 7 months after surgery [60]. Pain persisting for more than 6 weeks in a non-diabetic patient with a properly sized implant must first raise suspicion for a preclinical infection. If the pain subsides upon administering a gram-positive antimicrobial, an infection would most probably be the cause. This would be confirmed if symptoms recur after antibiotic discontinuation. In that case, an urgent implant salvage revision would be recommended. In many cases, the biofilm coating the implant prevents antibiotics from complete microorganism eradication. Moncada and his group suggested magnetic resonance imaging to be an important diagnostic tool for chronic penile pain suspected to be due to excessively long IPP devices requiring surgical correction. Nevertheless, surgical intervention for non-infective chronic pelvic pain should be considered with caution. IPP revision for the treatment of chronic pain may be futile in some cases or furthermore exacerbate the complaint. 68% of 22 patients, who had an IPP revision or explant to relieve symptoms of chronic pelvic pain not related to a device infection or erosion, suffered from persistent pelvic pain despite surgical intervention. Pain relief was successful only when device malposition was the cause. The authors concluded that surgical intervention for pain was to be spared except in certain cases. Otherwise, alternative conservative options may be more beneficial for chronic pain following PPI.

Excessively, oversized implants whether in girth or length are better to be revised not just for the pain associated but moreover to avoid the risk for other complications as impending erosion or device malfunction (Fig. 12.17). Another absolute indication for surgical correction of persistent pain would be improper positioning as in cases of cylinder crossover. This highlights the importance of accurate surgical planning and device size selection by the surgeon during primary surgery.

Complications Associated with IPP Reservoirs

Over the years, the space of Retzius (SR) reservoir placement (RP) has been established as the traditional location for placement of reservoirs during three-piece prosthesis placement [83]. Nevertheless, a number of rare but occasionally life-threatening

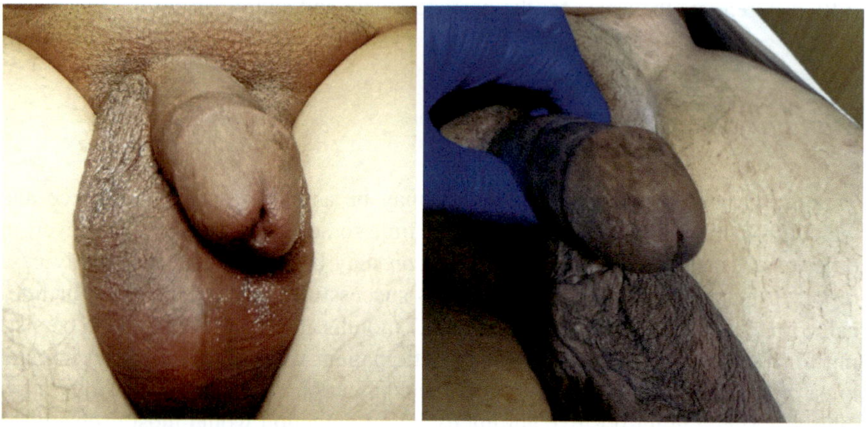

Fig. 12.17 Picture of an oversized malleable device stretching the tip of the glans bilaterally spreading the meatus open and causing chronic pain with the risk of urethral erosion (left). Postoperative picture after cylinder downsizing and repositioning combined with distal corporoplasty.(right) (Ragheb®)

complications have been reported that are associated with the RP in the SR. Possible complications are injury of the iliac vessels, injury of the epigastric vessels, compression of the iliac vein, bowel injury with development of bowel fistula, reservoir hernia, as well as intravesical dislocation of the reservoir. These complications occur most commonly in patients who underwent previous either intraperitoneal or extraperitoneal pelvic surgery [84–86]. The recent patient's preference of minimally invasive robot-assisted surgery has led to increasing numbers of robotic-assisted prostatectomies, cystectomies, or rectum resections, because the peritoneal veil is not restored after robotic surgery scar formation and adhesions in the space of Retzius hinder SR reservoir placement [85, 86].

SR implantation is always done "blindly" by relying on the tactile guidance of the surgeon's finger [83]. Therefore, a discrepancy may occur between the surgical estimate and the real anatomical distances in the pelvis of a particular patient, which may lead to injury of these structures. Although this is very rare, this risk has to be considered, not only by beginners but also high-volume implanters.

The most high-volume implanters are using ectopic high submuscular (EHS) reservoir location on a regular basis, and some have switched to it exclusively [87–89]. In the USA, where the highest volume of IPP in the world is performed, 75% of the implants are done by occasional implanters, individuals who do four or less per year [87]. These abundant but infrequent implanters have been slower to embrace the newer locations for RP [87, 88]. Recently developed low-profile reservoirs have been placed in non-traditional spaces, termed "ectopic" while others may prefer synonymous designations such as "alternative" or "submuscular" locations [87].

In the recent review article Dr. Wilson and colleagues conclude: "The worst that can happen following EHS RP is a visible or palpable reservoir. That particular reservoir was superficial and much too lateral where the abdominal muscles have no bulk. We believe the Pfannenstiel incision deflected the clamp laterally. Nevertheless, after 3 months capsule formation made it much less obvious; the shallow location did not affect the mechanical performance of the inflatable implant and the patient did not request repair" [87].

The main parameter in evaluating HSM RP is definitely patient satisfaction [4, 8]. In general, satisfaction with respect to reservoir placement includes the following aspects: palpability, pain, general satisfaction, complications, device difficulties, and location. Only six studies have evaluated these criteria (Table 12.1) [85, 90–94]. There were various locations for reservoir placement – including SR, HSM, lateral extraperitoneal (lateral), and subcutaneous. The working group of A. Morey from the University of Texas has published 2 retrospective studies: the first study investigated the patient reported outcome in 146 patients who had undergone HSM reservoir placement in IPP with different types of devices. Patient-reported satisfaction was 96% for the IPP devices; 80% of the reservoirs were impalpable for the patient [9]. In a larger study from 2018, the same group evaluated 560 patients who had undergone either HSM or SR. Presence of pain or herniation was queried from the cohort. Pain or herniation was reported by 4 and 4 patients, respectively in the HSM group and by 0 and 3 patients in the SR group. However, there was a higher rate of deep pelvic complications in the SR group ($n = 3$) than in the HSM group ($n = 0$) (Table 12.2) [90].

The prospective PROPPER study evaluated data of only Boston Scientific (formerly AMS) device implantations, in which PR had been placed in a SR location in

Table 12.2 List of the studies on HSM RP

Reference	Follow-up in months	Number of subjects	Outcomes measures	Summary
Pagliara, Viers [93], Urology Practice	Mean 25.6 (1.9–93.6)	560 1st time reservoir	Pain/herniation	619 HSM (IPP – Coloplast® and AMS® 344, AUS 275) 2009–2016
			Deep pelvic complications (vascular/ bladder)	8/399 1st time HSM revised – 4 for pain, 4 for herniation
				6/161 1st time SOR revised – 3 for herniation, 3 for deep pelvic complications
Garber and Bickell [94], Urology	7–11	7 (1 explanted early)	Palpable herniation	Subcutaneous reservoir 8/1000 Coloplast® IPP single surgeon, 1/8 explanted for infection, other 7 not palpable by patient or surgeon
		Average BMI 39		
Singla, Siegel [90], J Urol	Mean 23	294	Herniation	294 AUS (HSM 154, SOR 140)
			Deep pelvic complications	No demographic difference
				No pain
				1/140 SOR – herniation
				1/140 SOR – spontaneous bladder rupture unrelated to reservoir
				No problems with HSM
				No difference in continence rates
Karpman, Brant [85], J Urol (prospective)	Mean 17.8	744	Herniation	PROPPER study – AMS 700® IPP devices only
			Palpable	3/572 SOR – 81% very satisfied, 2 herniation, 1 capsular contracture
			Satisfaction rate	2/172 HSM – 85.9% very satisfied, 2 herniation
				Palpability was not an issue
Chung, Morey [92], Urology	Mean 3.2	146	Palpability	Mixed AMS700®, Coloplast Titan® and AUS
			Bother	146 cases, single surgeon
				80% not palpable by patient
				9/146 bothered but only 2 underwent revision
				2 AUS herniation
				Self-reported patient satisfaction 97% AUS, 96% IPP

Table 12.2 (continued)

Reference	Follow-up in months	Number of subjects	Outcomes measures	Summary
Osmonov et al. (2020) IJIR [91]	Mean 28	142	Palpability	Coloplast Titan OTR prosthesis with exclusive use of the "Clover Leaf" reservoir, single surgeon
			Bother	88% of the patients with ectopic HSM RP and 81% with traditional SR RP were satisfied with their implant. Of the patients with HSM RP, 64.3% ($n = 45$; BMI range: 18.5–28.8) reported that they were able to feel their reservoir by palpation immediately after surgery. Palpability disappeared in 80% of the patients in this group (BMI >26.5) after capsule formation at 3 months post-surgery

221 and in an HSM location in 55 patients. The patients reported overall satisfaction in 81% and 85.9%, respectively; herniation occurred in 0.5% in the SR group and in 1% in the HSM group. An important outcome was that the PR palpability and auto-inflation were not an issue in this group of patients (Table 12.1) [3]. In the first single surgeon European paper on HSM RP, the authors observed four (3.3%) cases grade III b Clavien-Dindo complications, which resulted in revision [8]. Distribution was as follows: infected device ($n = 4$), scrotal hematoma ($n = 2$), scrotal seroma ($n = 1$), and scrotal skin fistula ($n = 1$). 88% of the patients with ectopic HSM RP and 81% with traditional SR RP were satisfied with their implant. Of the patients with HSM RP, 64.3% ($n = 45$; BMI range: 18.5–28.8) reported that they were able to feel their reservoir by palpation immediately after surgery. Palpability disappeared in 80% of the patients in this group (BMI >26.5) after capsule formation at 3 months post-surgery [91]. Accordingly, to the current ESSM positions statements on penile prosthesis based on "Oxford levels of evidence" (Level 2, Grade C), HSM RP can be considered as an alternative method of RP during IPP implantations [95]. Moreover, palpability of the HSM reservoir does not seem to be a significant factor for revision surgery (Level 2, Grade C) (Fig. 12.18) [95].

Findings of all published studies (Table 12.2) suggest that the HSM RP is safe, efficacious, and accompanied by excellent patient satisfaction even if the reservoir is initially palpable or visible. However, the patient does not request revision and is as satisfied as with SR RP. Ectopic reservoir placement's only possible complications are visibility or palpability of the component. The fact that patients are not requesting revision upon discovery of these complications bodes well for the future of ectopic placement supplanting traditional space of Retzius.

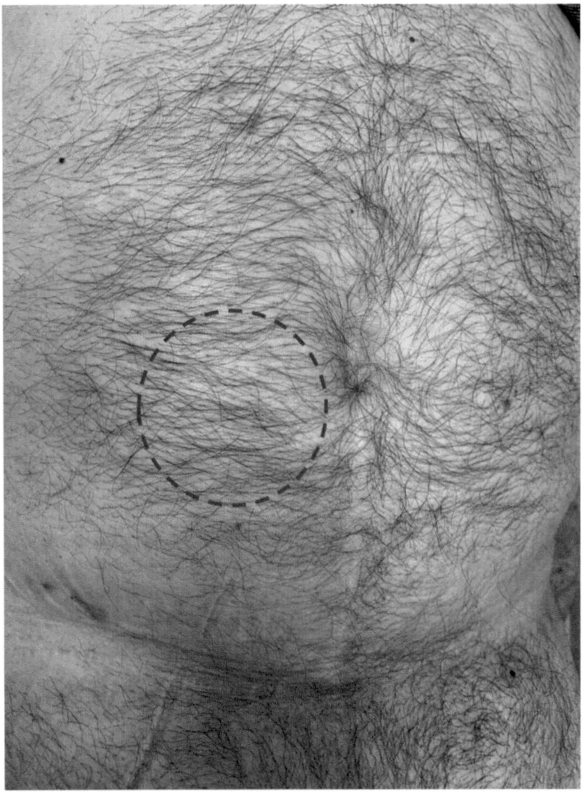

Fig. 12.18 Nonvisible but palpable HSM RP reservoir (marked area) during follow-up (Osmonov®)

References

1. Scott FB, Bradley WE, Timm GW. Management of erectile impotence. Use of implantable inflatable prosthesis. Urology. 1973;2(1):80–2.
2. Wolter CE, Hellstrom WJ. The hydrophilic-coated inflatable penile prosthesis: 1-year experience. J Sex Med. 2004;1(2):221–4.
3. Fishman IJ, Scott FB, Light JK. Experience with inflatable penile prosthesis. Urology. 1984;23(5 Spec No):86–92.
4. Trost LW, McCaslin R, Linder B, Hellstrom WJ. Long-term outcomes of penile prostheses for the treatment of erectile dysfunction. Expert Rev Med Devices. 2013;10(3):353–66.
5. Henry GD. Historical review of penile prosthesis design and surgical techniques: part 1 of a three-part review series on penile prosthetic surgery. J Sex Med. 2009;6(3):675–81.
6. Henry GD, Donatucci CF, Conners W, Greenfield JM, Carson CC, Wilson SK, et al. An outcomes analysis of over 200 revision surgeries for penile prosthesis implantation: a multicenter study. J Sex Med. 2012;9(1):309–15.
7. Kim DS, Yang KM, Chung HJ, Choi HM, Choi YD, Choi HK. AMS 700CX/CXM inflatable penile prosthesis has high mechanical reliability at long-term follow-up. J Sex Med. 2010;7(7):2602–7.
8. Mirheydar H, Zhou T, Chang DC, Hsieh TC. Reoperation rates for penile prosthetic surgery. J Sex Med. 2016;13(1):129–33.

9. Shaw T, Garber BB. Coloplast titan inflatable penile prosthesis with one-touch release pump: review of 100 cases and comparison with genesis pump. J Sex Med. 2011;8(1):310–4.
10. Kavoussi NL, Viers BR, VanDyke ME, Pagliara TJ, Morey AF. "Stiction syndrome": non-operative management of patients with difficult AMS 700 series inflation. J Sex Med. 2017;14(9):1079–83.
11. Garber BB, Khurgin JL, Stember DS, Perito PE. Pseudo-malfunction of the Coloplast Titan inflatable penile prosthesis One-Touch release pump. Urology. 2014;84(4):857–9.
12. Bickell M, Manimala N, Parker J, Steixner B, Wiegand L, Carrion R. Floppy glans syndrome: pathogenesis and treatment. Sex Med Rev. 2016;4(2):149–56.
13. Ziegelmann MJ, Alom M, Bole R, Kohler T, Trost L. Modified glanulopexy technique for supersonic transporter deformity and glanular hypermobility in men with penile prostheses. J Sex Med. 2018;15(6):914–9.
14. Morey AF. Reconstructing penile supersonic transporter (SST) deformity using glanulopexy (glans fixation). J Urol. 2005;174(3):969.
15. Wilson SK. Penile prosthesis implantation: pearls, pitfalls, and perils. In: Hellstrom WJG, editor. Male infertility and sexual dysfunction. New York: Springer; 1997. p. 529–48.
16. Mulhall JP, Kim FJ. Reconstructing penile supersonic transporter (SST) deformity using glanulopexy (glans fixation). Urology. 2001;57(6):1160–2.
17. Wilson SK. Surgical techniques: modeling technique for penile curvature. J Sex Med. 2007;4(1):231–4.
18. Ball TP Jr. Surgical repair of penile "SST" deformity. Urology. 1980;15(6):603–4.
19. Hirsch IH, Moy ML. Glandular-tunical stabilization to repair SST deformity of the inflatable penile prosthesis. Tech Urol. 2000;6(3):212–4.
20. Minhas S. Urethral perforation during penile implant surgery: what to do? J Sex Med. 2017;14(7):867–9.
21. Mulcahy JJ. The prevention and management of noninfectious complications of penile implants. Sex Med Rev. 2015;3(3):203–13.
22. Steidle CP, Mulcahy JJ. Erosion of penile prostheses: a complication of urethral catheterization. J Urol. 1989;142(3):736–9.
23. Carlos EC, Sexton SJ, Lentz AC. Urethral injury and the penile prosthesis. Sex Med Rev. 2019;7(2):360–8.
24. Hsu GL, Brock G, Martínez-Piñeiro L, von Heyden B, Lue TF, Tanagho EA. Anatomy and strength of the tunica albuginea: its relevance to penile prosthesis extrusion. J Urol. 1994;151(5):1205–8.
25. Vollstedt A, Gross MS, Antonini G, Perito PE. The infrapubic surgical approach for inflatable penile prosthesis placement. Transl Androl Urol. 2017;6(4):620–7.
26. Anaissie J, Yafi FA. A review of surgical strategies for penile prosthesis implantation in patients with Peyronie's disease. Transl Androl Urol. 2016;5(3):342–50.
27. Wilson SK, Cleves MA, Delk JR 2nd. Long-term followup of treatment for Peyronie's disease: modeling the penis over an inflatable penile prosthesis. J Urol. 2001;165(3):825–9.
28. Shaeer O. Management of distal extrusion of penile prosthesis: partial disassembly and tip reinforcement by double breasting or grafting. J Sex Med. 2008;5(5):1257–62.
29. Kaufman JL, Chang BB, Shah DM, Koslow AR, Leather RP. Acute arterial insufficiency of the male genitalia. Ann Vasc Surg. 1991;5(4):370–4.
30. Harris CF, Mydlo JH. Ischemia and gangrene of the penis. J Urol. 2003;169(5):1795.
31. Wilson SK, Mora-Estaves C, Egydio P, Ralph D, Habous M, Love C, et al. Glans necrosis following penile prosthesis implantation: prevention and treatment suggestions. Urology. 2017;107:144–8.
32. Weiner DM, Lowe FC. Surgical management of ischemic penile gangrene in diabetics with end stage atherosclerosis. J Urol. 1996;155(3):926–9.
33. Yildirim A, Basok EK, Basaran A, Tokuc R. Gangrene of the distal penis after implantation of malleable penile prosthesis in a diabetic patient. Adv Ther. 2008;25(2):143–7.

34. Mulcahy JJ. Long-term experience with salvage of infected penile implants. J Urol. 2000;163(2):481–2.
35. Houlihan MD, Köhler TS, Wilson SK, Hatzichristodoulou G. Penoscrotal approach for IPP: still up-to-date after more than 40 years? Int J Impot Res. 2020;32(1):2–9.
36. Kramer A, Chason J. Residents at the University of Maryland Medical System provide insight to learning infrapubic approach for IPP surgery: relative benefits but novel challenges exposed in first 15 cases. J Sex Med. 2010;7(3):1298–305.
37. Otero JR, Manfredi C, Wilson SK. The good, the bad, and the ugly about surgical approaches for inflatable penile prosthesis implantation. Int J Impot Res. 2020;
38. Xie D, Nicholas M, Gheiler V, Perito D, Siano L, Kislinger I, et al. A prospective evaluation of penile measures and glans penis sensory changes after penile prosthetic surgery. Transl Androl Urol. 2017;6(3):529–33.
39. Palmisano F, Boeri L, Cristini C, Antonini G, Spinelli MG, Franco G, et al. Comparison of infrapubic vs penoscrotal approaches for 3-piece inflatable penile prosthesis placement: do we have a winner? Sex Med Rev. 2018;6(4):631–9.
40. Jorissen C, De Bruyna H, Baten E, Van Renterghem K. Clinical outcome: patient and partner satisfaction after penile implant surgery. Curr Urol. 2019;13(2):94–100.
41. Montague DK. Penile prosthesis implantation: size matters. Eur Urol. 2007;51(4):887–8.
42. Mondaini N, Ponchietti R, Gontero P, Muir GH, Natali A, Caldarera E, et al. Penile length is normal in most men seeking penile lengthening procedures. Int J Impot Res. 2002;14(4):283–6.
43. Deveci S, Martin D, Parker M, Mulhall JP. Penile length alterations following penile prosthesis surgery. Eur Urol. 2007;51(4):1128–31.
44. Montorsi F, Rigatti P, Carmignani G, Corbu C, Campo B, Ordesi G, et al. AMS three-piece inflatable implants for erectile dysfunction: a long-term multi-institutional study in 200 consecutive patients. Eur Urol. 2000;37(1):50–5.
45. Wang R, Howard GE, Hoang A, Yuan JH, Lin HC, Dai YT. Prospective and long-term evaluation of erect penile length obtained with inflatable penile prosthesis to that induced by intracavernosal injection. Asian J Androl. 2009;11(4):411–5.
46. Osterberg EC, Maganty A, Ramasamy R, Eid JF. Pharmacologically induced erect penile length and stretched penile length are both good predictors of post-inflatable prosthesis penile length. Int J Impot Res. 2014;26(4):128–31.
47. Gentile G, Franceschelli A, Massenio P, Tuccio A, Cocci A, Divenuto L, et al. Patient's satisfaction after 2-piece inflatable penile prosthesis implantation: an Italian multicentric study. Arch Ital Urol Androl. 2016;88(1):1–3.
48. Lee KC, Brock GB. Strategies for maintaining penile size following penile implant. Transl Androl Urol. 2013;2(1):67–73.
49. Savoie M, Kim SS, Soloway MS. A prospective study measuring penile length in men treated with radical prostatectomy for prostate cancer. J Urol. 2003;169(4):1462–4.
50. Haliloglu A, Baltaci S, Yaman O. Penile length changes in men treated with androgen suppression plus radiation therapy for local or locally advanced prostate cancer. J Urol. 2007;177(1):128–30.
51. Munding MD, Wessells HB, Dalkin BL. Pilot study of changes in stretched penile length 3 months after radical retropubic prostatectomy. Urology. 2001;58(4):567–9.
52. Habous M, Giona S, Tealab A, Aziz M, Sherif H, Abdelwahab O, et al. Penile length is preserved after implant surgery. BJU Int. 2019;123(5):885–90.
53. Levine LA, Rybak J. Traction therapy for men with shortened penis prior to penile prosthesis implantation: a pilot study. J Sex Med. 2011;8(7):2112–7.
54. Pahlajani G, Raina R, Jones S, Ali M, Zippe C. Vacuum erection devices revisited: its emerging role in the treatment of erectile dysfunction and early penile rehabilitation following prostate cancer therapy. J Sex Med. 2012;9(4):1182–9.
55. Dalkin BL, Christopher BA. Preservation of penile length after radical prostatectomy: early intervention with a vacuum erection device. Int J Impot Res. 2007;19(5):501–4.

56. Henry GD, Kansal NS, Callaway M, Grigsby T, Henderson J, Noble J, et al. Centers of excellence concept and penile prostheses: an outcome analysis. J Urol. 2009;181(3):1264–8.
57. Ralph DJ, Garaffa G, Muneer A, Freeman A, Rees R, Christopher AN, et al. The immediate insertion of a penile prosthesis for acute ischaemic priapism. Eur Urol. 2009;56(6):1033–8.
58. Henry G, Houghton L, Culkin D, Otheguy J, Shabsigh R, Ohl DA. Comparison of a new length measurement technique for inflatable penile prosthesis implantation to standard techniques: outcomes and patient satisfaction. J Sex Med. 2011;8(9):2640–6.
59. Pryor MB, Carrion R, Wang R, Henry G. Patient satisfaction and penile morphology changes with postoperative penile rehabilitation 2 years after Coloplast Titan prosthesis. Asian J Androl. 2016;18(5):754–8.
60. Moncada I, Martínez-Salamanca JI, Jara J, Cabello R, Moralejo M, Hernández C. Inflatable penile prosthesis implantation without corporeal dilation: a cavernous tissue sparing technique. J Urol. 2010;183(3):1123–6.
61. Weinberg AC, Pagano MJ, Deibert CM, Valenzuela RJ. Sub-coronal inflatable penile prosthesis placement with modified no-touch technique: a step-by-step approach with outcomes. J Sex Med. 2016;13(2):270–6.
62. Egydio PH, Kuehhas FE, Sansalone S. Penile length and girth restoration in severe Peyronie's disease using circular and longitudinal grafting. BJU Int. 2013;111(4 Pt B):E213–9.
63. Sansalone S, Garaffa G, Djinovic R, Egydio P, Vespasiani G, Miano R, et al. Simultaneous penile lengthening and penile prosthesis implantation in patients with Peyronie's disease, refractory erectile dysfunction, and severe penile shortening. J Sex Med. 2012;9(1):316–21.
64. Rolle L, Ceruti C, Timpano M, Sedigh O, Destefanis P, Galletto E, et al. A new, innovative, lengthening surgical procedure for Peyronie's disease by penile prosthesis implantation with double dorsal-ventral patch graft: the "sliding technique". J Sex Med. 2012;9(9):2389–95.
65. Rolle L, Falcone M, Ceruti C, Timpano M, Sedigh O, Ralph DJ, et al. A prospective multicentric international study on the surgical outcomes and patients' satisfaction rates of the 'sliding' technique for end-stage Peyronie's disease with severe shortening of the penis and erectile dysfunction. BJU Int. 2016;117(5):814–20.
66. Egydio PH, Kuehhas FE. Penile lengthening and widening without grafting according to a modified 'sliding' technique. BJU Int. 2015;116(6):965–72.
67. Egydio PH, Kuehhas FE. The Multiple-Slit Technique (MUST) for penile length and girth restoration. J Sex Med. 2018;15(2):261–9.
68. Gaffney CD, Pagano MJ, Weinberg AC, Small AC, Kuehas FE, Egydio PH, et al. Lengthening strategies for Peyronie's disease. Transl Androl Urol. 2016;5(3):351–62.
69. Miranda-Sousa A, Keating M, Moreira S, Baker M, Carrion R. Concomitant ventral phalloplasty during penile implant surgery: a novel procedure that optimizes patient satisfaction and their perception of phallic length after penile implant surgery. J Sex Med. 2007;4(5):1494–9.
70. Borges F, Hakim L, Kline C. Surgical technique to maintain penile length after insertion of an inflatable penile prosthesis via infrapubic approach. J Sex Med. 2006;3(3):550–3.
71. Hakky TS, Suber J, Henry G, Smith D, Bradley P, Martinez D, et al. Penile enhancement procedures with simultaneous penile prosthesis placement. Adv Urol. 2012;2012:314612.
72. Li CY, Kayes O, Kell PD, Christopher N, Minhas S, Ralph DJ. Penile suspensory ligament division for penile augmentation: indications and results. Eur Urol. 2006;49(4):729–33.
73. Horton CE, Vorstman B, Teasley D, Winslow B. Hidden penis release: adjunctive suprapubic lipectomy. Ann Plast Surg. 1987;19(2):131–4.
74. Kim JJ, Kwak TI, Jeon BG, Cheon J, Moon DG. Effects of glans penis augmentation using hyaluronic acid gel for premature ejaculation. Int J Impot Res. 2004;16(6):547–51.
75. Shaeer O. Shaeer's glans augmentation technique: a pilot study. J Sex Med. 2012;9(12):3264–9.
76. Wilson SK, Delk JR, Mulcahy JJ, Cleves M, Salem EA. Upsizing of inflatable penile implant cylinders in patients with corporal fibrosis. J Sex Med. 2006;3(4):736–42.
77. Wallen JJ, Madiraju SK, Wang R, Henry GD. Implementation of length expanding inflatable penile prosthesis is not sufficient to prevent postsurgical penile shortening. Asian J Androl. 2018;21(1):98–100.

78. Mulhall JP, Jahoda A, Aviv N, Valenzuela R, Parker M. The impact of sildenafil citrate on sexual satisfaction profiles in men with a penile prosthesis in situ. BJU Int. 2004;93(1):97–9.
79. Chew KK, Stuckey BG. Use of transurethral alprostadil (MUSE) (prostaglandin E1) for glans tumescence in a patient with penile prosthesis. Int J Impot Res. 2000;12(3):195–6.
80. Reinstatler L, Shee K, Gross MS. Pain management in penile prosthetic surgery: a review of the literature. Sex Med Rev. 2018;6(1):162–9.
81. Gritsenko K, Khelemsky Y, Kaye AD, Vadivelu N, Urman RD. Multimodal therapy in perioperative analgesia. Best Pract Res Clin Anaesthesiol. 2014;28(1):59–79.
82. Moncada I, Hernández C, Jara J, Hernández L, Lafuente J, Lledó E, et al. Buckling of cylinders may cause prolonged penile pain after prosthesis implantation: a case control study using magnetic resonance imaging of the penis. J Urol. 1998;160(1):67–71.
83. Henry G, Hsiao W, Karpman E, Bella AJ, Carrion R, Jones L, et al. A guide for inflatable penile prosthesis reservoir placement: pertinent anatomical measurements of the retropubic space. J Sex Med. 2014;11(1):273–8.
84. Levine LA, Hoeh MP. Review of penile prosthetic reservoir: complications and presentation of a modified reservoir placement technique. J Sex Med. 2012;9(11):2759–69.
85. Karpman E, Brant WO, Kansas B, Bella AJ, Jones LA, Eisenhart E, et al. Reservoir alternate surgical implantation technique: preliminary outcomes of initial PROPPER study of low profile or spherical reservoir implantation in submuscular location or traditional prevesical space. J Urol. 2015;193(1):239–44.
86. Perito P, Wilson S. The history of nontraditional or ectopic placement of reservoirs in prosthetic urology. Sex Med Rev. 2016;4(2):190–3.
87. Wilson SK, Simhan J, Osmonov D. Should occasional implanters learn ectopic placement of IPP reservoirs? Int J Impot Res. 2020;32(4):371–8.
88. Tausch TJ, Morey AF, Zhao LC, Knoll P, Simhan J, Scott JF, et al. High submuscular versus space of Retzius placement of inflatable penile prosthesis reservoirs: results of a surgeon survey. Can J Urol. 2014;21(5):7465–9.
89. Wilson SK, Henry GD, Delk JR Jr, Cleves MA. The mentor Alpha 1 penile prosthesis with reservoir lock-out valve: effective prevention of auto-inflation with improved capability for ectopic reservoir placement. J Urol. 2002;168(4 Pt 1):1475–8.
90. Singla N, Siegel JA, Simhan J, Tausch TJ, Klein A, Thoreson GR, et al. Does pressure regulating balloon location make a difference in functional outcomes of artificial urinary sphincter? J Urol. 2015;194(1):202–6.
91. Osmonov D, Chomicz A, Tropmann-Frick M, Arndt KM, Jünemann KP. High-submuscular vs. space of Retzius reservoir placement during implantation of inflatable penile implants. Int J Impot Res. 2020;32(1):18–23.
92. Chung PH, Morey AF, Tausch TJ, Simhan J, Scott JF. High submuscular placement of urologic prosthetic balloons and reservoirs: 2-year experience and patient-reported outcomes. Urology. 2014;84(6):1535–40.
93. Pagliara TJ, Viers BR, Scott J, Morey AF. Extended experience with high submuscular placement of urological prosthetic balloons and reservoirs: refined technique for optimal outcomes. Urol Pract. 2018;5(4):293–8.
94. Garber BB, Bickell M. Subcutaneous placement of inflatable penile prosthesis reservoirs. Urology. 2016;88:93–6.
95. Osmonov D, Christopher AN, Blecher GA, Falcone M, Soave A, Dahlem R, et al. Clinical Recommendations From the European Society for Sexual Medicine Exploring Partner Expectations, Satisfaction in Male and Phalloplasty Cohorts, the Impact of Penile Length, Girth and Implant Type, Reservoir Placement, and the Influence of Comorbidities and Social Circumstances. J Sex Med. 2020;17(2):210–37.

Chapter 13
Intraoperative Complications of Penile Prosthesis Surgery

Hussain M. Alnajjar and Asif Muneer

Introduction

Implantation of a penile prosthesis that is a surgical option for end-stage erectile dysfunction has been reported to be associated with patient satisfaction rates as high as 90% [1]. Although internationally reported prosthesis infection rates of 4% are accepted, high-volume centres should have infection rates less than 2% [2]. However, intraoperative complications often lead to malfunctioning implants, risk of erosion and urethral injury as well as patient dissatisfaction. Therefore, these complications require identification and intraoperative management to ensure a satisfactory outcome. Recognition of complications intraoperatively provides the best opportunity to reduce the risk of infection, erosion or later revision of the prosthesis.

Recognised intraoperative complications are infrequently reported. The British Association of Urological Surgeons (BAUS) penile prosthesis national audit evaluated 1071 penile prosthesis procedures and reported intraoperative complications such as urethral injury (0.7%, $n = 7$), corporal perforation (1.1%. $n = 12$) and cross-over (0.6%, $n = 6$) [3]. However, an Italian study of a total of 353 penile prosthesis cases in 2016 reported only 2 (0.6%) intraoperative complications [4]. This may not accurately reflect the actual rates as correction of the complication intraoperatively often does not lead to adverse outcomes and therefore does not require recording.

H. M. Alnajjar
Institute of Andrology, University College London Hospital, London, UK

Division of Surgery and Interventional Science, UCL, London, UK

A. Muneer (✉)
Institute of Andrology, University College London Hospital, London, UK

Division of Surgery and Interventional Science, UCL, London, UK

NIHR Biomedical Research Centre, University College London Hospital, London, UK
e-mail: Asif.muneer@nhs.net

E. P. Miranda, J. P. Mulhall (eds.), *Penile Implant Surgery*,
https://doi.org/10.1007/978-3-030-82363-4_13

The aim of this chapter is to discuss the most common intraoperative complications during penile prosthesis insertion and how to troubleshoot these complications. It is also important to consider how to recognise and prevent these complications in order to increase patient satisfaction and avoid long-term issues with the prosthesis problems. Careful patient preparation, counselling and managing patient expectations prior to surgery is critical.

This chapter will cover the common intraoperative complications and provide an explanation on how to perform safety checks to recognise the complication and correct the situation.

Intraoperative Complications

Urethral Injury

Urethral injury is located at the level of the distal urethra during penile remodelling in Peyronie's disease or during the distal dilatation of scarred corpora or in cases of previous extensive penile surgery. This is due to the difficult dilatation in the presence of scarred corpora, and it can be relatively easy, to advance the dilators through the fibrotic tissue and lead to inadvertent urethral perforation. When faced with a difficult dilatation, the use of Rossello dilators can help, and it is important to ensure that during this manoeuvre, the direction of dilatation is kept lateral and away from the urethra. If there is still difficulty in advancing the dilators, then a further circumcoronal incision can be used to deglove the penis and perform a second corporotomy incision over the area of resistance to allow safer distal dilatation.

Additionally, using Hegar dilators as opposed to the more pointed Brooks dilators reduces the risk of perforation and urethral injury when faced with extensive fibrosis in the corpora. Brooks dilators provide less resistance during dilatation and are therefore at a higher risk in causing a perforation if not used cautiously. When performing this step, squeezing the fossa navicularis between the non-dominant index finger and thumb and protecting the urethra from the advancing dilator can reduce the risk of distal urethral injury. During penile modelling for cases with extensive Peyronie's disease, the area of the fossa navicularis should also be firmly squeezed to avoid a perforation. The presence of blood or visualisation of the dilator at the tip of the meatus indicates a distal urethral perforation. Furthermore, seeing a gush of fluid from the meatus after injecting irrigating solution into the corporotomy also confirms a urethral perforation.

Proximal urethral perforations often occur during the exposure of the corpora and urethra or when the corporotomies are performed. These injuries can be readily identified and repaired via the same penoscrotal incision and are usually not associated with microbial contamination. Therefore, it is acceptable to proceed with implantation of the prosthesis if the urethral perforation can be repaired in a watertight approach [5, 6].

How to Deal with the Complication

If primary closure is possible for a distal urethral injury, it may be attempted. However, small distal injuries usually heal without the need for a repair and heal over a catheter. Implantation of a penile prosthesis should be aborted at this stage and a 14 Fr Foley catheter should be left in situ for 2 weeks to allow the urethra to heal. A peri-catheter urethrogram can be performed before removal of the catheter to ensure adequate healing of the urethra. If the urethral injury is noted after inserting the prosthesis, then the prosthesis should be explanted as leaving a prosthesis in situ with a concomitant distal urethral injury increases the risk of prosthesis infection. Delayed penile prosthesis implantation should take place after at least 3 months. A single malleable prosthesis cylinder may be placed on the contralateral side to maintain the space in cases of unilateral urethral injuries that are adequately repaired with no communication between the corpora [5]. A longer rear tip extender may be placed in the ipsilateral crus, away from the perforation site to facilitate future redo surgery.

If the urethral injury was sustained with diathermy, it is important to excise any tissue with thermal injury as this can lead to delayed tissue necrosis with risk of a urine leak. Once the edges of the defect have been freshened up, the defect can be sutured in at least two layers using braided absorbable 5-0 or 4-0 sutures in a tension-free and watertight fashion. Adjacent dartos tissue can be used as a flap to protect the anastomosis and reduce the risk of a urine leak which can lead to prosthesis or wound infection. Placement of a suprapubic catheter to divert the urine is also a reasonable option [6].

Corporal Crossover

Cylinder or corporal crossover involves one or both cylinders perforating the midline corporal septum and passing through to the contralateral corpus cavernosum. Cylinder crossover can occur in either the proximal or in the distal corpora cavernosa. The septum of the corporal bodies is thin and fenestrated predisposing it to a midline perforation during a difficult dilatation. A safe approach to prevent crossover is to always direct the dilators away from the midline. Table 13.1 shows indicators of crossover during corporal dilation.

Table 13.1 Indicators of corporal crossover

Instrument contact 'clinking' during simultaneous dilatation
Unable to insert second cylinder easily
Foley catheter misalignment to one side
Discrepancy in corporal measurements
Penile tilt during cylinder inflation

Postoperative cylinder crossover can present with penile deformity and shortening with a new angulation of the erect penis. This requires a further surgical correction and repositioning of the cylinders; it is therefore important to identify and correct this complication at the time of primary insertion of the penile prosthesis. Patients can also present with penile pain during cylinder inflation or difficulty in prosthesis inflation.

Once distal crossover has been identified during the intraoperative setting, the dilatation needs to be redone and cylinder placement corrected. Although the signs of distal cylinder crossover can be subtle and missed intraoperatively by the operating surgeon, it becomes obvious in the postoperative period once a capsule has formed around the cylinders with the aforementioned complications – Fig. 13.1. Surgeons should remember that if the prosthesis does not look correct at the end of the procedure, then they should question the cylinder position.

Proximal corporal crossover is usually secondary to dense corporal fibrosis or technical error. This complication ensues when the proximal part of the first cylinder is inserted through the corporal septum and passed through into the contralateral crus, leading to difficulty with the placement of the second cylinder. This complication can occur when the operating surgeon does not follow the lateral deviation of the crus during proximal dilation [5, 7].

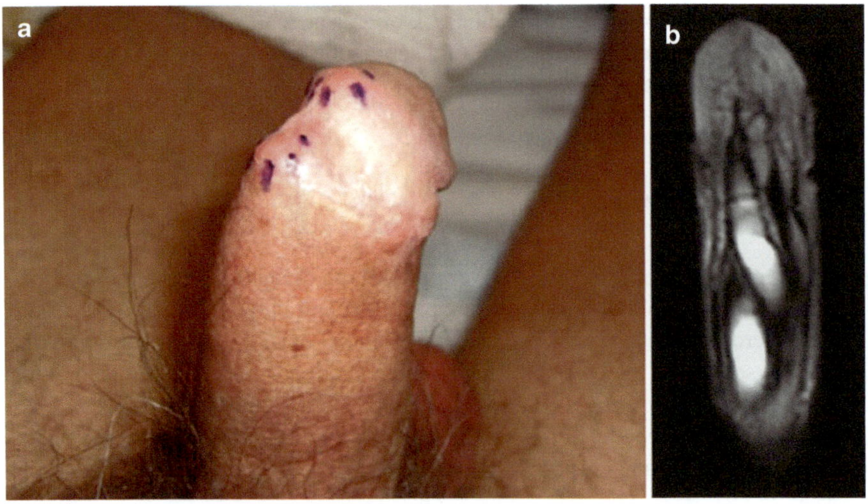

Fig. 13.1 (**a**) Distal crossover, note the tips of the prostheses are marked showing right to left crossover. (**b**) MRI image showing distal crossover. (Permission from Springer Prosthetic Surgery in Urology)

How to Deal with the Complication

Both cylinders should be removed and a dilator placed in the corpora which has been dilated successfully. The contralateral corpora should then be re-dilated ensuring to follow a dorsolateral course – Fig. 13.2. The Furlow is then inserted into the re-dilated cavity whilst keeping a dilator in the contralateral corpus. The Keith needle is then passed through using the Furlow but the cylinder is not yet inserted into the corpus cavernosum. The dilator is now removed and the second needle is passed through the glans penis using the Furlow and the Keith needle [5]. Once both needles are placed, it is then that the cylinders can be pulled through. This prevents inadvertent distal perforation of the cylinder by the needle if one cylinder is pulled into the dilated corpora and the needle for the second cylinder is misdirected.

Proximal crossover is managed using a similar technique to distal crossover. When placing the dilators in each proximal crus simultaneously, an 'American football goal post' sign should be observed which indicates that the dilatation is equal and excludes crossover or perforation – Fig. 13.3.

Proximal or Crural Perforation

Proximal perforation during corporal dilatation often occurs if there is proximal corporal fibrosis. This complication is a result of forceful downward dilatation by the operating surgeon. If proximal perforation is unrecognised intraoperatively, the

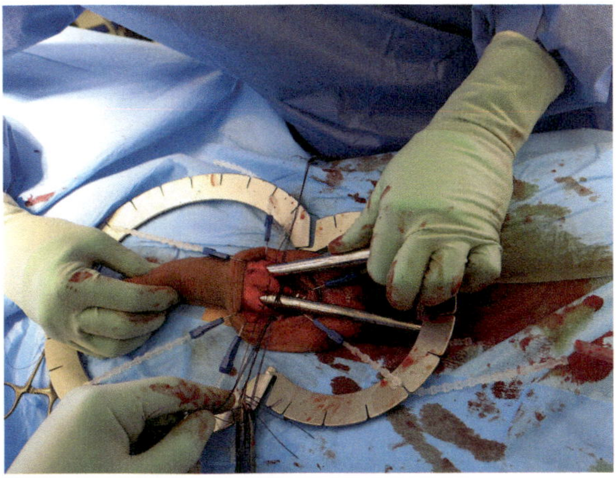

Fig. 13.2 Correction of intraoperative crossover. The Hagar is place in the right corpora and a new channel is created and re-dilatation follows a dorsolateral course on the contralateral side. (Image from Prosthetic Surgery in Urology)

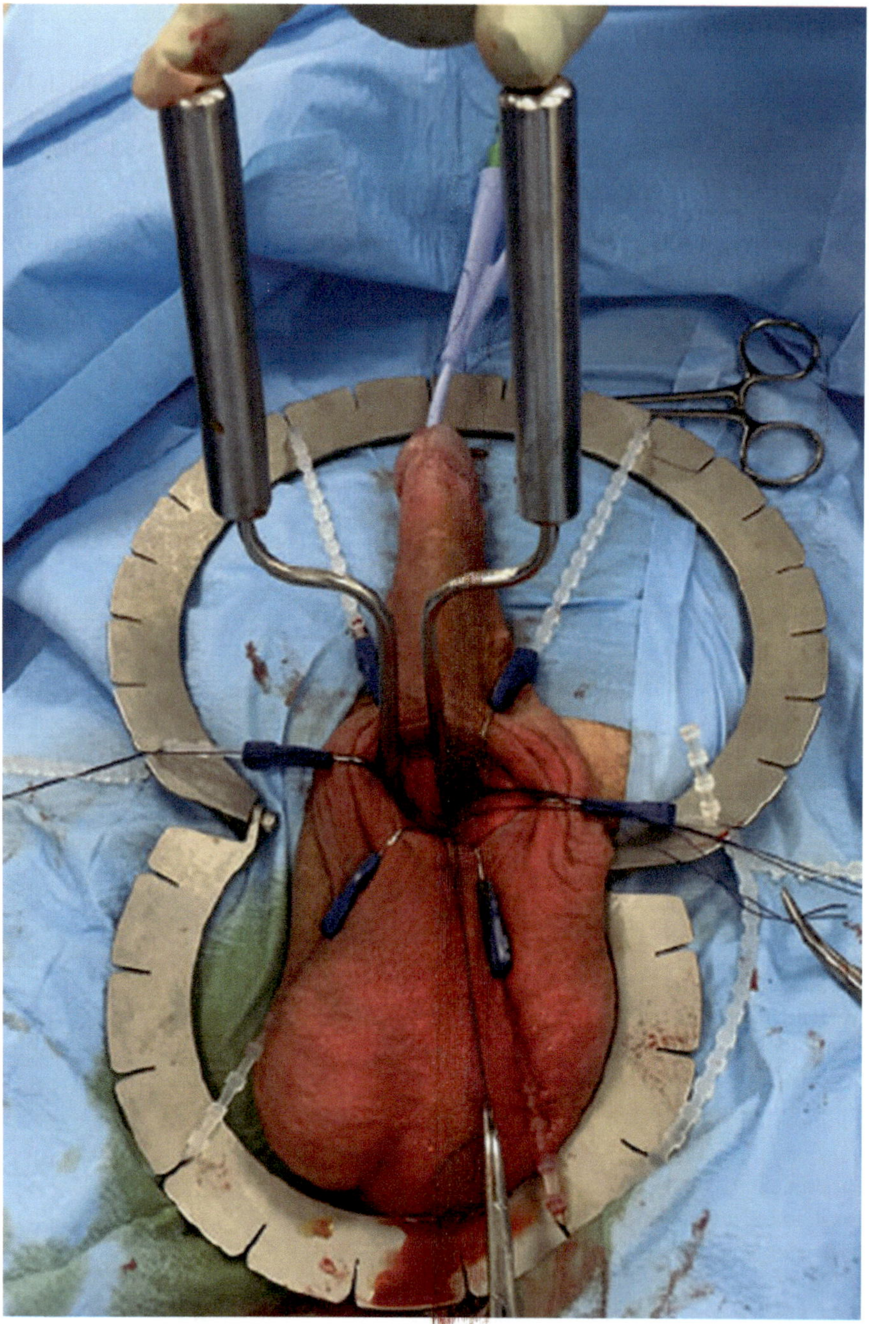

Fig. 13.3 'American goal post sign' indicating symmetrical bilateral proximal dilatation with no crossover or crural perforation

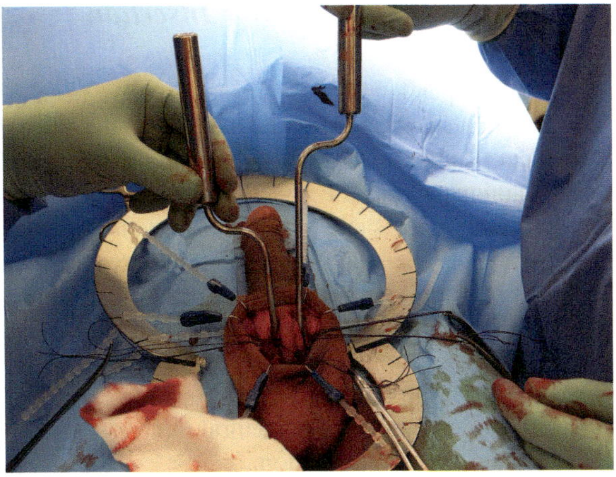

Fig. 13.4 Asymmetrical Brooks dilation demonstrating proximal perforation on the patient's right

patient will develop postoperative complications such as perineal pain or shortening of the cylinder on the perforated side due to migration of the cylinder. This complication can be prevented by avoiding the use of narrow-calibre dilators (<9 mm) [7]. Direct closure of the perforation via a perineal approach or the use of a 'windsock' graft is not advised due to high rate of postoperative infection [8, 9]. This complication is recognised when the dilator pushes through without the normal resistance encountered at the ischiopubic ramus, furthermore discrepancy in the dilators' length when Brooks dilators are simultaneously inserted into the proximal crura – Fig. 13.4.

How to Deal with the Complication

Wilson described a technique which avoids the cylinder base from migrating into the proximal perforation. The rear tip extender (RTE) sling technique negates the need to close the defect directly or the use of a graft [10]. The normal side is measured using a Furlow to evaluate the total length of the cavity and the required measurement for the cylinder and RTE. A non-absorbable suture (0 Prolene) is placed through the lateral wall of the proximal tunica albuginea at the level of the corporotomy, passed through the proximal end of the RTE and subsequently placed through the medial wall of the tunica albuginea. Cylinders are inserted in a standard approach and the corporotomies are closed. The glans guide sutures are held on tension to prevent the RTE from exiting through the proximal defect (the perforation). The implant is fully inflated and the sling suture is tied, preventing the proximal aspect of the cylinder migrating proximally. Postoperatively the patient is advised to avoid sexual intercourse for at least 12 weeks, to allow time for the development of fibrosis around the base of the cylinder which will fix the cylinder into place [9].

Injuries Related to Reservoir Insertion

Traditionally, penile prosthesis reservoirs have been placed in the space of Retzius (extra-peritoneal) in patients who have not undergone previous pelvic surgery. Blind placement of a reservoir during a penoscrotal approach is a relatively straightforward technique during IPP insertion in the hands of high-volume surgeons. An ideal reservoir placement is one where the reservoir is impalpable, is non-visible and does not autoinflate. The risk of autoinflation is reduced with the use of lockout valves and ensuring that the lockout valve in Coloplast implants do not lie adjacent to pelvic bone. Serious complications such as bladder, bowel or external iliac vessel injury can be catastrophic if not recognised, albeit these are rare. Bladder and bowel perforation may go unidentified intraoperatively. The presence of visible haematuria may be sign of bladder or urethral injury, whereas postoperative ileus or peritonitis indicates bowel perforation.

During blind insertion of the reservoir in the space of Retzius, the surgeon should always drain the bladder before puncturing the transversalis fascia to reduce the risk of inadvertent bladder injury.

Blind reservoir placement, in cases of prior prostatectomy or other pelvic surgery, has been reported to be associated with significant vascular and visceral injury [11, 12]. Robotic prostatectomy usually requires an intraperitoneal approach, and the peritoneal veil in the pelvis is not re-established; this leads to bowel migration to the prevesical space, increasing the risk of bowel injury during a blind approach. Coupled with the possibility of vascular injury, there is the risk of iliac vein compression, resulting in deep venous thrombosis and lower limb oedema [13, 14]. Vascular complications can be prevented by staying medial during the perforation of the superficial inguinal ring. Consequently, a second incision and an open placement of a reservoir under direct vision are recommended in cases where previous pelvic surgery has been performed. Another option is the ectopic placement of the reservoir in a space developed superficial to the fascia transversalis. The index finger is placed through the superficial inguinal ring above transversalis fascia and a space is created by blunt dissection, aiming to the ipsilateral shoulder. This space is then widened and extended towards the shoulder using a ring clamp. This approach can be used if comorbidity of a second incision is undesirable. In a large prospective multicentre study, Henry et al. reported that radical prostatectomy is the most common primary aetiology of penile implant surgery. Furthermore, patients treated with radical prostatectomy were more likely to have the reservoir placed in a submuscular location [15].

How to Deal with the Complication

In cases of bowel injury, all the components of the implant should be treated as infected and removed. A laparotomy and surgical repair of the bowel injury is always required with the help of colorectal surgeons due to the risk of peritonitis. In cases of bladder injury, they often only require prolonged catheterisation, as the bladder usually heals spontaneously if there is no intraperitoneal communication, whereas in cases of intraperitoneal bladder injury, a laparotomy and two-layer bladder repair is required. The prosthesis does not necessarily need to be explanted, and the reservoir can be repositioned on the contralateral side of the bladder injury.

Infrequently, in the postoperative period bladder injury may present only with irritative lower urinary tract symptoms and recurrent urinary tract infections. Diagnostic cystoscopy is the investigation of choice to rule out bladder injury, whereas a computed tomography (CT) scan of the abdomen and pelvis is mandatory to rule out a suspected bowel injury.

Complications During Closure of the Wound

Once the cylinders have been inserted, the corporotomy closure should be performed carefully to prevent needle perforation of the cylinders. Performing a corporotomy between stay sutures allows a tie over closure at the end and avoids the need for a continuous closure with a needle close to the cylinders.

Similarly, the implant tubing is at risk of perforation during the layered closure of the incision, and one technique described as the 'Harrier' technique helps to keep the tubing safely away from the suture during wound closure [16].

Conclusion

Careful patient selection, preoperative counselling and surgical planning whilst setting realistic patient expectations are crucial in penile prosthesis surgery. It is important for the implanting surgeon to be familiar with all the previously discussed intraoperative complications and to be able to confidently troubleshoot each one of them when faced with such challenges. Despite various advancements in surgical technique and prosthetic device design, intraoperative and postoperative complications may still ensue. It is therefore, essential that both the surgeon and the patient should be well prepared and accepting to deal with such complications, if they arise.

References

1. Shah T, Wang R. A review of factors affecting patient satisfaction with inflatable penile prosthesis. Sex Med Rev. 2020:S2050-0521(20)30035-4.
2. Carvajal A, Benavides J, García-Perdomo HA, Henry GD. Risk factors associated with penile prosthesis infection: systematic review and meta-analysis. Int J Impot Res. 2020;32(6):587–97.
3. Muneer A, Fowler S, Ralph DJ, Summerton DJ, Rees RW, BAUS Section of Andrology, Genitourethral Surgery. UK practice for penile prosthesis surgery: baseline analysis of

the British Association of Urological Surgeons (BAUS) Penile Prosthesis Audit. BJU Int. 2020;127:326–31.
4. Pescatori E, Alei G, Antonini G, Avolio A, Bettocchi C, Bitelli M, Boezio F, Cai T, Caraceni E, Carrino M, Colombo F, Conti E, Corvasce A, Dehò F, Fiordelise S, Ghidini N, Italiano E, La Pera G, Liguori G, Maretti C, Mondaini N, Natali A, Negro C, Palmieri A, Palumbo F, Paradiso M, Polito M, Pozza D, Silvani M, Tamai A, Timpano M, Utizi L, Varvello F, Vicini P, Vitarelli A, Franco G. INSIST-ED: Italian Society of Andrology registry on penile prosthesis surgery. First data analysis. Arch Ital Urol Androl. 2016;88(2):122–7.
5. Levine LA, Becher E, Bella A, et al. Penile prosthesis surgery: current recommendations from the international consultation on sexual medicine. J Sex Med. 2016;13:489–518.
6. Anele UA, Le BV, Burnett AL. Suprapubic cystostomy for the management of urethral injuries during penile prosthesis implantation. Sex Med. 2014;2:178–81.
7. Karpman E. Management of distal and proximal penile prosthesis crossover. J Sex Med. 2016;13:1008–12.
8. Mulcahy JJ. Crural perforation during penile prosthetic surgery. J Sex Med. 2006;3:177–80.
9. Stember DS, Kohler TS, Morey AF. Management of perforation injuries during and following penile prosthesis surgery. J Sex Med. 2015;12(7):456–61.
10. Wilson SK. Rear tip extender sling: a quick and easy repair for crural perforation. J Sex Med. 2010;7:1052–5.
11. Deho F, Henry GD, Marone EM, Sacca A, Chiesa R, Rigatti P, Montorsi F. Severe vascular complication after implantation of a three-piece inflatable penile prosthesis. J Sex Med. 2008;5:2956–9.
12. Karpman E, Sadeghi-Nejad H, Henry G, et al. Current opinions on alternative reservoir placement for inflatable penile prosthesis among members of the sexual medicine society of North America. J Sex Med. 2013;10:2115–20.
13. Levine LA, Hoeh MP. Review of penile prosthetic reservoir: complications and presentation of a modified reservoir placement technique. J Sex Med. 2012;9:2759–69.
14. Brison D, Ilbeigi P, Sadeghi-Nejad H. Reservoir repositioning and successful thrombectomy for deep venous thrombosis secondary to compression of pelvic veins by an inflatable penile prosthesis reservoir. J Sex Med. 2007;4:1185–7.
15. Henry GD, Karpman E, Brant W, Christine B, Kansas BT, Khera M, Jones L, Kohler T, Bennett N, Rhee E, Eisenhart E, Bella AJ. The who, how and what of real-world penile implantation in 2015: the PROPPER Registry baseline data. J Urol. 2016;195(2):427–33.
16. Muneer A. 'Harrier' technique to close a penoscrotal incision following insertion of an inflatable penile prosthesis. Ann R Coll Surg Engl. 2017;99(5):414.

Chapter 14
Medicolegal Impacts of Penile Implant Surgery

Caleb Natale, Gabe Leinwand, Michael Polchert, and Wayne J. G. Hellstrom

Introduction

Erectile dysfunction (ED) is a condition that has a prevalence of 2% in men under 40 and up to 86% in men 80 and older [1]. Up to 30 million men in the United States and 150 million men worldwide are estimated to suffer with ED [2]. There are a number of treatment options for men with ED. The gold standard for patients without adequate response to medical or vacuum treatment of ED is placement of a penile prosthesis. Inflatable penile prostheses (IPPs) were introduced in 1973 and have undergone multiple innovations in design and manufacturing since that time. Boston Scientific and Coloplast currently produce the majority of the devices inside the United States. The satisfaction rates of penile prosthesis implantation are quoted as being over 90% [3]. Although these devices have a high level of satisfaction, there are recognized risks associated with implantation of a penile prosthesis. It is essential that appropriate informed consent is obtained prior to penile prosthesis implantation, with patients understanding the risks of device failure, infection, bleeding, pain, or injury to the urethra, the penis, or surrounding structures, as well as other risks. In addition to appropriate informed consent, there is preoperative antimicrobial guidance published by the American Urological Association (AUA) [4]. Most complaints in litigation aimed at physicians after implantation of a penile prosthesis are due to incomplete counseling and documentation prior to the procedure. Herein we discuss the medicolegal considerations of implantation of penile prostheses.

C. Natale · G. Leinwand · M. Polchert · W. J. G. Hellstrom (✉)
Department of Urology, Tulane University School of Medicine, New Orleans, LA, USA
e-mail: cnatale@tulane.edu; gleinwan@tulane.edu; mpolchert@tulane.edu; whellst@tulane.edu

E. P. Miranda, J. P. Mulhall (eds.), *Penile Implant Surgery*,
https://doi.org/10.1007/978-3-030-82363-4_14

Considerations in Pre- and Postoperative Counseling

The implantation of a penile prosthesis is a viable option for the treatment of ED that offers men and transgender patients the option to generate an erection on demand. Primary risks include those from infection, alterations in penile appearance, and risk of device malfunction or failure, all of which can require reoperation. Patients and their partners may choose to attempt alternative treatments prior to opting for penile prosthesis implantation due to concerns about reversibility and invasiveness. AUA guidelines note that patients should be informed of all ED treatment options. It is valid and appropriate in some circumstances to begin treatment with any option, including IPP [5]. After prosthesis removal, a patient's penis will not generally be reliably responsive to other modalities of ED treatment.

According to the AUA Clinical Guidelines on Erectile Dysfunction [5], there are several reported adverse events in the early peri- and post-operative period associated with penile prosthesis implantation: penile edema or hematoma (23 studies: range 0.2% to 13.4%; mean 3.4%); corporal injury (11 studies: range 0.06% to 6.2%; mean 2.3%); urethral injury (9 studies: range 0% to 3.1%; mean 1.2%); acute urinary retention (9 studies: range 0% to 4.2%; mean 2.0%); and crural injury (7 studies: range 0.02% to 4.0%; mean 1.5%). These adverse events often resolve with observation and complications are rarely serious. However, it is important that prospective prosthetic patients be made aware of these operative risks and are provided realistic expectations. Physician-patient communication is central to any medical procedure. Physicians should always carefully follow an informed consent process, as suggested by the AUA clinical guidelines, the latest literature, and clinical best practices to minimize risks and maximize benefits of any treatment. It has been cited that in litigation proceedings, patients often allege they would not have undergone the procedure if they had been properly informed of all the associated risks [6].

In 2008, the Sexual Medicine Society of North America (SMSNA) published a supplement to guide counseling prior to informed consent [7]. A first consideration will be the selection of the appropriate penile implant for the patient, including evaluation of ease of use and appearance. Time courses for expected postoperative pain, the general healing process, and the required post-implantation abstinence period prior to intercourse must also be clearly stated. Setting realistic preoperative expectations and proper documentations of these interactions are vital procedural components of any penile prosthesis surgery [8]. In practice, certain psychological factors may indicate that patients are poor surgical candidates. The "CURSED" patient mnemonic ("Compulsive/obsessive, Unrealistic, Revision, Surgeon Shopping, Entitled, Denial, and Psychiatric") may guide clinicians in identifying patients who do not display sufficient reserves to manage complications [9]. Considering that this mnemonic is not all-inclusive, surgeons should trust their intuition in determining appropriate surgical candidates. It is important for the physician to derive a sense of patient expectations prior to undergoing the procedure. This can lead to a more individualized preoperative discussion of risks, benefits, and expectations.

Medical Malpractice in Urology

Across all medical specialties, physicians are aware of the increasing threat of medical malpractice lawsuits, though surgeons are more often implicated in medical malpractice than non-surgical specialties [10]. In order to prove malpractice, plaintiffs must have evidence for the following four criteria: (1) physician duty to act, (2) breach of physician's duty, (3) incurred damages, and (4) damages caused by breach of duty [11].

Compared with other surgical and non-surgical fields, urology has been reported to have a moderate to high risk of medical malpractice suits [12]. Studies indicate that a practicing urologist will be implicated in between 1 and 2 claims over the course of his/her career [6, 13, 14]. A recent survey of practicing urologists identified 63% of respondents who had been linked to a medical malpractice lawsuit a median of 2.1 times [13].

Studies examining medical malpractice in urology from insurance company data records estimate that claims related to surgery comprise somewhere between 40% and 60% of lawsuits filed by patients [15, 16]. Other foundations for medical practice claims include missed diagnoses, as well as improper treatment, failure to obtain proper consent, and equipment failure [15–17]. In an analysis of data obtained from the Physicians Insurance Association of America from 1985 to 2004, diagnostic errors and improper procedure performance are cited as the top two foundations for legal action against urologists [18]. During this 22-year period, researchers found that penile prostheses comprised 10% of total claims attributed to procedural error, below only those claims attributed to prostate surgery (13%); circumcision and vasectomy procedures accounted for 3% and 6% of claims, respectively. Another study analyzing negligence cases filed against urologists over a 4-year period found that penile prosthesis-related allegations represented 11.8% of claims [15].

There are no published studies that have identified metrics or proxies to predict urologists' risk of malpractice claims being filed against them with respect to procedures that they perform. The importance of honesty, transparency, and clear communication is critical when mistakes do occur [11]. The potential for lawsuits may correlate with the phenomenon of defensive medicine, which is defined as medical behaviors that avoid physician liability without providing increased benefits to the patient [19, 20]. Defensive medicine practices have been grouped into two behaviors in the literature – "assurance" and "avoidance" behaviors – respectively referring to increased test ordering and referral of high-risk patients [21]. In a 2006 survey of practicing urologists, a majority (58%) indicated that they often consider referring difficult cases, and 60% also replied that they decided to limit the scope of their practice [13]. The authors of that report asserted that the pervasive medical malpractice environment contributed to the prevalence of defensive medical practices.

Legal Proceedings

Across all medical specialties, most medical malpractice claims do not ever go to trial. Based on surveys collected from practicing urologists, it was estimated that 16.7% of claims went to trial, and only 21.2% of claims that went to trial were finalized with a payment to the plaintiff (3.5% overall) [13]. In limited international studies of urologic medical malpractice, physicians have been found to be at fault in 27% and 26.5% of filed lawsuits in France and South Korea, respectively [22, 23].

Clinical Considerations and Recommendations

Beyond qualifications and experience, failures in clinical "soft skills," such as clear and empathetic communication, can play a large role in patient dissatisfaction, potentially leading to a malpractice claim. One large retrospective study attempted to identify "high risk" urologists based on unsolicited patient complaints filed at hospitals and medical clinics. Researchers evaluated 1,516 complaints filed against 268 urologists over the course of 4 years [24]. Dissatisfaction regarding inadequate treatment and care accounted for the largest percentage (40%) of filed complaints, while complaints regarding "soft skills" in the subcategories of failures in communication, access and availability, and concern for patient and family comprised 56% of the complaints. The study also demonstrated that a small number of urologists in their cohort were associated with an outsized proportion of patient complaints. It was found that 125 (47%) urologists were associated with no complaints, while 30 (11%) urologists were associated with half of the patient complaints [24] (Fig. 14.1).

Both the initiation and results of medical malpractice lawsuits are dependent on many factors out of a physician's control. As such, physicians should be very clear in voicing realistic expectations and risks to their patients to minimize legal liability. Literature supports that it is most often a breakdown in communication which prompts patients to begin a conversation with legal counsel [6, 25]. Studies emphasize that proper communication, including adequately answering a patient's questions and full disclosure of medical errors, may reduce malpractice risk [26–28]. Urologists must also be diligent in proper documentation of patient interactions.

Surgeons must remain current on relevant clinical and scientific advances published in the urologic literature. Use of clinical guidelines published or approved by the AUA is recommended, but physicians must be aware that these clinical guidelines cannot be used as legal "standard of care" in court [11, 29]. If an adverse event does occur, in order to provide the best care for their patients and minimize the risk of any legal action taken against them, physicians should provide a clear explanation and have an open line of communication with patient and family [11]. In the case of a noted adverse event, it is also incumbent upon the physician to notify their hospital risk management officer immediately.

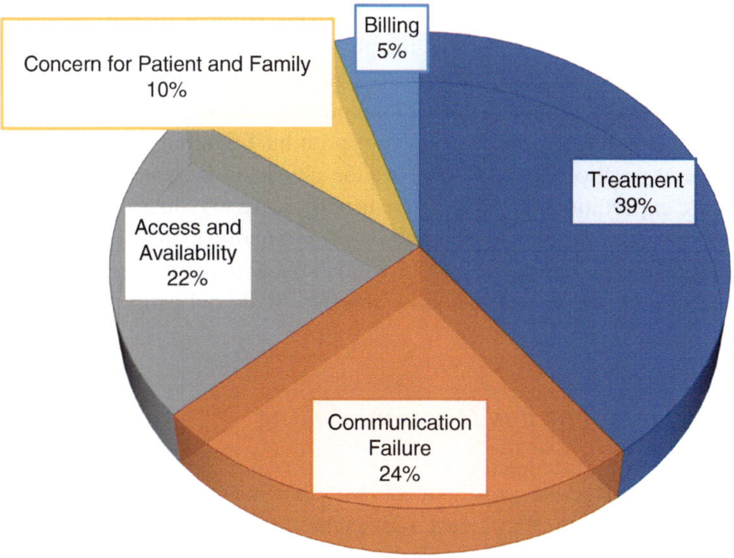

Fig. 14.1 Proportion of 1,516 patient complaints, separated by complaint category, filed against 268 urologists over a 4-year period [24]

Common Complaints Leading to Litigation After Penile Prosthesis Implantation

Informed Consent

The process of attaining informed consent represents an opportunity for building the physician-patient relationship, managing patient expectations, and reviewing the risks and benefits associated with surgery. It is the responsibility of the clinician to determine if the patient is appropriate for the surgery. The consenting process should take place in a low-stress environment, and the patient must be given the opportunity to inquire about any concerns. The physician should assess the patient's understandings of the risks and benefits of the procedure. Patients at higher risk for complications or dissatisfaction may require a more prolonged and thorough consent process [30]. Somewhat unique to penile prosthesis implantation is potential benefit of including the partner in the consent process, specifically in clarifying the goals of surgery, as the use of the prosthetic device requires a willing partner [30]. Sunaryo et al. conducted a legal database review of penile prosthesis medical malpractice cases, reporting that informed consent was an issue in 31.7% (13/41) of claims [31]. Complaints included that the device implantation was not indicated and that alternative treatment options were not adequately explained or provided prior to the procedure (e.g., vacuum erection device (VED) or intracorporal cavernosal injections (ICI)). In one example, an Oregon appellate court upheld a lower court ruling [32] that a physician failed to comply with the state's informed court statute [33]. The court found evidence that the physician did not discuss the risk of infection or the failure rate of the prosthesis with the patient, which were considered material risks and warranted a medical malpractice action [32]. While the provision of appropriate informed consent will not prohibit litigation against the clinician, good consent practices serve to improve the physician-patient relationship and set appropriate expectations [34, 35]. These usually serve to reduce the risk of malpractice lawsuits [36, 37]. The documentation of preoperative counseling and consenting are crucial to defending against litigation should a claim be filed [8]. An adage discussed in practice is, "if it is not documented, it did not happen."

Surgical Technique and Decision-Making

There are several penile prosthetic devices that are commercially available for implantation. Clinicians may select a device based on a variety of factors, including patient preference, surgical experience and comfort, and procedure indication, among others. Surgical implantation can be accomplished through either the infrapubic, penoscrotal, or subcoronal approach, each with their advantages [38]. Standard reservoir placement was traditionally considered for the space of Retzius or the extraperitoneal space [39]. More recent techniques have allowed for placement in "ectopic" locations [40]. Device choice, specifically, may be related to risk of litigation. In the Sunaryo et al. review of 41 claims, 42.9% of cases involving malleable implants were decided in favor of the plaintiff, compared to no cases involving inflatable prostheses being decided in favor of the plaintiff [31]. Notably, malleable devices are associated with lower patient satisfaction [40, 41]. An analysis of total national practice patterns showed that overall surgical use of IPP compared to malleable prostheses decreased to 25:1 in 2012 [42]. Interest in malleable devices may be increasing, as emphasis on lower-cost devices favors this alternative [43].

With considerable variability in devices and procedures, it is imperative that surgeons practice skilled surgical technique and intraoperative decision-making. In a review of urological malpractice suits, cases of malpractice after penile prosthesis surgery noted that surgical technique was the central issue in cases leading to payout [36]. Cited breaches of duty include a variety of deficiencies in surgical technique, among other failures (Table 14.1). In comparison, the most common central issues of urological cases leading to payout, overall, were issues of consent. It is imperative that clinicians receive adequate training and experience in penile prosthesis surgery in residency and continued training and experience throughout their practice. An outcome analysis comparing groups of patients treated by low-volume surgeons compared to a single high-volume surgeon noted improved outcomes in the form of reduced operative time, prolonged device survival, longer median cylinder length, and fewer iatrogenic complications in the group treated by the high-volume surgeon [44]. An analysis of the case logs obtained from the American Board of

Table 14.1 Most common breaches of duty and damages alleged by plaintiffs in malpractice cases (adapted from [31])

Primary breaches of duty		Alleged damages	
Failure in performing surgery	20	Complete impotence	7
Improper device placement	5	Partial penectomy	4
Sizing errors	4	Death	2
Bowel perforation	3	Partial numbness	2
Vein laceration	2	Loss of length	2
Urethral perforation	1	Bladder dysfunction	1
Failure to diagnose and treat	7	Gastrointestinal dysfunction	1
Surgical complication	5	Pain	1
Failure to perform total explant	3	Orgasm dysfunction	1
Device failure	2		
Failure to provide informed consent	2		
Removal of inflated Foley catheter	1		
Contraindicated prescription of vacuum erect assist device	1		

Urology found that, while high-volume urologists performed a disproportionate percentage of penile prostheses implantation surgeries, 75% of prostheses were still placed by surgeons who complete fewer than five of these procedures per year [42]. Considering that a high proportion of penile implant surgeries are being performed by infrequent implanters and that surgical technique is the most commonly cited central complaint in cases decided in favor of the plaintiffs, surgeons performing few penile implant procedures should ensure appropriate training and technical skill when performing this potentially litigious procedure. Simulation training courses may provide an opportunity for building the surgeon's knowledge and confidence necessary to perform penile prosthetic procedures [45]. Similar courses aimed at practicing urologists could provide opportunities to maintain or enhance optimal surgical technique when placing IPPs.

Attentive and thorough patient follow-up is also a necessity. An Ohio court found a physician negligent [46] after the physician failed to detect a laceration to the urethra sustained during implant surgery. The physician also failed to diagnose complications of that procedure after the patient complained of intense pain in his genitals during two visits to the hospital that the patient made postoperatively. The patient required four subsequent surgeries to remove the device, repair the laceration, and mitigate complications related to accumulated scar tissue. The court normally will not find fault with the presence of intraoperative or postoperative complication so long as they are not caused by gross negligence and addressed in a reasonable manner according to the standard of care. For instance, a district court in Rhode Island decided in favor of the defendant [47] in a case alleging malpractice in the intraoperative and postoperative periods when a plaintiff developed a bulge on the left side of his penis and constant pain in the scrotum and penis. The court noted that despite the claims of malpractice, the mild deviation of the prosthesis and the subsequent postoperative inflation maneuvers to readjust the device fell within the standard of care. Importantly, the court decision hinged upon the experience and credibility of the expert witnesses. In this case, the court found the testimony of the defendant's expert witness to carry decidedly more weight than that of the plaintiff.

The decision rendered in the previous legal case underscores the importance of expert witnesses in the determination of malpractice related to surgical technique or decision-making. The AUA policy statement concerning expert witness testimony in liability cases suggests that the qualifications for expert witness testimony include being active in the field of urology, having at least 5 years of clinical practice after completing residency/fellowship training, proficiency in the area of clinical practice, and expertise with texts, journals, guidelines, and other sources that establish the applicable standard of care [48]. While it is difficult to measure expertise, Sunaryo et al. utilized measures of years of experience, scholarly impact (as measured by h-index), and academic vs non-academic practice setting position to compare urologist expert witnesses found within 299 jury verdict and settlement reports [49]. Expert witnesses testifying on behalf of the defendants were more likely to be academic faculty, slightly younger with fewer years of experience, and with a higher scholarly impact. Notably, plaintiff witnesses were more likely to testify multiple times. Overall, the authors found that the expert witnesses for both the prosecution and the defense had a mean of greater than 30 years of experience, with an average of 35.7 years and 32.2 years of experience for urologists testifying on behalf of the plaintiffs and the defendants, respectively.

Infection

Infection is an inherent risk in any surgery, including penile implant surgery. Reported infection risk ranges between 1% and 4% [50]. Infection risk has been correlated with length of surgery [34]. The most implicated organism in infection of IPPs has traditionally been staphylococcus epidermidis, although gram negatives, anaerobes, and fungal organisms, as well as multi-organism infections, can be the culprits of infections [28]. Being that the avoidance of device contamination requires fastidious technique, it has been suggested that lower-volume implanters may have less experience in cases of malpractice where infection was a noted complication [8]. Physicians should be sure to follow appropriate guidelines on antibiotic treatment and be cognizant of early signs of infection for appropriate patient care. Given recent evidence that microorganisms identified in penile prosthesis infection cases are not adequately covered by the AUA and European Association of Urology guidelines, surgeons should also consider organisms that fall outside these recommendations. Guidelines should be updated to include a broader microorganism profile [51]. Sunaryo et al. observed that a large percentage of malpractice cases brought to trial after penile implant surgery involved postoperative infection [31]. The authors proposed that a possible deficiency in patient education concerning infection risk could have contributed to a high rate of cases involving infection being brought to trial.

Malpractice cases decided in favor of the plaintiffs have typically represented practice which deviated from the standard of care. A Florida court decided [52] against a surgeon who placed a second penile implant into an infected penile scrotal area and then failed to remove the implant despite signs of worsening infection to the point of gangrene. The patient lost a portion of his penis as a result. In another example, a Georgia court decided in favor of the plaintiff [53] after the court discovered the defendant failed to recognize that the plaintiff had developed a chronic infection. The patient developed severe signs of infection necessitating hospitalizations after undergoing a surgery for Peyronie's disease complicated by urethral injury and urethro-cutaneous fistula. Long-term complications of the case included permanent sexual dysfunction.

Conclusion

The basic inflatable penile prosthesis design has not fundamentally changed in more than half a century. There are well-known risks in the surgical placement of penile prostheses including infection, pain, hematoma, injury to genitourinary tract, and need for further surgery. The most common complaint in litigation aimed at a urologist after placement of penile prosthesis is lack of appropriate counseling. There is a published, patient-focused document from the SMSNA that allows for complete preoperative counseling that would minimize litigation [54]. Surgical decision-making error has been demonstrated to lead to the highest proportion of payouts to plaintiffs in litigation after penile prosthesis placement. Prior to placement of penile prosthesis, it is incumbent on the surgeon to have adequate training and experience to manage intraoperative hurdles. If the surgeon is adequately trained and the patient is well informed on expectations of the procedure, the overall risk of successful litigation is low.

Acknowledgements We give special thanks to Jessica Daigle for her assistance in the preparation and submission of this chapter.

References

1. Prins J, Blanker MH, Bohnen AM, Thomas S, Bosch JL. Prevalence of erectile dysfunction: a systematic review of population-based studies. Int J Impot Res. 2002;14(6):422–32. https://doi.org/10.1038/sj.ijir.3900905.
2. McKinlay JB. The worldwide prevalence and epidemiology of erectile dysfunction. Int J Impot Res. 2000;12(Suppl 4):S6–S11. https://doi.org/10.1038/sj.ijir.3900567.

3. Akdemir F, Okulu E, Kayıgil Ö. Long-term outcomes of AMS Spectra® penile prosthesis implantation and satisfaction rates. Int J Impot Res. 2017;29(5):184–8. https://doi.org/10.1038/ijir.2017.16.
4. Lightner DJ, Wymer K, Sanchez J, Kavoussi L. Best practice statement on urologic procedures and antimicrobial prophylaxis. J Urol. 2020;203(2):351–6. https://doi.org/10.1097/JU.0000000000000509.
5. Burnett AL, Nehra A, Breau RH, et al. Erectile dysfunction: AUA guideline. J Urol. 2018;200(3):633–41. https://doi.org/10.1016/j.juro.2018.05.004.
6. Hickey JD, Cowan J. Risk management and medicolegal issues in urology. BJU Int. 2000;86(3):271–4. https://doi.org/10.1046/j.1464-410x.2000.00291.x.
7. SMSNA. Penile prosthesis information form. Burnsville: Sexual Medicine Society of North America; 2008. http://www.smsna.org/V1/images/SMSNAIPP_policy.pdf
8. Henning J, Waxman S. Legal aspects of men's genitourinary health. Int J Impot Res. 2009;21(3):165–70. https://doi.org/10.1038/ijir.2009.4.
9. Trost LW, Baum N, Hellstrom WJ. Managing the difficult penile prosthesis patient. J Sex Med. 2013;10(4):893–907. https://doi.org/10.1111/jsm.12115.
10. DeVille K, Goldberg D, Hassler G. Malpractice risk according to physician specialty. N Engl J Med. 2011;365(20):1939–40. https://doi.org/10.1056/NEJMc1111003.
11. Sherer BA, Coogan CL. The current state of medical malpractice in urology. Urology. 2015;86(1):2–9. https://doi.org/10.1016/j.urology.2015.03.004.
12. Jena AB, Seabury S, Lakdawalla D, Chandra A. Malpractice risk according to physician specialty. N Engl J Med. 2011;365(7):629–36. https://doi.org/10.1056/NEJMsa1012370.
13. Sobel DL, Loughlin KR, Coogan CL. Medical malpractice liability in clinical urology: a survey of practicing urologists. J Urol. 2006;175(5):1847–51. https://doi.org/10.1016/S0022-5347(05)01021-9.
14. Kaplan GW. Malpractice risks for urologists. Urology. 1998;51(2):183–5. https://doi.org/10.1016/s0090-4295(97)00633-x.
15. Kahan SE, Goldman HB, Marengo S, Resnick MI. Urological medical malpractice. J Urol. 2001;165(5):1638–42.
16. Perrotti M, Badger W, Prader S, Moran ME. Medical malpractice in urology, 1985 to 2004: 469 consecutive cases closed with indemnity payment. J Urol. 2006;176(5):2154–7. https://doi.org/10.1016/j.juro.2006.07.024.
17. Badger WJ, Moran ME, Abraham C, Yarlagadda B, Perrotti M. Missed diagnoses by urologists resulting in malpractice payment. J Urol. 2007;178(6):2537–9. https://doi.org/10.1016/j.juro.2007.08.040.
18. Hsieh MH, Tan AG, Meng MV. Medical malpractice in American urology: 22-year national review of the impact of caps and implications for contemporary practice. J Urol. 2008;179(5):1944–9. https://doi.org/10.1016/j.juro.2008.01.061.
19. Loughlin KR. Medical malpractice: the good, the bad, and the ugly. Urol Clin North Am. 2009;36(1):101–vii. https://doi.org/10.1016/j.ucl.2008.08.006.
20. Calikoglu EO, Aras A. 'Defensive medicine among different surgical disciplines: A descriptive cross-sectional study. J Forensic Leg Med. 2020 Jul;73:101970. https://doi.org/10.1016/j.jflm.2020.101970. Epub 2020 May 5. PMID: 32442116.
21. Renkema E, Ahaus K, Broekhuis M, Tims M. Triggers of defensive medical behaviours: a cross-sectional study among physicians in the Netherlands. BMJ Open. 2019;9(6):e025108. Published 2019 Jun 25. https://doi.org/10.1136/bmjopen-2018-025108.
22. Papillon F, Cormier L, Legeais D. Risque médico-légal en urologie: analyse d'un portefeuille d'assurés auprès d'une compagnie d'assurances française entre 2009 et 2018 [Medico-legal risk in urology: Analysis of a portfolio of insured persons by a French insurance company between 2009 and 2018]. Prog Urol. 2019;29(1):18–28. https://doi.org/10.1016/j.purol.2018.10.002.
23. Shin SH, Kim SY, Jang SG, Lee W. Analysis of closed medical litigation in urology. Investig Clin Urol. 2017;58(5):317–23. https://doi.org/10.4111/icu.2017.58.5.317.

24. Stimson CJ, Pichert JW, Moore IN, et al. Medical malpractice claims risk in urology: an empirical analysis of patient complaint data. J Urol. 2010;183(5):1971–6. https://doi.org/10.1016/j.juro.2010.01.027.
25. Vincent C, Young M, Phillips A. Why do people sue doctors? A study of patients and relatives taking legal action. Lancet. 1994;343(8913):1609–13. https://doi.org/10.1016/s0140-6736(94)93062-7.
26. Levinson W, Roter DL, Mullooly JP, Dull VT, Frankel RM. Physician-patient communication. The relationship with malpractice claims among primary care physicians and surgeons. JAMA. 1997;277(7):553–9. https://doi.org/10.1001/jama.277.7.553.
27. Tsimtsiou Z, Kirana P, Hatzimouratidis K, Hatzichristou D. What is the profile of patients thinking of litigation? Results from the hospitalized and outpatients' profile and expectations study. Hippokratia. 2014;18(2):139–43.
28. Benson JS, Coogan CL. Urological malpractice: analysis of indemnity and claim data from 1985 to 2007. J Urol. 2010;184(3):1086–235. https://doi.org/10.1016/j.juro.2010.05.034.
29. Boscolo-Berto R. Legal claims and bias in creating clinical practice guidelines: which step in which direction? Int J Urol. 2010;17(5):498. https://doi.org/10.1111/j.1442-2042.2010.02501.x.
30. Trost L. Consenting the patient for penile implant surgery. J Sex Med. 2020;17(1):4–6. https://doi.org/10.1016/j.jsxm.2019.10.002.
31. Sunaryo PL, Colaco M, Terlecki R. Penile prostheses and the litigious patient: a legal database review. J Sex Med. 2014;11(10):2589–94. https://doi.org/10.1111/jsm.12649.
32. Wenger v. Oregon Urology Clinic, P.C., 102 Ore. App. 665, 796 P.2d 376, 1990 Ore. App. LEXIS 873 (Court of Appeals of Oregon August 1, 1990, Filed).
33. 677.097 Procedure to obtain informed consent of patient., ORS § 677.097 (The Oregon Annotated Statutes is current through the 2019 and 2020 Regular Session. Some sections may have multiple variants due to amendments by multiple acts. Revision and codification by the Legislative Counsel are updated as available, see ORS 173.111 et seq. For sections pending codification by the Legislative Counsel, see Newly Added Sections in the Table of Contents.)
34. Scherzer ND, Dick B, Gabrielson AT, Alzweri LM, Hellstrom WJG. Penile prosthesis complications: planning, prevention, and decision making. Sex Med Rev. 2019;7(2):349–59. https://doi.org/10.1016/j.sxmr.2018.04.002.
35. Kramer AC, Schweber A. Patient expectations prior to Coloplast titan penile prosthesis implant predicts postoperative satisfaction. J Sex Med. 2010;7(6):2261–6. https://doi.org/10.1111/j.1743-6109.2010.01799.x.
36. Chason J, Sausville J, Kramer AC. Penile prosthesis implantation compares favorably in malpractice outcomes to other common urological procedures: findings from a malpractice insurance database. J Sex Med. 2009;6(8):2111–4. https://doi.org/10.1111/j.1743-6109.2009.01317.x.
37. Stelfox HT, Gandhi TK, Orav EJ, Gustafson ML. The relation of patient satisfaction with complaints against physicians and malpractice lawsuits. Am J Med. 2005;118(10):1126–33. https://doi.org/10.1016/j.amjmed.2005.01.060.
38. Montague DK, Angermeir KW. Surgical approaches for penile prosthesis implantation: penoscrotal vs infrapubic. Int J Impot Res. 2003;15(Suppl 5):S134–5. https://doi.org/10.1038/sj.ijir.3901089.
39. Levine LA, Hoeh MP. Review of penile prosthetic reservoir: complications and presentation of a modified reservoir placement technique. J Sex Med. 2012;9(11):2759–69. https://doi.org/10.1111/j.1743-6109.2012.02807.x.
40. Levine LA, Becher EF, Bella AJ, et al. Penile prosthesis surgery: current recommendations from the international consultation on sexual medicine [published correction appears in J Sex Med. 2016 Jul;13(7):1145]. J Sex Med. 2016;13(4):489–518. https://doi.org/10.1016/j.jsxm.2016.01.017.
41. Bayrak O, Erturhan S, Seckiner I, Ozturk M, Sen H, Erbagci A. Comparison of the patient's satisfaction underwent penile prosthesis; Malleable versus Ambicor: single center experi-

ence. Arch Ital Urol Androl. 2020;92(1):25–9. Published 2020 Apr 6. https://doi.org/10.4081/aiua.2020.1.25.
42. Oberlin DT, Matulewicz RS, Bachrach L, Hofer MD, Brannigan RE, Flury SC. National practice patterns of treatment of erectile dysfunction with penile prosthesis implantation. J Urol. 2015;193(6):2040–4. https://doi.org/10.1016/j.juro.2014.11.095.
43. Trost L. Future considerations in prosthetic urology. Asian J Androl. 2020;22(1):70–5. https://doi.org/10.4103/aja.aja_103_19.
44. Henry GD, Kansal NS, Callaway M, et al. Centers of excellence concept and penile prostheses: an outcome analysis. J Urol. 2009;181(3):1264–8. https://doi.org/10.1016/j.juro.2008.10.157.
45. Lentz AC, Rodríguez D, Davis LG, et al. Simulation training in penile implant surgery: assessment of surgical confidence and knowledge with cadaveric laboratory training. Sex Med. 2018;6(4):332–8. https://doi.org/10.1016/j.esxm.2018.09.001.
46. Bailey V. Emiliio C. Chu, M.D., Inc., 80 Ohio App. 3d 627, 610 N.E. 2d 531 (Ohio Ct. App. 1992).
47. Gautieri v. U.S., 167 F. Supp. 2d 207, 209 (D.R.I.2001).
48. American Urological Association. Expert witness testimony in medical liability cases. Available at: http://www.auanet.org/about/policy-statements/testimony-in-medical-liability-cases.cfm. Accessed 16 June 2020.
49. Sunaryo PL, Svider PF, Jackson-Rosario I, Eloy JA. Expert witness testimony in urology malpractice litigation. Urology. 2014;83(4):704–8. https://doi.org/10.1016/j.urology.2013.11.045.
50. Narang GL, Figler BD, Coward RM. Preoperative counseling and expectation management for inflatable penile prosthesis implantation. Transl Androl Urol. 2017;6(Suppl 5):S869–80. https://doi.org/10.21037/tau.2017.07.04.
51. Gross MS, Phillips EA, Carrasquillo RJ, et al. Multicenter investigation of the microorganisms involved in penile prosthesis infection: an analysis of the efficacy of the AUA and EAU guidelines for penile prosthesis prophylaxis. J Sex Med. 2017;14(3):455–63. https://doi.org/10.1016/j.jsxm.2017.01.007.
52. Weinstock Kurzer, M.D., 03 FJVR 1-44, 2002 WL 32128165 (Fla. Cir. Ct. 2002).
53. Hyde v. Toole, 8 Nat. J.V.R.A. 12:12, 1000 WL 183947.
54. SMSNA. Penile Prosthesis Information Form. Available online at: https://www.smsna.org/V1/images/SMSNAIPP_policy.pdf.

Index

E. P. Miranda, J. P. Mulhall (eds.), *Penile Implant Surgery*,
https://doi.org/10.1007/978-3-030-82363-4

GPSR Compliance

The European Union's (EU) General Product Safety Regulation (GPSR) is a set of rules that requires consumer products to be safe and our obligations to ensure this.

If you have any concerns about our products, you can contact us on ProductSafety@springernature.com

In case Publisher is established outside the EU, the EU authorized representative is:

Springer Nature Customer Service Center GmbH
Europaplatz 3
69115 Heidelberg, Germany

Batch number: 10732090

Printed by Printforce, the Netherlands